FORENSIC NEUROPSYCHOLOGY CASEBOOK

FORENSIC NEUROPSYCHOLOGY CASEBOOK

Edited by
ROBERT L. HEILBRONNER

THE GUILFORD PRESS
New York   London

© 2005 The Guilford Press
A Division of Guilford Publications, Inc.
72 Spring Street, New York, NY 10012
www.guilford.com

Printed in the United States of America

This book is printed on acid-free paper.

Last digit is print number: 9 8 7 6 5 4 3 2 1

Library of Congress Cataloging-in-Publication Data

Forensic neuropsychology casebook / edited by Robert L. Heilbronner.
  p. cm.
  Includes bibliographical references and index.
  ISBN 1-59385-185-5 (hardcover: alk. paper)
  1. Forensic neuropsychology—Case studies. 2. Clinical
neuropsychology—Case studies. I. Heilbronner, Robert L.
  RA1147.5.F669 2005
  614′.1—dc22

                                                2005008519

About the Editor

Robert L. Heilbronner, PhD, is a board-certified clinical neuropsychologist practicing in Chicago. He is the Director of the Chicago Neuropsychology Group and Codirector of the Forensic Neuropsychology Institute. Dr. Heilbronner has faculty appointments at Northwestern University School of Medicine and the University of Chicago Hospitals, Pritzker School of Medicine. He is a Fellow of the Division of Clinical Neuropsychology of the American Psychological Association and of the National Academy of Neuropsychology. Dr. Heilbronner has published in peer-reviewed journals and books, and has presented on clinical and forensic neuropsychology issues at national and international meetings. He has also testified in a number of civil, criminal, and capital cases locally and nationally.

Contributors

Lidia Artiola i Fortuny, PhD, Independent practice, Tucson, Arizona

Bradley N. Axelrod, PhD, Psychology Section, John D. Dingell Department of Veterans Affairs Medical Center, Detroit, Michigan

William B. Barr, PhD, Departments of Neurology and Psychiatry, New York University School of Medicine, New York, New York

Lynn Bennett Blackburn, PhD, Department of Psychology, St. Louis Children's Hospital, St. Louis, Missouri

Kyle Brauer Boone, PhD, Department of Psychiatry, Harbor–UCLA Medical Center, Torrance, California

Paul L. Craig, PhD, Independent practice, and Department of Psychiatry and Behavioral Sciences, University of Washington School of Medicine, Anchorage, Alaska

Robert L. Denney, PsyD, U.S. Medical Center for Federal Prisoners and Forest Institute of Professional Psychology, Springfield, Missouri

Manfred F. Greiffenstein, PhD, Psychological Systems, Inc., Royal Oak, Michigan

Robert E. Hanlon, PhD, Division of Psychiatry and Law, Northwestern University School of Medicine, and Forensic Neuropsychology Institute, Chicago, Illinois

Robert L. Heilbronner, PhD, Chicago Neuropsychology Group and Forensic Neuropsychology Institute; Departments of Psychiatry and Behavioral Sciences and Physical Medicine and Rehabilitation, Northwestern University School of

Medicine; and Department of Psychiatry, University of Chicago Hospitals, Pritzker School of Medicine, Chicago, Illinois

George K. Henry, PhD, Los Angeles Neuropsychology Group, Los Angeles, California

Justin S. Huthwaite, PsyD, Department of Neurology, University of Alabama at Birmingham, Birmingham, Alabama

Paul R. Lees-Haley, PhD, Independent practice, Huntsville, Alabama

Mark R. Lovell, PhD, Sports Medicine Concussion Program, University of Pittsburgh Medical Center, Pittsburgh, Pennsylvania

Daniel C. Marson, JD, PhD, Department of Neurology, University of Alabama at Birmingham, Birmingham, Alabama

Michael F. Martelli, PhD, Concussion Care Centre of Virginia and Tree of Life, Glen Allen, Virginia

Michael W. Mayfield, JD, Murder Task Force, Office of the Cook County Public Defender, Chicago, Illinois

Kristie J. Nies, PhD, Independent practice, Kingsport, Tennessee

Jamie E. Pardini, PhD, fMRI and Sports Concussion Program, University of Pittsburgh Medical Center, Pittsburgh, Pennsylvania

Neil H. Pliskin, PhD, Department of Psychiatry, University of Illinois at Chicago, Chicago, Illinois

Lisa D. Stanford, PhD, Department of Psychiatry, University of Illinois at Chicago, Chicago, Illinois

James P. Sullivan, PhD, Veterans Affairs Medical Center, and independent practice, Tucson, Arizona

Jerry J. Sweet, PhD, Department of Psychiatry and Behavioral Sciences, Evanston Northwestern Healthcare, Evanston, Illinois

Preface

I have liked stories ever since I was a young boy. I think that is one of the reasons I became a psychologist. As a "trained listener" I have permission—and even a license—to listen to people tell their stories, to open themselves and reveal certain undesirable aspects of themselves that they would be loath to share with others. What a privilege. But I like telling stories too. Although trained to listen, I think that most psychologists like to tell stories about their patients and their lives. But we are restricted from doing so because of the privacy and confidentiality inherent in the work we do.

When I decided to pursue clinical neuropsychology as a specialty, knowing that the primary focus of work would be on assessment, I was initially worried that I would miss out on the stories to which I was privy with my therapy patients. Yet nothing could have been farther from the truth. As a clinical neuropsychologist, the clinical interview, although time limited compared to extended psychotherapy, provides a great vehicle for patients to tell their stories in a brief period of time. This context seems to provide even more momentum and opportunity for patients to self-disclose, thus further enriching those of us who enjoy the narrative tale. It is in the spirit of telling the narrative tale that this book was created.

As I considered writing a book documenting the tales of many of the brain-injured patients with whom I have worked (something that has been done by a number of other medical and mental health professionals for many years), it occurred to me that stories had not been written from the "other side of the couch," as it were—that is, the psychologist's, or in this case, the clinical neuropsychologist's, experience of the patient. Why would this be any less interesting? Indeed, myriad thoughts run through our minds during the interview and testing process: "How did this person come to be this way?"; "What does this person hope to accomplish by exhibiting such awkward behaviors?"; "How do this person's family members feel about him or her?" Indeed, as psychologists we have a whole host of reactions and, dare I say, "countertransference reactions" to our clients. Such thoughts and feelings about the person could certainly impact how we interact with him or her, interpret the test data, write the report, and so forth.

Until now, no one has really written about the phenomenological experience of the clinical neuropsychologist. In fact, there is a paucity of case studies in neuropsychology. Even truer, there is no material devoted to case studies in forensic neuropsychology. But go to any neuropsychology conference and stories abound about how this neuropsychologist testified in this or that case, how much money he or she makes from forensic activities, what this attorney asked during a deposition, etc. Indeed, some neuropsychologists who do forensic work even like to boast about their exploits, as if their report or testimony was *the* critical factor in the judge's or jury's decision to render a verdict—something that may happen on occasion, but far less often than many of us would like to think.

This text, perhaps the first of its kind in neuropsychology, uses the case study approach to facilitate insight into the mind of the forensic neuropsychologist so that the reader can begin to understand the thought process of the neuropsychologist as he or she ventures into the forensic domain. Read along as the expert examines a defendant on death row, as he travels by dog sled through the Arctic to evaluate schoolchildren injured in an airplane accident, or as she assesses a father and son who are both claiming damages following exposure to industrial toxins. These are rich stories written by some of the finest clinicians and scientists in our field today. I trust that the reader will find them intellectually stimulating as well as fun to read.

Topics were chosen to reflect the current scope of forensic neuropsychology practice. The sections are divided into civil (adult and pediatric) and criminal cases, because these appear to be the primary forensic arenas in which neuropsychologists have operated over the past decade. However, this does not mean that we are limited to these areas in the future. The chapters reflect the kind of work that neuropsychologists customarily (and not so customarily) do in their day-to-day practice. Also included at the end of the book is a special section entitled "Ask the

Experts." I invited three highly esteemed forensic colleagues to respond to questions that most of us have either not anticipated or have had to address without the benefit of consulting with an experienced colleague. I think that you will find a fair degree of consistency in the respondents' answers; yet there are also some obvious differences of opinion, reflecting divergent personal and philosophical approaches to forensic practice.

In choosing the present complement of authors, I wanted to ensure a sufficiently broad representation of individuals who are experts at managing the different kinds of forensic issues neuropsychologists are often asked to address. Readers who are familiar with forensic neuropsychological research, attendees of continuing professional education programs, and those experienced in forensic practice should recognize the names of many of the authors included in this volume. All of them bring to their topics a vast array of knowledge and experience acquired through their own research or clinical practice. Each chapter follows a recommended format, although contributors were allowed a fair degree of freedom and flexibility to write as they wished. Almost every one of them expressed a sense of relief and satisfaction in having created a piece of literature that did not have to follow specific journal requirements or other publication guidelines. I thankfully acknowledge the contribution and time commitment that each of them has made in preparing this book.

I am very grateful to the staff at The Guilford Press, who were very helpful at every stage of the publication process. I am particularly indebted to Rochelle Serwator and Anna Nelson—to Rochelle, for considering my initial proposal for this book, for her ongoing suggestions and support, and for allowing me free rein to choose the authors and topics; and to Anna, who was accommodating in all phases of the book's production. Thanks to my colleagues in Chicago and elsewhere who have provided peer consultation in some of the more difficult forensic cases in which I have been asked to serve as an expert. I thank my children, Sarah, Michael, and Jason, for their patience and willingness to forge ahead without me during those moments (e.g., bedtime) when I was downstairs in the basement office hard at work on this book. I will leave a copy for each of you on your respective pillows! Finally, I am indebted to my wife, Diane, for her tireless and unwavering support and words of encouragement throughout all aspects of our life together.

Contents

xiii

I

CIVIL CASES
Adult

1

Electrical Injury,
or "My Day at the Beach"

The background for this case dates back to 1993, when I was serving as Director of Neuropsychology and an Assistant Professor of Clinical Psychiatry and Neurology at the University of Chicago, Department of Psychiatry. At that time I was approached by Dr. Raphael Lee, a faculty member in the Department of Surgery, who by training was both a plastic surgeon and electrical engineer. I did not know Dr. Lee at the time, but I subsequently learned that he was an international expert on the diagnosis and peripheral nervous system treatment of electrical shock injuries. Dr. Lee called me on the phone, introduced himself, and stated that he had developed new techniques for treating the peripheral nervous system injuries associated with electrical shock burns. He noted, however, that many of the patients that he treated for electrical burns also seemed to have cognitive and neuropsychiatric complaints, despite the fact that there was no apparent electrical contact to the central nervous system during these injury scenarios. He invited me to attend his clinic and subsequently asked me if I wished to form a collaborative clinical and research team to study the manifestations of electrical shock injury. After reviewing the literature at that time, I noted that there were less than 10 studies investigating the cognitive sequelae of electrical injury—which was very surprising to me, given the fact that electricity had been around for

over a century. I subsequently wrote a review paper on that sparse literature in 1993, and that is how opportunistic clinical research careers can
get started. To my surprise, writing that one paper appeared to qualify
me as an "expert" in the area as far as attorneys were concerned. However, that initial collaboration grew into the University of Chicago Electrical Trauma Research Program, with a multidisciplinary team that
included primary team members from the fields of neuropsychiatry, plastic surgery, physiatry, physical therapy, occupational therapy, and pain
management. As part of this group, I have now evaluated over 250 elec-
trically injured patients and have written scientific articles and presented
our findings at national and international meetings. To my surprise,
there continues to be a limited understanding regarding the neuropsychological effects of electrical injury, and I consider myself very fortunate
to be contributing to new knowledge in this area.

BACKGROUND INFORMATION

I was first contacted by the patient's fiancée, who located me through the
new standard in this millennium: a Google-based search of the Internet.
The patient in this case, whom I refer to as "Mark Smith," was a 44-year-
old, right-handed Caucasian male who had sustained a life-threatening
electrical injury in 1995 while working at a construction site on a Caribbean island where he lived. Mr. Smith had not resumed employment
since his injury, and he was self-referred for an evaluation in the context
of his ongoing litigation against that island's power company. He and his
fiancée (whom I refer to as "Barb Jones") flew to Chicago for their evaluation. They brought medical records with them, which, along with my clinical interview with each of them, served as the primary basis for the background information in this case.

Mr. Smith was injured while working on a job site for a steel construction company during the fall of 1995, when a steel angle iron came
into close proximity or contact with an electrical power line that was
reportedly supposed to have been shut down by the local power company. As an aside, it has become increasingly understood that an individual does not have to come into direct physical contact with an electrified
power source in order to receive an electrical shock. If the individual
finds him- or herself in a position to become part of a "circuit," whereby
he or she is between the power source and the ground, especially when
near a conducting a material (e.g., a steel beam), then the electricity can

actually "arc" over to the individual. This appears to be what happened in this case. Witnesses reported hearing an explosion (further evidence of an arc injury, whereby the air between the individual and the power source becomes heated and produces an acoustic/vibratory explosion), then seeing Mr. Smith fall backward. Mr. Smith immediately stopped breathing. Cardiac and respiratory arrest after electrical shock are not uncommon because the electricity can disrupt the electrical rhythms of the heart. Mr. Smith's brother, a coworker, performed CPR on him for approximately 15 minutes before carrying him over his shoulder to descend from the beam where the injury took place to the ground.

The paramedics treated Mr. Smith's cardiac arrest with six defibrillations before transporting him to the island hospital. He was transferred by air ambulance to a hospital in southern Florida later that afternoon, where he remained for 18 days. On admission to this Florida hospital, Mr. Smith had a Glasgow Coma Scale score of 6. A computed tomography (CT) scan conducted on that day was normal, although an EEG was abnormal and interpreted as indicating an encephalopathy. Mr. Smith remained dependent on a ventilator for breathing for 1 week. He was treated for cardiomyopathy (left ventricular ejection fraction was between 25 and 30%), anoxic encephalopathy, rhabdomyolysis, potential renal failure, multiple fluid electrolyte abnormalities, second- and third-degree arc burns totaling 10% of his body surface area, pneumonia, and dysphagia. During this period, Mr. Smith was reported to be confused and have short-term memory problems. For example, he asked for his father, not remembering that he had passed away 1 year ago. He did not remember seeing his children at the hospital, nor did he remember their names.

Mr. Smith was subsequently transferred to a postacute rehabilitation hospital in Florida, where he remained as an inpatient for approximately 1 week and was followed as an outpatient for 4 months. At the time of his admission to the rehabilitation hospital, Mr. Smith demonstrated retrograde amnesia for events up to 1 year prior to his injury. He made semantic paraphasic errors in spontaneous speech, his thoughts were tangential, he had difficulty following two-step directions, and he was perseverative and had difficulty shifting attention. Therapy included training in the areas of swallowing, reading, writing, safety awareness, mobility, cognition, and communication. At the time of discharge, Mr. Smith continued to demonstrate problems with (1) planning, (2) maintaining concentration for 15 minutes in a highly distracting environment, (3) following his weekly schedule, (4) using his daily planner consistently to assist his memory difficulties, and (5) insight into his cognitive and physical limitations. A neuropsychological evaluation completed at that time (8 weeks postsurgery) indicated areas of difficulty with concentration, executive organization skills, memory, and initiation, accompanied by limited awareness of these deficits. Mr. Smith was described as disinhibited and agitated, with impaired intention and spontaneity. He was diagnosed with "dementia secondary to electric injury and anoxia with irritability, concentration difficulty, and spiritual preoccupation." For the next several years he was followed by a neurologist who diagnosed him with "residual bilateral cortical dysfunction," with no "major improvements" in his status. His reported deficits included poor recent memory, insomnia, headaches, ataxia, depression, and anxiety.

Over the course of the 4 years between Mr. Smith's electric and anoxic injury and when I first evaluated him, Mr. Smith's friends noted that he underwent significant personality changes, had persistent cognitive and neurological limitations, and demonstrated ongoing psychological adjustment issues. His fiancée reported a lack of sensitivity, initiation, and motivation that were not characteristic of his premorbid personality. "Donna Marx," Barb Jones's ex-roommate, reported that whereas Mr. Smith was very sociable and hard working before his injury, he now spent much of his time watching television and avoided socializing with others. She reported that Mr. Smith often got lost on his way to her apartment when he was alone, despite having been there many times. "John Connolly," a friend who had known Mr. Smith for 30 years, reported that Mr. Smith's mental (i.e., concentration, word-finding, reading, and memory) and physical capabilities were drastically reduced since his injury. Importantly, Mr. Smith never returned to work after his injury.

At the time of my evaluation of Mr. Smith, he reported neurological symptoms that included headaches, sleep disorder (only sleeps 0–3 hours per day due to "racing thoughts"), hypersensitivity to sunlight and to noises generated by motors of fans and blow dryers, loss of sense of smell and taste, numbness in his fingers, and needle-prick sensations in his skin. Cognitively, he reported difficulty with memory, concentration, and word finding, and retrograde amnesia for events up to about 1 month before his injury. He reported psychological symptoms that included sad mood, loss of appetite, and decreased libido.

Given this type of apparently devastating injury and extensive documentation via medical records and collateral interviews, the plaintiff's medical history and psychosocial background would be critical information necessary for any defense team to determine if there are alternative explanations for at least some component of Mr. Smith's current condition. This case, in which Mr. Smith was suing the power company, was no exception. His medical history was notable for a trauma to his right hand in 1960, which had required surgical treatment, and a car accident at age 5 with unspecified injuries. Mr. Smith denied any past psychiatric history but reported that he smoked one-third of a pack of cigarettes daily and that he had a history of alcohol use of six or more beers per day prior to his injury. This background was utilized by the defense team in a way that I describe shortly.

Ultimately, the most substantive and contentious aspect of the defense's position in this case related to Mr. Smith's preinjury level of functioning, as reflected by his educational and occupational history. The facts were that Mr. Smith had completed 12 years of education in a Florida public school system. At graduation, he had a cumulative grade-point average (GPA) of 2.53 and was ranked 100 in a class of 198. He reported that he had never received any special educational services, did better in math and business courses than in English classes, and actually graduated 1 year early in order to work full time. Mr. Smith also noted that he was skilled in chess before his injury. He reported that he had beat a Pennsylvania State Champion once, although he never participated in official competitions. After high school, he owned and operated a grocery/convenience store, which he expanded to sell T-shirts and animal feeds. Reportedly, he built up this business from a money-losing enterprise to a profitable business. In 1985 Mr. Smith entered the steel construction business and worked first as a sheet-metal mechanic, then as a foreman in various construction companies. He began his own construction company in 1988 and expanded this business to jobs in the Caribbean islands in the early 1990s. At the time of his injury, Mr. Smith and his brother co-owned a steel construction company. At the heart of the defense expert's position in this case was establishing the level at which Mr. Smith functioned prior to his injury and as suggested by his educational history.

NEUROPSYCHOLOGICAL EVALUATION

Behavioral Observations

Mr. Smith presented as a casually dressed, slender male of his stated age with good hygiene. He was accompanied to this evaluation by Ms. Jones, his fiancée; they had flown into Chicago the day before the evaluation.

Mr. Smith was alert and fully oriented. He did not demonstrate any gross motor abnormalities, though his motor and mental speed both appeared to be slow. His speech was fluent, with normal tone and volume. He did not demonstrate marked word-finding difficulties during the testing session. His thoughts were organized and logical. He often interjected information about himself that related to the question being asked. For example, when asked about years of education, Mr. Smith added that he had moved out of the family home at age 15 in order to distance himself from his parents' marital problems. Though slightly tangential, these remarks always related to the topic being discussed. Mr. Smith presented primarily with flat or shallow affect. He consistently spoke about his children (from a previous marriage) and fiancée without any prosody or facial expression, though the content of his speech suggested a strong emotional component.

Symptom Validity Testing

Due to the medical–legal nature of this case, Mr. Smith was given a test designed to assess the level of his effort (Victoria Symptom Validity Test). His performance indicated that he put forth his best effort, which was consistent with behavioral observations as well. Therefore, results of this evaluation were deemed valid representations of his level of neurocognitive functioning at that time. The neuropsychological tests administered and test scores are presented in Tables 1.1 and 1.2. Whenever possible, current data were compared to existing test scores from the evaluation conducted 2 months after his injury while at the rehabilitation

TABLE 1.1. Tests Administered

- Beck Depression Inventory
- Boston Naming Test
- California Verbal Learning Test
- Competency Rating Scale
- Gordon Diagnostic System
- Grooved Pegboard
- Impact of Event Scale
- Neuropsychological Symptom Checklist
- Posttraumatic Stress Diagnostic Scale
- Rey Complex Figure Test
- Stroop Color–Word Test
- Trail Making Test
- Verbal Fluency Test
- Victoria Symptom Validity Test
- Wechsler Adult Intelligence Scale–Revised
- Wechsler Memory Scale–Revised, Logical Memory and Visual Reproduction subtests
- Wide Range Achievement Test–Third Edition
- Wisconsin Card Sorting Test

TABLE 1.2. Test Results

WAIS-R	1/11/2000	12/95
	IQ score	IQ score
Full Scale	93	91[a]
Verbal Scale	99	96[a]
Performance Scale	84	86
Verbal Scale	Age-corrected scaled score	Age-corrected scaled score
Information	10	9
Digit Span	7	7
Vocabulary	11	9[a]
Arithmetic	12	9
Comprehension	12	10
Similarities	11	12
Performance scale		
Picture Completion	10	10
Picture Arrangement	7	7
Block Design	9	9
Object Assembly	6	7
Digit Symbol	5	7

WRAT-3	1/11/2000	12/95
	Standard score	Standard score
Reading	68	66
Spelling	58	55[a]
Arithmetic	83	83

	1/11/2000		12/95	
Confrontation Naming	BNT	$Z = -0.13$	BNT	$Z = -0.13$
Verbal Fluency	FAS	43rd %	CFL	25–75th %
	Animals	75th %		
Comprehension	WAB Auditory Comprehension	100% accuracy	MAE Aural	71st %
			MAE Reading	80th %
			MAE Token	67th %
Repetition	WAB	92% accuracy	MAE	15th %

CVLT	Raw	Z-score	Raw	Z-score
Trial 1	4	−2	4	2
Trial 5	11	−1	10	−2
Total	38	$T = 24$	43	$T = 31$
List B	5	−1	4	−2

(continued)

TABLE 1.2. *(continued)*

CVLT *(cont.)*	Raw	Z-score	Raw	Z-score
Short Delay Free Recall	6	–3	7	–2
Short Delay Cued Recall	9	–2	8	–2
Long Delay Free Recall	7	–2	7	–2
Long Delay Cued Recall	8	–2	9	–2
Recognition Hits	11	–4	16	1
False Positives	2	1	2	1
Discriminability	84%	–2	95%	0
WMS-R	Raw	%ile	Raw	%ile
Logical Memory I	18	24	19[a]	25
Logical Memory II	13	22	11[a]	17
% Retention	72%		58%	
Recognition	10/21			
Visual Reproduction I	34	59	36[a]	79
Visual Reproduction II	25	20	30[a]	48
% Retention	74%		83%	
Recognition	5/5			
RCFT	Raw	Z-score	Raw	Z-score
Copy	21.5	–3.11	25	–1.34
Immediate	15	–1.08	7.5	
Delay	14	–1.13		
Gordon Diagnostic System	Raw	Z-score	Raw	Z-score
Vigilance Hits	30	0.58		
Vigilance Commissions	0	0.46		
Vigilance Hit Reaction Time	450	–0.78		
Distractibility Commissions	6	–1.36		
Distractibility Reaction Time	510	–1.35		
Trail Making Test	Raw	T-score	Raw	T-score
Part A	59 seconds	30	44 seconds	34
Part B	107 seconds	40	122 seconds	34[b]
Stroop Color–Word Test	Raw	T-score	Raw	T-score
Word	59	26		
Color	56	34		
Interference	1.27	51		

(continued)

TABLE 1.2. *(continued)*

WCST	Raw	T-score or %ile	Raw	T-score or %ile
Categories Completed	6	>16%	6	>16%
% Errors	19	51	32	41
% Perseverative Responses	11	51	20	39
% Perseverative Errors	11	49	16	41
% Conceptual Level Responses	80	53	65	43
Trials to 1st Responses	80	53	65	43
Failure to Maintain Set	1	>16%	0	>16%
Learning to Learn	−1.52	>16%	−1.04	>16%
Grooved Pegboard	Raw	T-score	Raw	T-score
Dominant (Right)	96 seconds	29	76 seconds	37[b]
Nondominant (Left)	170 seconds	17	92 seconds	33

*Note.*WAIS-R, Wechsler Adult Intelligence Scale–Revised; WRAT-3, Wide Range Achievement Test–3; BNT, Boston Naming Test; CFL, FAS, Controlled Oral Word Fluency; WAB, Western Aphasia Battery; MAE, Multilingual Aphasia Examination; CVLT, California Verbal Learning Test; WMS-R, Wechsler Memory Scale–Revised; RCFT, Rey Complex Figure Test; WCST, Wisconsin Card Sorting Test.
[a]Reflects our scoring of existing data.
[b]Differs from 12/95 report due to different norms applied.

hospital, which in some instances differed from the scores reported in the original report because of scoring errors I detected and/or norm differences I applied to those data.

Summary of Test Findings

Mr. Smith was approximately 4 years postelectrical injury and cardiac arrest when I evaluated him. Prior to his injury, I estimated him to have been a man of average intellectual functioning, with a high level of self-motivation and a strong business sense, based on considerations such as his completing high school 1 year early in order to live on his own, finishing in the 51st percentile of his class, and developing a series of successful businesses.

The results of the neuropsychological evaluation indicated that Mr. Smith was a man of average general intellectual functioning who exhibited specific neuropsychological deficits. He demonstrated impaired reading and writing, slowed mental and motor speed, problems with planning and organization, and impaired memory, especially with initial learning of verbal information. By contrast, he demonstrated average abilities in problem solving, language, and visual memory. His attentional capacity was also average, except under conditions of environmental distraction, at which point his attention decreased to the low-average range.

Compared to the initial evaluation 2 months after his injury, Mr. Smith's level of functioning appeared to have changed only modestly. Neurocognitively, his scores on a test of problem-solving abilities improved from low average in 1995 to the average range. By contrast, his ability to identify verbal information in a multiple-choice format was average in 1995 but severely impaired when I tested him, reflecting increasing difficulty with encoding verbal information. His performance on a task of motor dexterity decreased from a low-average level to an impaired level currently, and the decline was more marked with his left, compared to his right, hand. Psychologically, a primary finding was that Mr. Smith's personality had changed since his injury. His friends described him as a motivated, hard-working, and sensitive individual prior to his injury; now he was a man who lacked drive, initiative, and social sensitivity. Furthermore, although Mr. Smith had complaints of sad mood, decreased libido, and loss of drive, accompanied by disturbances of sleep and appetite (possibly reflecting an underlying mood disorder), his outward presentation was characterized by flat or shallow affect, which I interpreted as a neurobehavioral alteration due to his brain injury. Though Mr. Smith was able to verbalize some of his difficulties, his insight into the magnitude of these difficulties appeared to be rather limited. Indeed, Mr. Smith was spending much of his time watching television, with limited insight into his changes and no real plan for the future.

From a diagnostic standpoint, Mr. Smith's complaints of somatic (i.e., needle-prick sensations in skin, loss of smell and taste, hypersensitivity to light and noise), cognitive (i.e., difficulty with memory, concentration, and word finding), and emotional (i.e., sadness, decreased libido) symptoms were consistent with symptoms reported by many survivors of electrical injury. However, the long-term outcome regarding neuropsychological function in patients with electrical injury was not well understood at that point in time, making it unclear to what extent Mr. Smith's neuropsychological deficits reflected sequelae of an electrical injury to the central nervous system versus some other explanation, such as anoxia. Indeed, it was clear that his clinical presentation, including his cognitive and neurobehavioral alterations, were entirely consistent with the changes that occur following an anoxic injury with extended cardiac arrest, as was the case for Mr. Smith. An outstanding scientific review on this topic had been published earlier in the year (Caine & Watson, 2000), which I relied upon heavily. Prognostically, given that Mr. Smith's current neurocognitive profile was not appreciably different from his abilities as assessed in 1995, it was my opinion that he had likely reached a plateau in his neurocognitive recovery and was not able to function at a vocational level commensurate with his previous level of functioning. I specifically recommended that he be referred to a neuropsychiatric specialist for pharmacological treatment of his amotivational syndrome and depression. Likewise, given his decreased insight into his difficulties as well as his cognitive problems, his decisions regarding important financial or medical issues would need to be monitored by a trusted family member or business partner.

THE DEFENSE EXPERT'S EXAMINATION

The defense expert in this case was an "assessment psychologist" with a board certification that was not part of any mainstream board certification group of which I was aware. The fact was that he was not a clinical neuropsychologist by training as defined by International Neuropsychological Society/Division 40 standards. Curiously, he belonged to a group practice that included a well-known neuropsychologist whose stamped signature appeared on the final report, although Mr. Smith and his fiancée claimed that they had never met this person as part of the assessment process. In a subsequent affidavit, the defense expert, himself a psychologist apparently in practice for many years, stated that he had prepared his report "in conjunction" with the well-known neuropsychologist. So, whether this was a supervisory relationship or a case in which the neuropsychologist's name was added to the report to lend credibility to the findings was unclear to me. But you can bet that the plaintiff attorney was going to get to the bottom of this!

The defense experts' 14-hour neuropsychological evaluation was conducted 1 month after my evaluation; the test scores are presented in Table 1.3. The experts concluded that Mr. Smith clearly "sustained neuropsychological and psychological injuries related to his electrocution and sustained anoxia" (which is, of course, curious because 'electrocution' implies death from electrical shock), and diagnosed him with "dementia (mild) due to sustained anoxia." They described his prognosis as "fair" and concluded that cognitively he was unlikely to make further

TABLE 1.3. Defense Expert's Test Results

Wide Range Achievement Test–3	Standard score	Grade level
Reading	68	4th
Spelling	53	2nd
Arithmetic	83	6th

Wechsler Memory Scale–III	Score	Subtest	Scaled score
Auditory Immediate	74	Logical Memory I	4
Visual Immediate	68	Logical Memory II	2
Immediate	65	Verbal Paired Associates I	7
Visual Delayed	78	Verbal Paired Associates II	7
Auditory Delayed	77	Faces I	8
Auditory Recognition Delayed	90	Faces II	2
General Memory	69	Family Pictures I	2
Working Memory	83	Family Pictures II	2
		Auditory Recognition Delay	8
		Spatial Span	7

Rey Complex Figure Test	Percentile		T-score
Copy	≤1		N/A
Time to Copy	≤1		N/A
Immediate Recall	31		45
Delayed Recall	7		35
Recognition	1		27

Category test			
Number of Errors	20		48

Wisconsin Card Sorting Test	Percentile		T-score
Categories Achieved (4)	11–16		N/A
Number of Errors	21		42
Perseverative Responses	6		35
Failure to Maintain Set	>16		N/A

Trail Making Test	Raw		T-score
A	56 seconds		30
B	118 seconds		35

(continued)

TABLE 1.3. *(continued)*

Stroop Color–Word Test		*T*-score
Word Score		< 20
Color Score		< 20
Color–Word Score		27
Interface		59
Finger Tapping Test		*T*-score
Dominant Hand		19
Nondominant Hand		26
Controlled Oral Word Association		
CFL	25–75th %	Normal
Categorical Fluency (Animals)		Normal
Luria–Nebraska Neuropsychological Battery		*T*-score
Motor Functions		47
Visual Functions		52
Receptive Speech		40
Expressive Speech		57
Memory Functions		52
Intellectual Processes		51

gains. Curiously, however, they also gave him two "rule-out" diagnoses: "learning disorder not otherwise specified" and "personality disorder not otherwise specified," and noted that there may be "preexisting factors such as early head injury and learning disability" that affected his test results. They recommended that "increasing his productive activity (i.e., working) would likely improve his psychological status, although they could offer no specifics as to how that would be accomplished, given Mr. Smith's prominent cognitive and neurobehavioral deficits.

As the trial grew closer, the defense expert(s) generated two addendums to their initial neuropsychological report that seemed an attempt to distance themselves from their initial conclusions (perhaps with some pressure from the defense attorneys in the case?) and place more emphasis on Mr. Smith's preinjury level of functioning, specifically implying that it was low due to his educational background. Indeed, he had low achievement scores on the Wide Range Achievement Test, and there was no record of him ever having taken the SAT exam in Florida. So the issue became, what was his baseline? It is important to reiterate (as I did to his attorneys) that Mr. Smith graduated high school 1 year early and began to work in a shop selling T-shirts, which he eventually grew into a substantial business. However, in their first addendum to their report, the defense experts reported that Mr. Smith had earned C's and D's during the first half of his freshman year in high school. By his junior and senior years, his performance had improved, and he had earned B's in physical science and business math. His overall grade point average was 2.5. Yet, in the conclusion to this first addendum, the defense expert still stated that Mr. Smith had a premorbid IQ estimate of 100 and that it was "unlikely" that he had suffered a significant learning disability, as previously postulated.

In a second addendum to the neuropsychological evaluation produced only 18 days later, the defense expert noted that he had contacted a "micrographics technician" at Mr. Smith's high school who confirmed that Mr. Smith's senior semester included three courses entitled "on-the-job training," which required him to leave school early to attend regular employment. These classes were felt to reflect vocational rather than academic orientation; if the grades he received in gym, shop, speech, drafting and other electives were "deleted," his grade point average would drop to somewhere around 2.0. The defense experts concluded that given the poor grades in the 9th grade and the "mediocre" grades in 10th–12th grades, coupled with a non-college track of studies, the earlier finding of preexisting learning disability "could not be ruled out." Thus, his difficulties with reading, spelling, and arithmetic were interpreted as related to both "his premorbid functioning and his injury." Yet the expert still concluded in the second addendum that the results of his neuropsychological evaluation "were not significantly affected by this added information." There seemed to be some waffling and inconsistency on the part of the defense expert, who appeared to be doing his best to cast some doubt, without overtly saying so, on Mr. Smith's acquired injuries.

TRIAL AND FOLLOW-UP COMMENTARY

One of the most fascinating aspects of this case was that Mr. Smith was living on a Caribbean island under British rule that still utilized the British legal system. I knew very little about this legal system, and I never gave it close consideration when I agreed to have Mr. Smith fly to Chicago and undergo his neuropsychological evaluation. I only subsequently learned that there would be no discovery depositions in this case. There would also be no settlement in advance of the trial, and a separate trial attorney from Mr. Smith's regular lawyers, a barrister, would be the person responsible for trying this case.

The next step in the pretrial process involved a quick trip to Miami to meet with Mr. Smith's attorneys, the barrister, and, over the telephone, the patient's fiancée, who was assuming all trial expenses for the case. Locked in a hotel room for 2 days, I educated these individuals about neuropsychology, electrical and anoxic injury, and how to respond to the defense experts' report.

This case presentation would not be complete without describing the trip to the Caribbean Island for the trial itself. I still fondly recall sitting for hours prior to the trial in the plaintiff attorney's office building overlooking the Caribbean Sea, with cruise ships coming in and out of the bay and snorkelers' heads bobbing in and out of the water as they explored the coral reef. However, before any of that occurred, I had been taken directly from the airport to a car driven by the judge ("His Lordship" in the British legal system) for the purpose of visiting Mr. Smith in his apartment that evening! Apparently, Mr. Smith was not going to be attending the trial, and His Lordship wanted to have a face-to-face meeting with him. To make matters even more interesting, the defense's expert (whom I had never met) was waiting in the car, and the three of us rode together to Mr. Smith's apartment. So there I was, in a car at night on a beautiful Caribbean island with His Lordship driving and myself and the defense expert sitting in the backseat together.

When we arrived at the apartment, Mr. Smith was sitting in the dark not wearing a shirt, with long unkempt hair, watching CNN. He got up to shake the judge's hand, said hello to me, and promptly turned to the defense expert and said in a voice devoid of prosody, "You sir, are a f— ing liar." The judge appeared particularly unnerved by this outburst, although the defense expert did not appear at all perturbed. When the three of us sat down to listen to His Lordship speak to Mr. Smith, the defense expert pulled out a Rey 15-item stimulus card (i.e., an effort test sometimes called the Malingering Memory Test) and asked His Lordship if he could give Mr. Smith a "memory test" while we were sitting there in his living room. Now it was my turn to be shocked and surprised by this crude attempt on the part of the defense neuropsychologist to conduct some last-minute testing by which to be able to say that the patient was a malingerer. Interestingly, no effort tests were ever included in the defense expert's neuropsychological evaluation. In that moment I explained to His Lordship the inappropriate nature of this request, and he promptly asked the defense expert to sit quietly and not speak again.

The trial began the next day with His Lordship and the barristers wearing their powdered wigs in the small courtroom. I was the first witness called. His Lordship began asking me questions directly about why Mr. Smith had acted the way he had the night before (i.e., his appearance, his cursing), and I spent the next few hours in direct conversation with His Lordship, explaining how anoxic brain injury changes personality and social function, and how electrical injury can cause cardiac dysfunction. The defense barrister never had the opportunity to cross-examine me because the trial was dismissed for the day (it was a Caribbean paradise, after all). The case settled that evening in a very favorable way for Mr. Smith, and I had 2 hours to enjoy the beach before flying back to the United States. I have stayed in touch with Mr. Smith and his fiancée, and I am saddened (but not surprised) to say that the large settlement they received did not lead to any change in behavior or lifestyle for Mr. Smith. The money has been set aside to care for him when he is older.

LESSONS LEARNED

Aside from the opportunity to spend time on a beautiful Caribbean island, this case taught me about the British legal system and the importance of maintaining objectivity and high standards when doing medical–legal work.

It is also very important to review the relevant scientific literature regarding the condition you are evaluating (in this case electrical injury and anoxic brain injury) as you conduct your evaluation and prepare for court proceedings. Finally, it is critical to administer your neuropsychological tests in a standardized fashion under appropriate circumstances, and not attempt last-minute test administrations in a plaintiff's home in an effort to advocate for your client. You will quickly lose credibility in the eyes of your colleagues and court if you attempt to do so.

REFERENCE

Caine, D., & Watson, J. D. (2000). Neuropsychological and neuropathological sequelae of cerebral anoxia: A critical review. *Journal of the International Neuropsychological Society, 6,* 86–99.

2

Workers' Compensation and Traumatic Brain Injury

BRADLEY N. AXELROD

My interest in clinical neuropsychology was motivated by a need to understand the cognitive process involved in clinical cases. I was awed by the power of the brain to control specific functions as seen in the focal cognitive deficits following a gunshot wound or the resilience observed in individuals recovering from strokes. The amazing functions of the brain are equaled by the force of the psyche to minimize deficits, as seen in Alzheimer's disease, or to create them, as is the case of individuals with schizophrenia or depressive disorders. My transition from evaluating patients seeking information for clinical care to evaluating patients in the forensic setting developed from my interest in wishing to see a broader spectrum of patients. The variety of patients I encountered in my clinical position at the Department of Veterans Affairs was enhanced when I began seeing patients referred for forensic assessment. Over the years, I have been repeatedly intrigued by the commonality of the combined influence of cognition and affect on neuropsychological functioning, regardless of the source of the referral. I believe that if one is a good clinician, the skills should be applicable in all settings.

RECEIPT OF REQUEST
FOR NEUROPSYCHOLOGICAL EVALUATION

I had the opportunity to perform a neuropsychological evaluation with "Mr. Fred Bentler" in May 2003. The referral request and scheduling of Mr. Bentler for the evaluation was routine. Typically, requests for independent evaluation of workers' compensation cases are generated by the claims adjuster or nurse case manager. Adjusters are typically workers' compensation insurance company employees who monitor claims and make decisions about the appropriateness of evaluations and treatments. Nurse case managers are typically hired by the insurance company in an effort to maximize the employee's care following a work-related injury. I received a telephone call from Mr. Bentler, asking to be seen for a neuropsychological evaluation. The date for the evaluation was made, and I was told that Mr. Bentler would be there at the appointment time. This was the first referral I had received from this particular case manager.

PREEVALUATION INFORMATION

I encourage referring agents to provide me with as much information as possible regarding medical treatment at the time of an injury, in the emergency room and acute care, rehabilitation and extended care, and prior relevant evaluations including neuropsychological, psychological, neurological, and psychiatric assessments. Because we know that the best predictor of future behavior is past behavior, I find the review of academic transcripts, standardized test results, and preaccident mental health records also to be of interest. In the case of workers' compensation, additional information pertaining to a claimant's employment history provides insight into the individual's persistence with employment, frequency (or lack thereof) of claims, and working relationships with others.

Mr. Bentler's arrival was preceded by a small set of records. The medical records included the police report; emergency room records from the hospital where Mr. Bentler was initially seen on the day of the accident; a neuropsychological evaluation report that was conducted 7 months prior to my assessment; and a psychiatric evaluation. Although not the backbreaking box of records often made available for an evaluation, the content of the relatively few items is likely the best sample of what any neuropsychologist might wish to have. Prior to seeing Mr.

Bentler, I knew that I would have independent information regarding his injury on the day of the accident as well as information related to his cognitive and emotional status.

BACKGROUND INFORMATION

Background Information about the Injury from the Patient

Fred Bentler was a 39-year-old single, right-handed, black skilled laborer who had obtained 14 years of schooling in a Caribbean country. He was the belted driver of his employer's Chevrolet Cavalier on a morning in June 2002. There was a passenger in the front seat of his car. As he waited at a red traffic light at a busy intersection, he suddenly felt the impact of another vehicle rear-ending his car, noting that the vehicle was an ice truck. Mr. Bentler did not hear the truck approaching, nor did he see it in his rearview mirror. He believes that he might have lost consciousness for a few seconds. His last memory is of feeling the impact and striking the windshield with his head. He next recalls the driver of the ice truck asking him if he was alright. Mr. Bentler recalls that he felt "out of it" at that time.

Mr. Bentler reported that emergency personnel arrived on the scene and helped him to get out of his car. They took him to the side of the road, where he sat down and "gained his composure." Because his car was still drivable and contained his equipment for work, he drove himself and his passenger to Sinai Grace Hospital. Mr. Bentler recalls being given a number of tests and X-rays. He was given medication for pain and a neck brace and was then discharged home.

The following day, Mr. Bentler recalled that he was "stiff throughout [his] body." He also related that he was unable to turn his head because of severe neck pain that radiated down his back and right arm. He experienced low back pain and intermittent numbness in his right foot. Two weeks after the incident, Mr. Bentler reportedly experienced blurred vision.

In July 2002, a few weeks after the accident, Mr. Bentler began physical therapy for back pain; he continued with the treatment three times weekly for 6 months. After little benefit had been observed 6 months following the beginning of treatment, he underwent magnetic resonance imaging (MRI) scans of his back and head. He claims that he was diagnosed with a lumbar disc injury and head trauma. At that time, his treating physician referred Mr. Bentler for surgical evaluation. The surgeon recommended the use of a back brace in hopes of delaying required surgery. By the time of his evaluation, Mr. Bentler was continuing to see his treating physician once monthly. The treatment at that time included ongoing use of the back brace and refills for prescriptions of Tylenol #3 and 800 mg of Motrin for pain control.

In February 2003, 7 months after the automobile accident, Mr. Bentler began 1-hour sessions of outpatient cognitive rehabilitation on a weekly basis in response to many reported complaints. He was still attending regularly by the time I saw him 3 months later, in May 2003. He related that the rehabilitation treatment typically included the reading and analysis of complex problems.

Current Symptoms

During my clinical interviews I inquire about three domains relative to current symptoms. Specifically, I am interested in ongoing physical concerns, cognitive difficulties, and emotional changes. At the time of his neuropsychological evaluation, Mr. Bentler reported that he continued to experience the primary physical symptoms of neck and upper back pain that radiated down his right arm and the right side of his back. Two months prior to the assessment, he reportedly began experiencing the new sensation of pain on the left side of his neck. He claimed to lose feeling intermittently in either his left or right hand. He also had experiences in which his legs or feet were moving but he had no feeling that this was happening. In addition to neck pain, Mr. Bentler reported low back pain and complained of unremitting headaches that reportedly worsened with reading and extended concentration but improved with rest. Mr. Bentler related that his sense of smell was significantly diminished and that food tasted either too salty or too sweet.

Cognitively, he reported being more forgetful than he used to be and having difficulty understanding directions to a location, remaining attentive, and following the plot in a television show. He also claimed to have a stutter that began after the incident.

From an emotional point of view, Mr. Bentler reported being more irritable, easily angered, and less tolerant of others by the time I saw him. As he was reportedly a semiprofessional athlete (e.g., cricket, soccer, track), he had become despondent about being unable to play sports with his children. He claimed that he was not sleeping more than a few minutes at a time and that he remained awake watching television until 3:00 or 4:00 A.M. He would then go to bed, sometimes sleeping between 5:00

A.M. and 7:00 A.M.. He related that his appetite was diminished and that his weight had fluctuated. His libido was depressed in comparison to before the accident.

Background Information about Mr. Bentler's Personal History

Mr. Bentler's medical history prior to the motor vehicle accident was reportedly significant only for treatment of conjunctivitis in 2000. He denied any personal or familial mental health or substance abuse treatment. He admitted to drinking alcohol occasionally, but denied drinking more than one drink at those times.

Mr. Bentler was raised in the Caribbean. He claimed to have obtained a high school diploma while in his country. He stated that he was double promoted (i.e., skipped one grade) when he was in school. After high school, he attended college for 2 years but did not complete a degree. Mr. Bentler reported obtaining good grades and excelling in all of his classes when he was in school.

Vocationally, Mr. Bentler was a police officer for 11 years in his home city. He moved to New York in 1993. After working as a construction worker for a few years, he relocated to Michigan in 1999, where he reported obtaining certification as a nursing assistant. He subsequently sought employment as a postal worker and as a nursing assistant. At the time of his injury, Mr. Bentler had been working for himself, performing residential plastering and painting. He stated that he had been doing that work "for a number of years" at the time of the accident, although that could have been only as long as 3 years.

On a typical day since the accident, Mr. Bentler reported that he awakened between 5:00 and 7:00 A.M. and spent much of his day watching television. However, he found that he had to place himself in positions that provided relief from back pain. He stated that he did not do his own grocery shopping or cooking; a friend did his laundry, cleaned his home, and tended his lawn.

Background Information about the Injury from the Medical Records

The emergency room records from the initial hospital indicated that Mr. Bentler's vehicle "was rear-ended at low speed." At the time he was seen at the hospital, he complained of low back pain that was worse on his right side. The diagnoses of cervical and lumbar strains were offered. Importantly, Mr. Bentler denied a loss of consciousness at the scene of the accident and subsequently. Therefore, this finding contradicts his report in the clinical interview in which he claimed to have experienced an episode of altered consciousness.

An initial neuropsychological evaluation was performed with Mr. Bentler in October 2002, only 4 months after the accident. A brief summary will provide the general impressions I had prior to evaluating him. The first neuropsychological evaluation revealed intellectual functioning in the high end of the low-average range, with relative difficulties on tasks of perceptual organization, cognitive flexibility, and executive functioning. Memory, language, and motor skills were within normal limits. Mr. Bentler's emotional presentation was considered consistent with someone who was trying to present himself in an overly positive light, while simultaneously reporting dysphasia, fatigue, agitation, and health concerns. The concluding diagnosis was that Mr. Bentler's presentation was consistent with cognitive deficits and psychological distress relating to the June 2002 motor vehicle accident. It was recommended that he participate in cognitive rehabilitation. The possibility for a referral for psychiatric consultation and/or psychotherapy was left open.

EVALUATION DAY

Mr. Bentler arrived on time for his appointment in May of 2003, 11 months after the motor vehicle accident. He had driven himself to the appointment, which involved a 45- to 50-minute trip. Mr. Bentler was about 6 feet tall and likely about 220 pounds. He entered the office and walked by himself without assistance into the interview room; he did not use a cane, nor did he favor one leg over another. As he made his way to the interview room, I spoke informally with him to ensure that he was aware of the length of the appointment. He smiled amiably and in a good-humored manner about the assessment procedure. Because he had undergone an evaluation 7 months ago, he mentioned that he knew that the neuropsychological evaluation would take much of the day.

During the interview, Mr. Bentler responded to my questions without needing clarification. He offered coherent responses and concisely explained the circumstances of the accident, his subsequent treatment, ongoing difficulties, and background information. Rarely did I need to ask him follow-up questions, because his responses were thorough without straying from the topic. Qualitatively, his speech had an accent consistent with his upbringing in the Caribbean islands. He spoke at a slow rate, but otherwise produced normal volume, articulation, and prosody. Although Mr. Bentler claimed during the interview that he acquired a stutter after his work-related car accident, no stutter, or any other language abnormalities, occurred during the interview or evaluation. During the assessment, he followed the neuropsychological task instructions without requiring any assistance. Throughout the day, Mr. Bentler was stoic. He offered little spontaneous speech and refused to engage in casual conversation. He presented with a blunted and restricted range of affect. Contrasting with his initial amiable manner, his mood was despondent and sullen throughout much of the evaluation. He was unresponsive to humor—something I attempt to evaluate informally in all of my assessments.

Allow me to digress momentarily to discuss what I believe is an important aspect of every evaluation, regardless of how the referral makes its way to my office. Foremost in my mind is that all individuals, no matter what their history, should be treated in the same manner as I would want myself or my family members to be treated. I would not tolerate a clinician who disrespects me or otherwise treats me poorly. I find it incredible when referred claimants tell me that they were "yelled at" by clinicians to whom they were sent for independent examinations. The rationale for such behavior is unclear. A second factor guiding my interaction with patients is in keeping with my understanding of my duty as a neuropsychologist. Regardless of the source of the referral, my role is to obtain the most accurate understanding of the referred individual's cognitive and emotional state. Optimal rapport is required to obtain optimal test performance. It may be difficult to convince someone who has been "ordered" to see me that I aim to be as accurate as possible in assessing his or her abilities. Despite a person's suspicion and doubt, my interviews serve the purpose of not only obtaining information but also establishing rapport to optimize performance. I always attempt to make patients feel at ease when participating in an evaluation. Offering appropriate humor and sincere interest in the individual assist in moderating the discomfort that is often reported prior to an evaluation.

Given Mr. Bentler's overall behavioral presentation during the interview, the evaluation, and when interacting during breaks, I believed that his task performance was accurate and reliable. However, his mood and affect certainly offered some concern that his performance on the cognitive tasks might not reflect his optimal performance level.

TEST RESULTS

Validity and Response Bias

Whether referred to as incomplete effort, diminished motivation, inattention, exaggeration, fictitious behavior, or malingering, the level of a patient's motivation must be incorporated into an evaluation. As the reader can see from the test results section below, I often incorporate discussions of effort testing throughout the report. Measures of motivation are available in examining aspects of the WAIS, Rey Auditory Verbal Learning Test, Trail Making Test (TMT), and WCST. In addition to examining the specialized scoring for those measures, my reports discuss the relative patterns of performance across measures within the same cognitive domain. Of course, the content of responses cannot be minimized; it is a treasure trove of information. It is my preference to first address the primary scores obtained from each measure, followed by relevant findings as related to effort testing, and finally an examination across different measures within the same domain (e.g., different memory tests). In addition, results are presented in a separate section for tests that explicitly detect less than full effort, such as the Test of Memory Malingering or the Warrington Recognition Memory Test.

Mr. Bentler's performance on the two subtests (Words and Photos) of the Warrington Recognition Memory Test fell in the severely impaired level. His performance, which was 72% correct for words and 68% for faces, fell just above a research-derived cutoff (64%), below which few patients with moderate-to-severe brain injury fall. These scores do not "scream" intentionally poor performance, but they were significantly lower than his average performance on the WMS-R and the mildly impaired performance on the other memory measures. Therefore, his scores raised the possibility of poor motivation or incomplete effort in performing these tasks.

Cognitive Functioning

The specific findings from the evaluation appear in the second column in Table 2.1. At the time of the evaluation, I did not have at my disposal the information from the October 2002 evaluation, aside from Wechsler Adult Intelligence Scale–III (WAIS-III) IQ scores. With that in mind, try to evaluate the 2003 assessment on its own, without glancing at the results from 7 months earlier.

TABLE 2.1. Test Results

	October 2002	May 2003
Intellectual functioning		
Wechsler Adult Intelligence Scale–III		
Full Scale IQ	89	89
Verbal IQ	91	95
Performance IQ	86	81
Verbal Comprehension	96	94
Perceptual Organization	82	86
Working Memory	94	95
Processing Speed	86	
Academic achievement		
Wide Range Achievement Test–3 (WRAT-3)		
Reading	87	90
Spelling	96	93
Math	86	91
Memory		
Wechsler Memory Scale–III	WMS-III	WMS–Revised
Immediate	98	90
Delayed	93	82
Auditory Recognition Delay	95	
Rey Complex Figure Test		
Immediate		79
Delayed		78
List Learning	WMS-III	Rey AVLT
Total over trials	100	79
Recall	100	70
30-minute delay	100	82
Recognition Memory	110	55
Executive functioning		
Trail Making Test		
Part A	115 (19 seconds)	72 (43 seconds)
Part B	79 (101 seconds)	73 (124 seconds)
Wisconsin Card Sorting Test		
Conceptual level responding	86	78
Perseverative responses	86	76
Number of categories	2	0
Verbal Fluency (COWAT)	106	112
Motor tests		
Finger Tapping–dominant	106 (55 taps)	< 50 (26.6 taps)
Finger Tapping–nondominant	118 (58 taps)	< 50 (22.6 taps)

Note. Results are expressed as standard scores.

Looking at the results, Mr. Bentler's level of intellectual functioning fell in the high end of the low-average range, consistent with the evaluation that occurred only 4 months postincident. He demonstrated significantly higher verbal skills relative to his performance abilities. His current performance is consistent with estimations of intellectual functioning based on demographic information alone (estimated Full Scale IQ = 99 ± 12) and based on his performance on a complex reading task, the North American Adult Reading Test (estimated Verbal IQ = 90). Mr. Bentler demonstrated average verbal comprehension and working memory skills, with his perceptual organization skills falling in the low-average range. Using an arithmetic algorithm of subtest scores sensitive to diminished effort on the WAIS-III revealed a low probability (33%) that Mr. Bentler had poor motivation.

Academic achievement, evaluated with the Wide Range Achievement Test–3 (WRAT-3), revealed average sight-reading, spelling, and arithmetic computation skills, consistent with his level of intellectual functioning.

Memory functioning revealed immediate recall of newly learned material to fall in the low end of the average range (standard score; SS = 90), consistent with his WAIS-III performance. Following a 30-minute delay, his performance fell slightly lower, in the low-average range (SS = 82). Mr. Bentler was fully oriented to time, date, and location. On the Rey Complex Figure Test, Mr. Bentler's performance fell in the mildly impaired range after both a brief delay and again 30 minutes later. His initial performance on a difficult list learning task also fell in the mildly impaired range. At first, he remembered six (average performance) of the 15 words, recalling nine words (mild impairment) after the fifth trial. His recall after a brief (n = 6) and 30-minute (n = 8) delay fell in the mildly impaired and low-average ranges, respectively. Oddly, his recognition was poor, correctly identifying only 10 of the 15 words. Overall, Mr. Bentler's performance demonstrated memory functioning that generally fell in the mildly impaired range, apparently worse than the reported intact memory functioning from his prior evaluation. No verbal–visual difference among the tests was noted.

Mr. Bentler's performance on tests of cognitive flexibility ranged from the mildly impaired range to the average range. His ability to perform a simple connect-the-dots test of psychomotor speed was mildly impaired. When the task became more difficult, requiring rapid alternation between cognitive sets (e.g., numbers and letters), his performance remained in the mildly impaired range. However, an analysis of the relative performance on the two tasks revealed that Mr. Bentler's difficulty was one of slow motor speed and not impaired cognitive flexibility (Trail Making Test B ÷ Trail Making Test A = 2.88). Mr. Bentler performed in the high-average range on tests of verbal fluency. Finally, his performance on the Wisconsin Card Sorting Test (WCST) revealed some unusual performance patterns. Although he appeared to understand the task demands, Mr. Bentler's performance was often haphazard and careless. He benefited minimally from the examiner's feedback and, at times, failed to continue to respond accurately after performing correctly for five or more trials. His performance is consistent with poor effort or attention when performing this task.

Motor testing revealed severely impaired fine motor speed and finger dexterity, bilaterally, relative to age, gender, and education peers. His performance fell below testable limits.

Emotional Functioning

On the Postconcussive Syndrome Questionnaire, Mr. Bentler responded to more symptoms than did 99.5% of the medical patients upon whom the questionnaire was standardized. He reported comparably high levels of psychological, cognitive, and somatic concerns and indicated that almost one-half of his psychological and cognitive symptoms were worsening in severity over time. The somatic complaints of back pain, headaches, and constipation were also reportedly worsening. The worsening of symptoms, be they neurological, psychiatric, or somatic, is inconsistent with the expected recovery from an incident that occurred at a single time point. This finding is particularly relevant if the incident occurred 1 year earlier.

The results from the Minnesota Multiphasic Personality Inventory–2 (MMPI-2) appear in Figure 2.1 in the solid line. The validity configuration revealed a valid profile, but one in which Mr. Bentler attempted to minimize his current psychological symptoms while at the same time reporting moderate levels of emotional distress. Individuals with this profile typically come from lower socioeconomic backgrounds and are quite defensive about admitting to having psychological problems. My configural interpretation of the clinical scales revealed an individual who feels inadequate, lacks self-confidence, and is often anxious and self-critical. He is typically viewed by others as being socially withdrawn, dysphoric, dependent, and occasionally confused. Individuals with this profile are rarely agitated. However, when met with heightened distress,

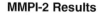

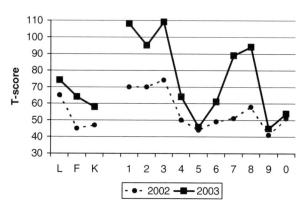

FIGURE 2.1. Results from the Minnesota Multiphasic Personality Inventory–2. (Buthcher, Dahlstrom, Graham, Tellegen, & Kaemmer, 1989).

they may become restless, overbearing, demanding, excitable, and short-tempered. Poor marital adjustment is seen with this profile. Overall, this clinical profile is felt to reflect more of a longstanding personality style than a reaction to a specific stressor. The interpretation of his profile seemed consistent with that reported in the neuropsychological evaluation that preceded mine by 7 months.

Conclusions

The findings of Mr. Bentler's neuropsychological evaluation revealed that his scores on most of the tasks fell within normal limits, consistent with his evaluation in October 2002. He otherwise presented with mild impairment on some tasks of new learning and executive functioning. Motor functioning was severely impaired. Mr. Bentler's memory difficulties were not noted in the evaluation 7 months earlier, and his performance on the executive and motor functioning tasks were reportedly worse than they had been the first time he was tested. His test results suggested a decline in cognitive functioning since October 2002, 7 months before the evaluation with me. Performance on a number of tasks sensitive to poor effort was also suggestive of such a finding. However, the results were not consistent across all measures. I believe that Mr. Bentler's presentation was more probably indicative of inattention and distractibility, or perhaps unconscious factors, than it was an intentional exaggeration or fabrication of deficits.

With regard to his emotional functioning, Mr. Bentler reported being easily fatigued, depressed, self-critical, anxious, easily overwhelmed, and passive. His profile is consistent with individuals with a longstanding personality style in which they respond to stressors with an increase in the above symptoms. Treatment for this condition is best achieved via psychotropic medication and psychotherapy that focuses on teaching assertiveness, relaxation, and self-esteem building.

In summary, Mr. Bentler's presentation was not consistent with the deficits observed in patients following a traumatic brain injury. I believed that his subjective experience of cognitive difficulties resulted from decreased cognitive efficiency secondary to heightened psychiatric distress. As his distress worsens, so would his mood, physical complaints, and claims of cognitive difficulties. In fact, his relative worsening of performance in comparison to the evaluation from 7 months earlier speaks to increasing distress. The diagnosis of undifferentiated somatoform disorder (300.81) with cognitive and pain complaints was offered. Certainly pain disorder (307.89) might be included in the differential. However, my "read" of Mr. Bentler was that his concerns were as focused on his perceived cognitive changes as they were on his pain complaints.

The following recommendations were made:

1. Medical treatment should be based on objective clinical findings rather than subjective complaints. That approach to treatment was offered to reduce the "doctor shopping" typically observed in individuals with this presentation.

2. Cognitive rehabilitation is not clinically indicated. Clearly, in contradiction with the prior neuropsychologist, Mr. Bentler's primary benefit would result from the positive psychological effects of having individual attention and not from the cognitive training per se.

3. There appeared to be no cognitive or psychological contraindications for full-time competitive employment. In fact, a return to a more active lifestyle, even on a part-time or volunteer basis, would likely assist in lifting his mood and self-esteem.

4. In terms of mental health treatment, a referral for psychiatric evaluation and possible treatment are recommended. In addition, goal-directed psychotherapy focusing on stress management, assertiveness training, and relaxation is recommended.

There was no indication that his affective state resulted from the motor vehicle accident in June 2002.

Upon completion of my report, it was mailed to the nurse case manager without fanfare. I heard nothing about the consequences my evaluation had on Mr. Bentler's benefits, medical treatment, or mental health care. The next conversation regarding Mr. Bentler was initiated 1 year later by an attorney who informed me that Mr. Bentler's trial was approaching, and my services were going to be needed. I was never called to testify in a deposition on this case.

TRIAL PREPARATION

The call from the attorney, "Mr. Thomas," requested that I clear my schedule for a specific day about 3 weeks later. He related that Mr. Bentler was offered a settlement from workers' compensation, but he refused the offer. Consequently, he had hired an attorney to represent his interests in litigation. The workers' compensation company had hired the attorney who called me. He told me the dates the trial was to begin, so that I could make arrangements to be available around that time. The actual start date of the trial was postponed twice, an occurrence that is common in the legal system.

Prior to testifying, Mr. Thomas and I spent 30 minutes on the telephone discussing my findings and thoughts about the now-plaintiff, Fred Bentler. I summarized my finding that indicated that Mr. Bentler had a condition in which stress increases his interpretation of pain and cognitive difficulties. Although cognitive deficits were observed, they did not directly result from the effects of a cerebral concussion, but were an expression of his varied attention and overall emotional distress.

Mr. Thomas asked if my opinions would change if I knew that between the time of the first neuropsychological evaluation and the time I saw Mr. Bentler, he experienced a number of unrelated personal stressors. Specifically, Mr. Bentler's wife discovered that not only had he been having an affair, but that he had a child with the other woman. She reportedly filed for divorce. Further, he had a third family back in his home country. In addition, he was in ongoing discussions with the Immigration and Naturalization Service (INS), who wished to deport him. I did not believe that the additional information altered my conclusions but, in fact, strengthened them. I agreed that any of those issues, individually and certainly in combination, could increase Mr. Bentler's distress level, thus exacerbating his cognitive and physical complaints.

Then Mr. Thomas asked if my opinions would be altered if I were told that Mr. Bentler was observed to lie down on a stretcher at the scene of the accident, but when told that he would be billed the cost of the ambulance ride, he stood up and stated that he would drive himself to the hospital. My interpretation? Well, my gut reaction was that maybe Mr. Bentler was attempting to fabricate ailments from the time of the accident. I took another look at the test data and did not find that this new information altered my conclusions.

Finally, Mr. Thomas asked if I had received the raw test data from the other neuropsychologist. I told him that I had not. He had apparently requested that those data be forwarded to me for my review prior to the trial date. The phone conversation ended and Mr. Thomas told me that he would be in touch.

On the day before I was to testify, weeks after the original date, Mr. Thomas telephoned to confirm that I was still available to testify at trial. After a few formalities, he asked if I had ever come up against the plaintiff's attorney. The name was unfamiliar, as was his law firm. "Interesting," said Mr. Thomas, "as he appears to have quite an ax to grind with you." Mr. Thomas then proceeded to tell me that in his opening statement, the plaintiff's attorney warned the jury that my testimony would soon be irrelevant. He stated, "You will see Dr. Axelrod fall apart during cross-examination, as I have revealing information that will discredit him." Gulp. I had not heard of this attorney and had no idea what information he might have that could be so damaging. Sure, I know that the primary intent of cross-examination is to discredit the witness by demonstrating poor credentials, inexperience, or incompetence. But it sounded as if the attorney indeed had a personal grudge, which raised my level of concern about testifying from "guarded" to "uneasy."

On the day I was scheduled to testify, there was to be one professional who was to appear before me. He was a physician who performed an examination focusing on Mr. Bentler's physical complaints of back and neck pain. As I sat in the courtroom, ready to acclimate myself to the setting, the plaintiff's attorney approached Mr. Thomas. The man was unfamiliar to me. They spoke briefly and then Mr. Thomas came over to me. He told me that it was requested that I wait in the hall and not be present during the proceedings. Although not uncommon for witnesses to be excused when others testify, it only served to allow me to fret about my own impending testimony. It also made me wonder for what reason the other attorney wished me to be absent. (I never figured out why that was the case, so I have no great answer to the questions running through my head at the time.)

There I was. Sitting on a long bench in the hall, waiting for my opportunity to testify. The time passed quite slowly. As I sat on the bench in the hallway, I watched people come and go throughout the courthouse hallway. The whole time, I wondered what information was going to be raised during my cross-examination that would be as damaging as indicated in the opening statement. At noon, the courtroom doors opened. Mr. Thomas told me that it was going longer than expected and that I should simply plan on returning to the courthouse the next day. He told me that if the other neuropsychologist's data had arrived, I should try to evaluate it before the following day. The data had not arrived, so my testimony would be based on my evaluation in isolation.

TRIAL TESTIMONY

On my second day at the trial, I was told that I would start first thing in the morning. Mr. Thomas called me to the stand and I was sworn in. The direct examination covered the information typically covered in most depositions or trial testimonies. My credentials and type of practice were presented, followed by the specific details of Mr. Bentler's background information, neuropsychological test results, and my conclusions. In providing results from Mr. Bentler's evaluation, I was asked if he presented with sequelae from a brain injury. Because I considered his cognitive difficulties the consequence of his affective state, I said that if he had sustained a brain injury, no persisting deficits were observed in my evaluation. "So why is his performance on some tests worse than they should be?" asked Mr. Thomas. My response involved a discussion of Mr. Bentler's affective presentation and the effect one's emotional state can have on cognitive test performance. Mr. Thomas then asked if one's wife discovered that you had a child out of wedlock, might that heighten one's affective state? He also asked if having difficulty with the INS might be stressful for the average individual. I responded to both questions. Approximately 90 minutes had zipped by, and it was time for the cross-examination.

In general, cross-examinations typically address three separate areas. First, the professional's credentials, education, employment, and source of referrals are addressed. Next, attempts to discredit the professional are made on the basis of the method of evaluation, use of tests, typographical errors in a report, and picayune details of the assessment. A third portion of a cross-examination usually delves more deeply into the report and findings, aiming to extract material that will bolster the case of the attorney questioning the professional. Thus, the first two-thirds of a deposition are often adversarial, with the goal of demonstrating poor training, knowledge, or ability.

Credential Review

My assessment of the cross-examination regarding Mr. Bentler was that it was not so much grueling as it was persistent. First, my credentials were examined. I was asked the expected questions regarding training, lack of prescription privileges in comparison to a physician, the extent of work with concussed patients (either too much or too little, depending on the expert), prior work with the current attorney, and so on. I was surprised that my fees for evaluation and for testimony appearance were not asked during cross-examination. I was told later by Mr. Thomas that the plaintiff's attorney had been stung by an earlier defense expert witness, who charged one-half of what the plaintiff's expert charged.

Critique of Neuropsychology Knowledge

The second section of the cross-examination concentrated on information pertaining to appropriate reliability, validity, and interpretation of neuropsychological test data in general. These issues, important for all neuropsychologists to know, were quite specific and seemed to be set in place in an effort to demonstrate my failure to adequately consider these in my examination.

The shift in the questions from credential review was obvious, with the first one being, "You failed to give the Halstead–Reitan Neuropsychological Battery, didn't you?" This type of question includes the assumption that the Halstead–Reitan Neuropsychological Battery is the only acceptable test battery. This type of question falls in the same category as "When did you stop beating your wife?" By only responding to the question, one fails to address the underlying assumption. Therefore, I stated the following: "I use a standardized collection of neuropsychological measures, each of which has been individually standardized and normed." "But you did not use a validated neuropsychological test battery in which the collection of tests has been demonstrated to work together in the detection of brain injury, did you?" Recognizing that the best response I could generate would alter the facts, I repeated that my test battery is composed of validated tests that can be used together. The attorney sighed loudly and moved onto other questions.

At one point, the plaintiff's attorney stated in a grand way, "Doctor. We know that you have done a lot of research in the neuropsychology field. Your vita lists numerous articles that might be relevant for some neuropsychologists. But for all of that research, I do not see a single article in which you assess cross-cultural issues of postconcussive syndrome in individuals who sustained a traumatic brain injury." I understood that the purpose of the question was to try to present an impression that my research does not apply to the type of case presented, as well as to suggest that my interpretation failed to address relevant cultural issues. Quickly flipping to the appropriate page and indicating where in the vita I was looking, I stated, "As can clearly be seen, I authored a presentation entitled 'Cross-Cultural Issues of Postconcussive Symptoms in Patients Following Traumatic Brain Injury.' " I was pleased that my response countered both intended purposes of his query. Not skipping a beat he countered with, "But your study did not evaluate patients from a Caribbean country, did it?" There was nothing to do at that point but to say that the study indeed did not include individuals from a Caribbean island. Although I did not "win" the series of questions, I believe that my response demonstrated my sensitivity to cultural issues as well as my commitment and familiarity with clinical research.

Later in the cross-examination, I was handed a reprint of a publication in which a 64-card version of the WCST was examined in a traumatic brain injury sample. The article, with which I was familiar, found that in an adult brain-injured sample, the 64-card version of the WCST did not generate standardized scores that were comparable to the full version of the WCST. The attorney paraphrased these findings, and I concurred that this was an accurate summary of the publication. "If the literature clearly argues against using the 64-card version of this test, then why was Mr. Bentler given only the first 64 cards in your evaluation?" Although not clearly explicated in the WCST administration manuals, most clinicians discontinue administration if no categories are obtained by the end of the 64th card. I stated so in response to his question. The attorney stated again, "But this study clearly states that such a procedure is inaccurate when evaluating traumatic brain injury . . . and the 64-card version should not be administered." As I sat in the courtroom, I thought back to my own studies of the 64-card WCST, which were consistent with the one presented by the attorney. I attempted to think of a way in which I could use that information to my advantage, but I was stymied. Even more so when he read from the WCST manual that the test ends "following the completion of six categories or when all 128 cards have been administered." I simply responded by noting that competent standards of clinical practice allows clinicians to discontinue the test after 64 cards. Only after returning home that evening did I replay that section of the questioning in my head. I suddenly realized that in the study presented, as well as in my own research, those patients who failed to complete one category by the end of 64 cards were omitted from the study. Consequently, in the relative silence and calm of my own home did I realize that had my response addressed that issue, I would have walked away from that line of questioning intact.

Evaluation of Report

Finally, the attorney focused on the conclusions reached in my evaluation. He asked numerous questions relating to whether or not a traumatic brain injury had occurred. At one point, I offered that as there was no loss of consciousness or posttraumatic amnesia, the likelihood for long-term deficits is negligible. He responded by asking, "Well, then, how fast does a car need to be going in an accident to create sufficient force to cause brain injury?" I answered, to the best of my ability, that brain injury is not measured by the speed of the car but by the performance of the individual on cognitive tasks. He asked about the utility of single photon emission computerized tomography (SPECT) scans in detecting brain injury. He also requested that I "educate the jury" as to why neuropsychology is more sensitive in detecting traumatic brain injury than an X-ray. For close to 30 minutes, I fielded questions about the strengths and weaknesses of neuropsychology in determining brain injury in individuals. Although not easy questions, I believe that any knowledgeable neuropsychologist would have been able to provide such information. I was abruptly told that he had no further questions.

Post-Testimony Analysis

I was initially surprised that the intense cross-examination "promised" to me never actually materialized. The next thought that came to mind related to his near-constant barrage of questions about traumatic brain injury. I strongly believe that Mr. Bentler presented with a psychiatric condition that was not caused, but could have been exacerbated, by the motor vehicle accident or by stressors in Mr. Bentler's personal life. It was surprising that his attorney focused exclusively on a potential concussion, setting aside any notion that Mr. Bentler's condition may have resulted from anything else. Clearly, his intent was to determine the presence of a brain injury and not to offer other reasonable causes to explain Mr. Bentler's poor cognitive performance.

While in the witness box, I reflected intermittently on the reaction of the jurors. Although I attempted to direct responses to them and not the attorneys, I was struck by the bland and bored expressions I saw. Eye contact was minimal, and many doodled on their pads of paper. I wondered whether the information I was providing was too obtuse, dull, or scientific to sustain their interest.

That evening, after replaying much of my testimony and the reactions (or lack thereof) of the jury, I began to doubt my ability to convince the jury of my position. I received a call the next morning from the case manager who had been present during the trial. She stated that she was convinced that my testimony was "well received" and that I "clearly swayed the jurors." I mentioned to her that I thought that the jury appeared deadpan, at best. She laughed and stated, "You have not seen too many juries, have you?"

TRIAL FEEDBACK

In my conversation with the case manager, she told me that the final arguments would occur on the following day and then the jury would deliberate. Although I know that it is unprofessional to seek to determine the outcome of a case, I could not help but consider how my testimony was received by the seemingly unresponsive jurors. I allowed for time to pass, did not receive any telephone calls, and assumed that the trial had finished.

Three days after I testified, I obtained the raw neuropsychological test data from the evaluation that had predated my evaluation. The data are presented in the left column of Table 2.1 and in the dashed line in Figure 2.1. It appeared that in comparison to the first evaluation, by the time I saw Mr. Bentler, he scored the same (e.g., WAIS-III, WRAT-3, and TMT-B) or significantly worse (e.g., list learning, TMT-A, WCST, and Finger Tapping) on the cognitive tasks. In addition, his emotional presentation was significantly more distraught compared to 7 months previous.

Although it made no difference in terms of the outcome of the case, I felt justified in my opinion that Mr. Bentler had suffered a psychiatric, and not neurological, condition.

Approximately 2 weeks after I testified, the case manager called me with the results of the case. She was most excited that the plaintiff's allegation of traumatic brain injury was dismissed by the jury. In contrast, they believed that his back and neck injuries were legitimate complaints. In their posttrail debriefing, the jurors stated that they found my testimony compelling and that they did not believe that any neurological injuries were sustained in the accident. In contrast, the physical injuries appeared more probable and more obvious. In terms of financial remuneration, the attorneys from both sides had agreed to a maximum compensation, regardless of the outcome of the trial. Although no compensation for brain injury was made, the jury supported the full amount of compensation for Mr. Bentler's physical injuries. The workers' compensation case manager was very pleased with the outcome, even though there would have been no difference financially if a brain injury was believed by the jury. She expressed to me how important it is to obtain an accurate and valid evaluation of a claimant to ensure that an appropriate outcome is achieved.

I spoke with Mr. Thomas a few months later. He expressed some dismay at what he saw as the loss of the case. However, he said that he gained some pleasure in the fact that Mr. Bentler did not receive compensation for a brain injury.

FINAL THOUGHTS

This evaluation offered a number of learning experiences, more in terms of the process of these assessments than the content of this specific case. First, just because an attorney "talks trash" to the jury about you does not mean that there is substance to the threat. In addition, treating each encounter with professionalism and honesty will work wonders in countering any personalized attempts to discredit. Further, speaking with confidence about what you know, as well as what you do not know, is typically well-received by the audience. Finally, the perceived interest of jurors during your testimony is not directly related to their assessment of your testimony. These findings were derived from real-life experiences and are typically not taught during the graduate training process.

Workers' compensation cases offer neuropsychologists the opportunity to provide treatment recommendations for an individual soon after an alleged injury. It is usually a pleasure to interact with nurse case managers who wish to work with the claimant in an attempt to find the best care and to facilitate a claimant's return to work. Although many of these individuals do return to work, there are many cases that progress, as this one did, into litigation. Regardless of the referral source, I attempt to offer a valid evaluation, based on my best understanding of the neuropsychological research, clinical interpretation, and professional experience.

REFERENCE

Butcher, J. N., Dahlstrom, W. G., Graham, J. R., Tellegen, A., & Kaemmer, B. (1989). *Manual for the restandardized Minnesota Multiphasic Personality Inventory: MMPI-2*. Minneapolis: University of Minnesota Press.

3

Symptom Validity Testing and Posttraumatic Stress Disorder

Nothing but the Truth

KRISTIE J. NIES

If clinical work is perilous, forensic work is deadly. I found out the hard way when I agreed to evaluate a woman with alleged posttraumatic stress disorder (PTSD). The attorney requested only symptom validity testing (SVT). To my credit, I held out for a diagnostic interview as well.

I had started a private practice 2 months prior to receiving this referral and was suspended in that happy place known (colloquially) as "insurance limbo"—that is, the 60- to 90-day period filled with anticipation of payment, dread of denial, and total inability to accurately gauge my financial health. I would like to say that I was driven to accept a legal case because I so strongly believe in our system of justice and the role of neuropsychology within it. The truth is, I was driven to accept just about any case at that time!

I am certain I was imagining the fees that could be collected for phone conferences, record review, consultations, depositions, and court appearances. I am certain that, because I was trying to establish a private practice, I was harried and slightly desperate. I am certain I was channeling my internship supervisor, who was prone to preach "answer the referral question and only the referral question." I am certain, in hindsight, that I should have paid attention to the niggling suspicion that being hired by a defense attorney involves more than sound clinical work and that SVT involves more than administering and scoring a test. We should view SVTs, in particular, as O'Connor (1999) views modifiers in the English language; as (to paraphrase) powerful tools that help give life to otherwise dull evaluations. "Think of these tools as weapons: load carefully, conserve ammunition, and always know where they're pointed." In this particular case, the weapon was eventually pointed at me.

PHILOSOPHICAL DIFFERENCES BETWEEN FORENSIC AND CLINICAL ASSESSMENTS

There are practical and logistical differences between forensic and clinical assessments. For example, consent forms vary. With forensic assessment, consent pertains to knowledge of the purpose of the evaluation, how long the evaluation could take, and how and by whom the information will be used. There is no confidentiality, HIPAA (Health Insurance Portability and Accountability Act) rules do not apply, and the examinee typically does not have access to the test results.

The contrast between these two types of assessments that appears most stark to me is in the nature of the relationship. There is no collaborative or even hierarchical role for the forensic practitioner. Indeed, the relationship is, at best, triangular, with "loyalty" due to the payor. The plaintiff, as a person, is almost irrelevant; the plaintiff, as a subject of controversy, is paramount.

Operating as a doctor in the absence of a doctor–patient relationship is more difficult than it may sound because of the degree of emotional restraint that must be practiced. Whereas the shades and nuances of my emotional response to someone's plight are vital in clinical work, they can be liabilities in forensic work. The explicit task is to conduct a thoroughly neutral and objective evaluation. The implicit task, at least for a defense-retained expert, is to provide evidence, if it is available, that an individual's injuries might not be as severe as claimed. The twin traces of sympathy and empathy must be held taut, because they can become tangled with the facts and steer the case in an unexpected direction.

I regard myself as a clinical neuropsychologist and as a psychotherapist. My goals, when serving in these roles, include helping people understand their cognitive deficits or their pain and suffering and guiding their healing process. I am typically not a naive person, but it never occurs to me to question the veracity of someone's claims in my clinical work. In my experience, people speak their truth, however distorted. I am aware that some patients have probably lied to me. Nevertheless, I tend to get sucked in every time I listen to a client's story, as though I were reading the engaging first chapter of a novel that I know will hold my attention rapt for days. These represent the intrapsychic barriers with which I have to contend when I am retained as an expert.

THE SPECIFIC CASE

This case was not really about SVT or PTSD. In very meaningful ways, for me and the plaintiff the case was about the truth. And although the legal system relies on the idea that fact can conform with reality, I suspect it is a myth.

I was contracted by an attorney from a prominent law firm to serve as a consultant and as an expert witness in a personal injury case. The issue of SVT was discussed in reference to neuropsychological evaluations. I explained that by using these particular assessment devices, a psychologist could determine whether someone was putting forth "good" (i.e., sufficient) effort. Verification of consistent effort would allow interpretation of the test scores as reliable and valid indicators of neural function/dysfunction. Detection of inconsistent effort, on the other hand, would raise questions as to the validity of the test results and self-reported symptoms.

The case on which this chapter is based was not about primary neuropsychological dysfunction, although the plaintiff was complaining of memory loss. She was seeking compensation for symptoms of PTSD; the referral question was quite simply "Is she lying about the extent or degree of her symptoms and limitations?" It was my opinion that SVT was one way to address this question.

I remember feeling very self-righteous about SVTs, which were new additions to the armamentarium of the neuropsychologist at that time, having recently discovered that about 30–50% of my patients (litigators and nonlitigators) were failing them. Initially, the high percentage of invalid test results confused me, and I thought I was interpreting the tests incorrectly. I soon found out that the percentage of patients failing the tests was consistent with estimates by others in the field. I was frustrated and outraged. I know I must have thought that "catching" people exaggerating their difficulties was a just cause. How dare someone exaggerate their claims or provide less than optimal effort when I was, after all, try-ing to help them?

I remember, in this case, feeling justified in using only an interview and the SVTs to render my opinion about the possibility that this woman was exaggerating her complaints. I did not believe I had to be an expert in PTSD to answer the question posed to me. Nor did I have to complete extensive memory testing or personality testing. In some ways, because of my implicit arrangement with the attorney, I was bypassing the issue of diagnosis altogether. My reticence, in this area, was not because I was without opinion. In fact, I promulgate the view that the criterion of sever-ity, crucial to all diagnoses, is often overlooked by zealous practitioners. I believe that people misinterpret normal variability of function as indica-tion of an abnormal condition. I was prepared to address this client's symptoms, armed with the knowledge that PTSD, as defined by DSM-IV, must involve a stressor considered extreme and a response considered intense.

I know now that the issue of SVT is far more complicated than my dichotomous mind can often grasp. Except for frank below-chance per-formance (e.g., < 50%), which reflects conscious distortion (i.e., malinger-ing), there are myriad possible causes of exaggerated deficits and/or insufficient effort. The cause may be "unconscious" and denote exaggera-tion rather than malingering, or it may reflect hostility, fatigue, or pain. Often, the cause eludes the patients themselves. I typically ask individuals who fail SVT if there is any reason I did not get their best performance. Invariably, they fail to understand why someone who has been in a coma for 3 months did better than they did on this task. They typically respond with platitudes regarding how hard they tried. Occasionally, I will get a response such as "the room was too warm" to explain the poor scores, but any allusion to poor effort is vehemently denied.

Record Review

I was provided with two notebooks of records with neatly tabbed sec-tions. This form of record keeping appeals to my obsessive–compulsive nature, and I interpret it as a sign of a courteous and conscientious attorney—or at least an overworked paralegal. No matter how specific the referral question, I believe a thorough record review is essential in foren-sic work. Although tedious, information pertinent to the case (e.g., drug seeking, history of interpersonal conflicts, underperformance on a job, frequent visits to a primary care physician for minor nontreatable ail-ments) may be found lurking between the pages. A comprehensive record review provides the background on which to place the current image of the plaintiff.

Contractual Information

My involvement in a forensic case usually rests, in part, on the acceptance of my fees. My hourly rate for any forensic activity (i.e., record review, consultation, deposition, appearance in court) is twice my clinical rate because it generally involves at least twice the aggravation. It took only one question for me to raise my forensic fees: "Ms. Nies [emphasis on the Ms.], you're not a real doctor now, are you?" It took only one denial of payment to implement my policy that fees are due and are not refundable 1 week in advance of the scheduled activity or the activity will be cancelled. These are the kinds of things that are not taught in graduate school.

BACKGROUND INFORMATION

Case History

"Ms. Carter" was a 35-year-old platinum-blond female with no visible scars, other than several strategically placed tattoos whose designs looked vaguely floral or sexual.

According to Ms. Carter, she had been brutalized in so many ways that I could not hold them all in my consciousness at one time. Drugs had ravaged her mind (i.e., past crack addiction); men had ravaged her body (i.e., rape and prostitution); circumstance had ravaged her womb (i.e., multiple pregnancies, multiple abortions, multiple sexually transmitted diseases); and the legal system, it seemed, had ravaged her spirit. Whereas I initially thought it a blessing to feel no connection to this woman, the issue of symptom exaggeration and even malingering started to fade in importance compared to the human response I could not inhibit. Suspicion, doubt, and cold clinical scrutiny were slowly replaced by compassion as I realized that her very survival, with respect not only to the accident but to her life, seemed miraculous. The rule of thumb for traumatic brain injury is that the outcome, ultimately, is not based solely on the type of injury but rather the type of brain (e.g., high vs. low intellect or healthy vs. diseased) that was injured. I believe the same concept is applicable to trauma. Recovery is contingent upon the type of relationship the traumatized person has to the sum total of his or her life experience. In other words, the canvas of Ms. Carter's life was the tragic context on which she interpreted the additional brushstrokes of the injury.

Diagnostic Interview

Interview Information

Ms. Carter appeared to understand the nature of our relationship and the nature of the evaluation. She readily signed the consent form presented to her. She indicated that the accident, which she was able to describe in some detail, occurred in April 2000. She had been working on a road crew as a "flagman." She was riding on a road grader to get from one site to the next when the step on which she was standing broke off of the truck, sending her to almost certain death (or some form of dismemberment) underneath either the wheels of the truck or the blade of the grader. However, she denied having any head injury or loss of consciousness as well as posttraumatic amnesia. She was taken to the hospital by ambulance, where she was simply X-rayed and then released home. She was expected to return to work after 3 days of rest, but was unable to complete job duties even after 2 weeks. Her stated complaints included pain, depression, paranoia, anxiety attacks, flashbacks, and nightmares. Her stated reason for being unable to return to work was her "nerves."

Ms. Carter reported problems with attention and memory. Examples included double checking to ensure that she had locked a door or turned off a faucet. She also said that she would often have to check to see if she had inadvertently left her car in gear or if she had set the emergency brake. She stated that her current husband said that she repeated herself constantly. She acknowledged misplacing objects such as her purse, wallet, car keys, phone, and money.

Ms. Carter also reported some functional limitations. She said that she was able to drive, but was "all over the road." She often forgot to take her medications, which included Celebrex and Zantac. She no longer engaged in hobbies such as gardening or going to movies, and she reported a complete disruption of her family life secondary to irritability. Ms. Carter indicated that all of these reported symptoms began subsequent to the accident.

Psychosocial History

Ms. Carter was raised with two brothers and one sister by her biological parents. She described her childhood as "rough" and acknowledged a history of physical and sexual abuse. There was no reported family history of workers' compensation claims or disability prior to the accident. She completed the 10th grade and dropped out of school to get married. She had three children. She was forced into prostitution by her husband, and eventually divorced him. She then began working on a city's road crew. Because of the accident she had received sick benefits for a time and then began receiving long-term disability payments. She could not tell me if she had applied for, or received, Social Security Disability payments— which raised the index of suspicion for me. There was no reported history of previous interaction with the law other than speeding tickets and the lawsuit related to the accident.

Medical–Psychiatric History

Ms. Carter denied past hospitalizations and major medical conditions such as hypertension and diabetes. She acknowledged intermittent back pain that occurred on a daily basis. On a scale from 0 to 10, her worst pain was rated as 6–7, and her least pain was rated as 1. Her pain on the day of the evaluation was rated as 1. Medications included Paxil, Klonopin, Remeron, Celebrex, and Zantac. Ms. Carter denied any history of neurotoxic exposure or head injury/loss of consciousness. She acknowledged a history of substance abuse that included excessive use of alcohol five days a week for 1 year and some use of crack cocaine during her 20s. There was no reported history of psychiatric illness/treatment prior to the accident and no reported family history of psychiatric or neurological illness.

Mental Status Examination

Ms. Carter was casually dressed and adequately groomed on the day of the evaluation. Her steady voice belied the anxiety and insecurity she expressed physically. She appeared restless (e.g., foot swing, bouncing leg) and frequently leaned forward with her hands on her knees when trying to make a point. Her affect was appropriate and her mood was anxious. There was no evidence of a formal thought disorder. Intellect was estimated as low average; however, formal assessment was not completed. Insight into her current situation was fair.

Ms. Carter described her mood as "really depressed." She acknowledged a persistent sad mood, disturbance of sleep onset and maintenance (sometimes secondary to pain), nightmares, variable appetite, weight gain, feelings of worthlessness, occasional fatigue, and a diminished ability to concentrate. She also acknowledged difficulty controlling excess anxiety and stated "I've stayed upset and have been nervous since the accident." She described feeling restless, irritable, and tense. She also reported avoiding people and believing that she was being followed every time she left her house. Symptoms of panic disorder were reported, including shakiness, increased heart rate, shortness of breath, nausea, and sweating that occurred three or four times per week and lasted 15–45 minutes. These episodes were distinct from "flashbacks," which were reported to occur three or four times per week and last 5–10 minutes. Ms. Carter indicated that she did not merely remember the accident but relived it as if she were on the pavement under the truck. When questioned, she denied any change in her appearance or position during these recollections. She stated "I just look like I'm staring off into space." She denied obsessions but acknowledged some mildly compulsive behavior (i.e., checking locks, faucets, etc.). She also denied suicidal/homicidal ideation and hallucinations.

Test Data

Ms. Carter was administered the Word Memory Test (WMT) and the Computerized Assessment of Response Bias (CARB). On the CARB she performed with good effort and 100% accuracy. On the WMT test, however, she performed in the abnormal range. Her scores on the effort components were within normal limits, but several of the scores on the memory components were abnormal. That is, her scores were very impaired on two of the very easy tasks, compared to a group of neurological patients, but entirely within the normal range on the two most difficult tasks. This pattern of performance (i.e., adequate effort but an unbelievable pattern of memory impairment) suggested possible coaching or perhaps an exaggerated response style.

Conclusions

My conclusion was that I could reach no conclusion. Even my standard interpretation of failed SVT performance (i.e., failure means inconsistent effort, which raises questions as to the validity of self-reported symptoms) did not apply.

Ms. Carter's performance on the WMT was abnormal. The abnormality, however, was not reflected on the effort component of the test; rather, it was reflected in a manner inconsistent with known injury/psychiatric disturbance, on the actual memory measures embedded within the test. It appeared that she had exaggerated her claims, at least with respect to the memory loss, albeit in a sophisticated manner—that is, without failing the effort portion of the test. The possibility that she had been coached could not be ignored or ruled out. The implication was that her entire presentation had been coached and that all of her claims may have been exaggerated.

Correspondence

Correspondence from the plaintiff's attorney to the defense attorney began in the usual fashion. An excerpt from a letter dated January 8, 2001, follows:

> Now that your clinical psychologist has had the opportunity to meet with my client, I will appreciate a report from her as soon as she reasonably can prepare it. Furthermore, I request that all notes, tests, any other forms, and other documents completed in the course of the evaluation by her or others at her office be attached to her reports so that I have every note and document associated with her evaluation.

After speaking with the defense attorney I readily complied with this request. I am accustomed to requests and court orders for records as well as intense scrutiny that might include line by line analysis of the report. One month later, I received a Notice to Take Deposition (telephone deposition), which stated that I was to bring with me "any and all records in my possession which relate to the plaintiff including, but not limited to, all notes and material which she has seen and/or relied upon in preparation for this deposition, regardless of the source of those materials."

I sent the following letter to the plaintiff's attorney to confirm the time allotted for a deposition:

> One hour has been scheduled per your request. We require pre-payment of $350.00 for the schedule time one week in advance. This is non-refundable unless cancelled one-week prior. . . . If additional time is necessary to complete the deposition, it will require rescheduling and an additional pre-payment.

Prior to the deposition, I had a 30-minute conference with the defense attorney. During this conference, I casually mentioned that although test findings were subtle, I had confidence in my conclusions, particularly since I had discussed the scores with one of the test's authors. The attorney slowly looked up from the legal pad on which he had been jotting notes and asked for clarification. I explained that I had communicated by e-mail with one of the authors to clarify some information in the manual.

Although I assured him that no identifying information had been revealed, he continued to fix a rather incredulous stare upon me and asked if I still had the e-mail correspondence. Time stood still. I knew that my future in the legal arena hinged on the answer to this question. I was hoping for a reprieve from the moral dilemma. I was praying for a bell to send me back to my corner of the ring before I took a hit. I said yes. That's when the trouble began.

The attorney then indicated that the e-mails were discoverable and therefore I was commanded to provide the plaintiff's attorney with them. When I objected, he voiced his concerns and stated he could not advise me in this matter and that, perhaps, I might need to hire my own attorney. In response to this challenge, on February 13, 2001, I wrote:

> To Whom It May Concern:
>
> I received a Notice to Take Deposition requesting that I provide "any and all records in her possession which relate to Ms. Carter and/or to this captioned case including, but not limited to, all notes and materials which she has seen and/or relied upon in preparation for this deposition, regardless of the source of those materials." I object to production of private electronic mail correspondence that relates to a test that was used in the evaluation of Ms. Carter.
>
> Please note that the opinions rendered regarding this case were mine. Also note that consultation with colleagues is a common and accepted practice. The release of the requested electronic information presents the following problems:
>
> 1. The individual with whom I corresponded will not give permission to release his communications. In fact, he objects very strongly to the release of the correspondence and the data contained therein. He provided information to me with the understanding that it was in strict confidence, as professional to professional communication.
> 2. Test scores were presented to him in an anonymous fashion without any history, and he was asked to clarify information presented in the test manual. In principle, we were discussing a hypothetical set of test results. Psychologists do not interpret results clinically without history. Any conclusions he drew were in the nature of seminar-based advice on general principles and not advice on a particular case, per se.
> 3. I ask that the electronic mail in question be viewed as private correspondence and not be considered part of the file. Symptom validity tests are an extremely valuable part of a psychologist's practice. The detection of insufficient/inconsistent effort is crucial to medical–legal proceedings as well as general clinical work. Detailed interpre-

tation of the test in question is something I cannot in good conscience simply release to an attorney.

If you choose to consider the correspondence as part of the file, I ask that it be viewed as sensitive information similar to raw data. I ask that I be allowed to send the information directly to another psychologist. Additionally, if necessary, I request that you enter a special order of protection into the legal case such that the materials will be guaranteed to be secure by the court during the course of the legal proceedings and will either be destroyed or returned to me at the end of the courts proceedings.

Thank you very much for your time and consideration. Please advise my office of how we are to proceed.

An excerpt from the immediate response, dated February 14, 2001, from the plaintiff's attorney to the defense attorney read as follows:

With respect to Dr. Nies's deposition that was scheduled to occur by telephone this Friday, 16 February, I am canceling the deposition. I suggest you contact Dr. Nies to let her know that the deposition will not go forward as scheduled. While I cannot rule out the possibility of her deposition in the future, I do ask that the $350.00 fee for her time be returned to us as soon as is reasonably possible as she is entirely to blame for this breach of legal and professional ethics.

I am very surprised at the content of her letter, To Whom It May Concern, a copy of which I received today. I must give serious thought about what course of action to pursue at this point, including legal action against her, and will discuss the matter with you soon.

I am distressed to learn at this late hour that another person was involved in Ms. Carter's evaluation. I vehemently disagree with Dr. Nies's various assertions and positions contained in her letter. Not only do I question the legitimacy of her claims, I also question her competency as a professional. I am giving thought to filing a motion to exclude her testimony in this case. I believe that would be appropriate relief under the circumstances. I have contacted the court reporter to cancel Friday's deposition. Of course, this action is necessitated by the content of Dr. Nies's letter, which reflects grossly inappropriate conduct.

Outcome

I was not threatened by this letter. I never consulted my attorney or my malpractice insurance carrier. In fact, I am still not sure what I could have been sued for. The plaintiff's attorney clearly did not like the implication of my letter and its relevant interpretation, but was protesting his innocence just a little too loudly. I was embarrassed. My limited role in this production had shifted to center stage and was being illuminated by a very unflattering light.

Because of my "bad behavior" I assumed that my tenure with the law firm that hired me was summarily over. Yet, February 19, 2001, I was notified that the case was set for trial. I sent the following letter:

> This is to confirm that I am expected to be presented as a witness at the trial in the above case. The trial date is April 9–12, 2001. I understand I am to be available either April 11th or April 12th.
>
> The charge for forensic activities, including live testimony, is $350.00 per hour inclusive of travel time. A $500.00 deposit is due one week prior to the trial date. This payment is nonrefundable unless the office is notified by April 2 that my presence is not required. Preparation time will also be billed to you at $350.00 per hour.

The following week I was contacted by the paralegal, who informed me that the case was settled out of court.

DID I EVER GET A CASE
FROM THAT LAW FIRM AGAIN?

I never heard from the firm again. Out of curiosity and to complete this chapter, I recently contacted the attorney who hired me. His statements were courteous. However, it was what he did not say that convinced me that his once warm professional interest had become tepid. He did not report a positive outcome of the case, he did not thank me for my work, and he did not say he looked forward to future collaboration. Yet I was paid for all the time I had put in on the case.

WHAT I LEARNED FROM MY INVOLVEMENT
WITH THE CASE

First, I learned that regardless of the high rates of monetary compensation, the overall cost of doing forensic work is prohibitive. Although I am in favor of stepping outside of my comfort zone on occasion, I found that veering from standard clinical practice is labor intensive. If I had wanted to traffic in jurisprudence, I would have become an attorney. Second, I learned that Oscar Wilde was right: "The truth is rarely pure and never simple." Truth is subjective and is more related to what someone needs to believe than it is to any objective test. Ms. Carter probably believed her claims as much as I believed mine. In psychotherapy, the truth is a gray area that can largely be ignored. Therapists encourage people to find their voice to speak their own truth; its correlation to anyone else's reality is often irrelevant. In forensic work, the truth is a darker shade of murky. The truth, the whole truth, and nothing but the truth is expected of witnesses. This oath of honesty does not budge for truth born of ignorance, disagreement, erroneous beliefs, or emotional distress. There was certainly no wiggle room for my truthful but untimely revelation.

I fault myself not for the wrong action as much as not knowing the right action. I was admonished by several colleagues for my behavior—not for the presumed breach of forensic protocol but for my stubborn insistence on being forthright. I was told I should have lied about the e-mails. I was told I was being overly virtuous, to no end. And although I agree that lying would have been the easier solution and would likely have preserved my relationship with the attorney, it also would have injured my relationship with myself. Character is often built on inconvenience and discomfort; ease rarely breeds integrity. I believe it is only when we are tested that we discern our true nature. As I write this, I am still not sure what the right action would have been. I am clear that I should not have lied. I am less clear about the degree of dishonor associated with omitting some of the truth. Perhaps the dark fact of my discussing scores with the test author need never have seen the light of day.

I learned several additional important lessons.

1. Forensic work does not play to my strengths except in cases of brain injury, when I am called to testify as a treating clinician. In these cases, I am called to defend my clinical work, not a priori assumptions of dishonesty.

2. I learned to guide the referral question. Referral sources, forensic and clinical, often do not know the questions they would like answered. I have learned that most individuals need assistance in articulating the issue they want addressed.

3. I learned that e-mail correspondence has evolved as a form of communication to the point of requiring legal protection. Most professionals now attach warnings, similar to the following, at the end of their correspondence.

> ***CONFIDENTIAL*** The information in this e-mail and any file trans-
> mitted with it is protected by state and federal law. Further disclosure of this
> information without prior written consent of the person whom it concerns
> is prohibited.

Whether this warning has any power in a court of law is a question I hope
never to have to answer.

    4. Most important, I came to believe that trauma is in the eye of the
victim. Although I understand that the identification of a causal relationship is necessary to assist in a determination of financial remuneration,
an individual's symptoms cannot be separated from his or her history.
Peter Levine, a noted expert on trauma, states, "Common occurrences
can produce traumatic aftereffects that are just as debilitating as those
experienced by veterans of combat or survivors of childhood abuse"
(1997, p. 45). He also states that recovery from a threat is determined by
the event, the context of the person's life at the time of the event, physical characteristics of the individual, a person's learned capabilities, the
individual's experienced sense of his or her capacity to meet danger, and
the history of success or failure in similar situations. Because we have the
ability to detect suboptimal performance, coaching, and malingering, it
does not mean that we can rate a person's degree of suffering or subjective level of despair.

WOULD I DO ANYTHING DIFFERENTLY NEXT TIME?

I hope there will not be a next time. I have become much more careful
about which cases I will consider. I complete comprehensive evaluations
in similar cases that include measures of pain, personality, and posttraumatic symptoms to get a full picture of a plaintiff's difficulties. Forensic
work, more than general clinical work, involves very real consequences
that can significantly, and sometimes unalterably, affect very real futures.
Such large decisions require consideration of a large number of data
points. Having said that, I do not believe that additional testing would
have been helpful, from a legal standpoint, in this case. The SVTs actually
served the purpose the defense attorney intended.

    I am no longer seduced by the glamour of SVTs. They began their
career as pretty sexy instruments. After a seemingly capricious and sometimes gaudy adolescence and young adulthood, I believe that they have
settled into a staid existence. Although not without continued contro-

versy, they continue to play an important role in neuropsychological evaluations.

WHAT CAN STUDENTS OR YOUNG PROFESSIONALS LEARN FROM MY INVOLVEMENT IN THIS CASE?

Pay attention to your barometer of discomfort before accepting a forensic case. Determine whether or not you can stomach the outcome. Prepare to be considered a pawn in a very large chess game and know that you may be insulted, blamed, or threatened if it suits the attorney and helps his or her case. You can protect yourself financially with strict policies regarding prepayment and cancellations. It is more difficult to protect your soul from wear and tear. Always know where the weapon is pointed. The bullet is not yours to take, so be prepared to duck.

I believe I gleaned something, even at this late date, from my involvement in the case. I was recently asked by a defense attorney to complete a neuropsychological evaluation of a woman who, prior to an alleged rape, had sustained a severe traumatic brain injury. I indicated that I could evaluate cognitive function and that I could determine degree of impairment. In shaping the referral question, it became apparent that the real issue was whether or not this woman had been competent to consent to sex. I found the idea of her competency invalidating her accusation reprehensible. Furthermore, I found the idea of false accusation equally reprehensible. Also, I am unaware of a literature that outlines the cognitive abilities necessary and sufficient to consent to have sex. After all, even people with otherwise good judgment sometimes make decisions they later regret. Needless to say, I declined the case.

REFERENCES

Levine, P. A. (1997). *Waking the tiger; healing trauma*. Berkeley, CA: North Atlantic Books.

O'Connor, P. T. (1999). *Words fail me*. New York: Harcourt.

4

Medical Malpractice, or "Up the Nose (and Brain) with an Endoscopic Hose"

ROBERT L. HEILBRONNER

I got involved in forensic practice like most other clinical neuropsychologists: first, as a treater and, over time, as a retained expert. It just seemed like the "natural course" of development emanating from my primary interest and experience working with patients with traumatic brain injury in a rehabilitation setting. I never would have anticipated that I would be doing as much forensic consulting as I currently do. I guess the ethics and high standards I have set for myself have paid off. Or perhaps it is because I like the challenge of defending my opinions and the process of teaching and educating attorneys, judges, and juries about brain dysfunction and neuropsychology. I'm not sure. Whatever the reason, I hope that forensic work will continue to be a source of satisfaction and income as I embark on the last 20 years, or so, of my professional life.

BACKGROUND INFORMATION

This case starts out like so many other forensic cases . . . with a telephone call from an attorney. It began something like this: "Dr. Heilbronner, my name is 'Alan Peterman' and I have a case that I'd like for you to consult on. My client 'Tracy Frizzle' underwent septorhinoplasty surgery 2 years ago that resulted in a cerebrospinal fluid [CSF] leak and aseptic meningitis. My client used to be a vital, energetic, 60-year-old woman, and now she is unable to do anything. She has ongoing complaints of dizziness, headaches, and vertigo; cognitive problems such as word-finding difficulties and short-term memory deficits; she is depressed and very angry, as you might expect." The attorney went on to say that he has never used a neuropsychologist before and is rather unfamiliar with the kinds of things someone like me might be able to offer. His client had been evaluated previously by two treating neuropsychologists and, at the very least, he needed someone like myself to assist him in understanding their test results and opinions. He had also retained a forensic psychiatrist (who had actually provided him with my name) and was hoping that, in tandem, we might be able to assist him in explaining the psychological damages to an arbitrator. The four defendants were the surgeon, his group practice, the hospital, and the medical malpractice insurance carrier.

Mr. Peterman regarded Mrs. Frizzle's physical complaints (e.g., dizziness and vertigo) as being the primary damages, but he wanted to have the psychological issues as kind of a "backup." He was quite clear that he wasn't trying to prove brain damage or the presence of any prominent cognitive difficulties. In fact, he was worried about possibly spoiling his case if she proved to be a malingerer on testing. I told him that I would be interested in consulting with him and that I would provide him with an honest and objective opinion. "Of course," he said, "that is how I prefer to operate." I have heard this claim before from many personal injury attorneys, many of whom are simply giving this principle lip service. Still, most credible attorneys actually do want the truth from their experts, so that they know how to evaluate the strengths and weaknesses of their case and perhaps to anticipate the kinds of responses they may get from the opposing side's expert. I got the sense that Mr. Peterman was a reasonable person who was really interested in trying to understand his client's condition. I also correctly anticipated that he would require a fair amount of education about neuropsychology and psychological disorders.

Before our conversation ended, Mr. Peterman asked me for the names of other attorneys with whom I had worked and wanted to know if it would be acceptable to me if he were to contact them to find out a little bit more about me. I had never been asked for references before (except during a deposition) but said that it would be fine with me. Besides, the names I gave him were those of attorneys who had appreciated the work that I had done in their cases! I faxed him my CV and fee schedule, as requested. Then I did not hear from him, which led me to think that he had either found someone else, was upset by my fees, or had decided not to pursue the psychological aspects of the case. About 3 weeks later, Mr. Peterman called to tell me that he had sat in during my courtroom testimony on another personal injury case about 2 weeks earlier. He said that I had done a fine job describing the plaintiff's condition to the jury and that he wanted me to provide the same kind of testimony in his case. I told him, that is the kind of information a neuropsychologist is able to provide, whether he used me or someone else. One week later, a box of records showed up at my office, including the requested retainer check. I guess he was actually impressed with my testimony, after all!

As records go, the box was fairly hefty. I didn't weigh it, but I felt a pain in my lower back as I carried it from the office to my car! From a financial perspective, such a large box of records is a good thing, especially to someone in independent practice. On the other hand, a comprehensive review of extensive records places an additional demand on the expert: It requires him or her to be on top of a lot of information—not so much to commit it to memory, but to be familiar with a lot of little details and seemingly unimportant facts that may prove to be very relevant to the outcome of the case. As an expert, I feel that it is important to be familiar with the case from beginning to end, at least from a neuropsychological perspective. That is one reason why it is important to obtain as many records as possible, including those from the plaintiff's premorbid history. Indeed, when rendering opinions about alleged changes in functioning after an injury, accident, or faulty surgery, it is important to have a basis for comparison. Of course, such records often do not exist or are otherwise unobtainable. In such instances, the practitioner must decide whether or not the patient's subjective report provides enough reliable and valid information. In the context of litigation, the patient's self-report may certainly be looked upon with some skepticism, especially by the opposing attorney or expert. When I review records, I don't usually take notes, choosing instead to highlight points. In this case, because of the voluminous records, I decided that taking notes would be helpful, keeping in mind that any written materials could be subpoenaed or at least be made available for review by all relevant parties.

Mrs. Frizzle's records included information pertaining to the surgery, her acute postrecovery period, follow-up appointments with treating physicians, and her participation in a number of therapies, including physical therapy, occupational therapy, and craniosacral manipulation. Her premorbid medical history was essentially unremarkable; as her attorney had described her, she was actually a vital and energetic 60+-year-old woman who enjoyed Rollerblading, writing, and acting. She was even anticipating entering into the Peace Corps a few weeks after the surgery, had it not gone awry. There was no premorbid history of alcohol or other drug abuse, smoking, or cardiovascular risk factors. Mrs. Frizzle had participated in psychological treatment over 15 years ago to assist her in adjusting to a divorce. In fact, she had seen this aging analyst on a number of occasions since then, including a couple of visits after the surgery, in order to assist her in coping with the psychological and emotional consequences of this event. Particular emphasis was placed on her strong resentment toward the doctor, who admitted fault but had never apologized to her for what happened.

As an aside, I was a candidate for sinus surgery about 3 years prior to becoming involved in this case. I chose not to go through with the procedure because I did not feel I had been adequately informed about the potential complications that might ensue, one of which included a CSF leak as a result of going too far into the nasal cavity and puncturing the cribiform plate. With hours to go before the scheduled surgery, I decided to put it on hold and try a more conservative course of treatment with some of the newer antihistamines that have proven to be successful for individuals with chronic sinusitis. The records indicated that Mrs. Frizzle had sought surgical consultation for liposuction, and the plastic surgeon (who was not an ear, nose, and throat specialist [ENT]) had offered to do sinus surgery while she was under anesthesia. She had agreed to do this because she had had many years of discomfort with her breathing, and she apparently felt a level of confidence in the doctor, who had informed her that he had done this type of surgery before on a number of occasions.

Even before I had evaluated Mrs. Frizzle, I already had more than a modicum of feelings about this case—some might call it "countertransference" (there's a term you don't commonly hear from a neuropsychologist!). Because of these personal issues, I really needed to be cognizant of the potential biases that might influence my interpretations and opinions, something we need to be aware of in any forensic case we undertake.

PREVIOUS EVALUATIONS

Mrs. Frizzle had been evaluated by a psychologist and neuropsychologist on two previous occasions. She underwent an initial psychological evaluation 11 months postsurgery, upon referral of her treating neurologist secondary to complaints of failing memory, word-finding problems, reduced attention and concentration, fatigue, and balance difficulties. She also reported pain in the back of her head and neck and sleep problems. Results of the evaluation revealed impaired attention and concentration and a lower than expected score on a test of abstract reasoning and concept formation. Testing strongly suggested that "there may be a neurological component to her compromised cognitive functioning." It was also the examiner's impression that Mrs. Frizzle's subtle cognitive deficits affected her emotional well-being. Personality test results suggested that she was prone to react under stress. She reported a considerable amount of situational anxiety and depression, helplessness, and feelings of hopelessness, but no suicidal ideations.

Mrs. Frizzle was evaluated by an American Board of Clinical Neuropsychology board-certified neuropsychologist 2 years postsurgery, upon referral of a second treating neurologist. At that time, she reported that she cried a lot, got dizzy, had vertigo and fell often, had pain in the back of her neck and in the "cerebellum," had difficulty with concentration and memory, and had trouble reading. An abbreviated evaluation was conducted because Mrs. Frizzle reportedly did not feel well during the second day of testing. Results did not support the presence of cognitive deficits; she scored in the average range or better on all the measures. Her personality profile was elevated, with a "conversion-V" pattern on the Minnesota Multiphasic Personality Inventory–2 (MMPI-2). The examiner reviewed the previous test results and did not find any evidence of cognitive deficits. Yet both evaluations revealed abnormal MMPI-2 profiles that reflected a person who presented with somatic complaints that are often better explained by psychological, rather than organic, etiologies.

When I serve as a forensic consultant, it is not always implicit that I will conduct, or even have the opportunity to conduct, a neuropsychological evaluation of the plaintiff in a civil case or a defendant in a criminal case. However, more often than not, after I review the records, I make the request to perform such an evaluation because it would provide a better foundation for my opinion(s). Moreover, it is in keeping with sound ethical principles, which state that "psychologists provide opinions of the psychological characteristics of individuals only after they have conducted an examination of the individuals adequate to support their statements or conclusions" (American Psychological Association, 2002, Ethical Standard 9.01). There have been occasions where I have not been allowed to examine a person in litigation. In such circumstances, at the outset of my report or Federal Rules of Evidence (FRE) opinions I make it clear that the opinions I have expressed are "based solely on a review of records, and I reserve the right to amend these opinions as new information is made available to me or after I have evaluated the client" (consistent with the recommendation of American Psychological Association Ethical Standard 9.02). I was accused of being unethical one time because I had rendered an opinion without examining the client—but this accusation was from the same attorney who had gone to court to file a motion effectively prohibiting me from performing an examination on his client!

NEUROPSYCHOLOGICAL EVALUATION

Interview Information

Mrs. Frizzle arrived for the evaluation on a Monday morning. Although she was a half-hour early, she was upset that I was not at the office to greet her. Thus, she started the day on a rather sour note, accusing me of changing the time and the office not being opened up so that she could sit down because she was so dizzy after walking from the bus to my office. I apologized for any miscommunication, politely offered her some water, then asked if she wanted to lie down on the couch in the waiting room until she felt ready to begin. She declined, preferring instead to begin the evaluation with the hope of completing it in a single day. At the outset of the interview, she stated, "I didn't like Dr. P. [the second evaluator], he's a control freak. I told him that I wasn't feeling well, and he was the one who wanted to discontinue the testing . . . not me. But he put in his report that I was the one who wanted to stop and that I was hysterical. Can you believe that? He's got no business practicing." Now I understood where some (but certainly not all) of her apparent hostility and anger had come from: she'd had a previous unpleasant experience with one of my neuropsychology colleagues. This perceived indignity was on top of feeling violated and abandoned by the physician who had performed the sinus surgery. I sympathized with Mrs. Frizzle, but told her that I know the neuropsychologist who examined her and I happened to regard him quite highly. I anticipated another hostile response, but she seemed appreciative of the fact that I could disagree with her in a forthright and noncondescending manner. The interview continued.

Mrs. Frizzle became rather tearful as she described the various ways in which her life had been affected by her symptoms. She said that because of her dizziness and poor equilibrium, she is very fearful of crossing the street, has problems getting into elevators, going up the stairs, and often falls when she has to bend over. She reported having fallen on a number of occasions, such that her body was "a mass of bruises." She added, "There isn't a day that doesn't go by that I don't bump into something." Mrs. Frizzle said that she has no sense of smell any longer. As a result, she has had several fires in her apartment and has burned teapots and pans. She said that she often walks away when she is cooking something and then forgets about it. In describing these and other events, Mrs. Frizzle became very teary and stated, "It's difficult for me to accept what has happened to me. I try to still be who I was and I just can't. I used to be psychologically strong and could weather a lot of stuff. I don't like being vulnerable and giving up control." She said that the only good thing that has come from all of this is that she has "learned to live with disorder." She stressed that she needs things to be more in control now more than ever. Mrs. Frizzle said that she "felt like a victim" and was disappointed that the doctor had never apologized to her. She added that others (including defense attorneys) are not "inside my head" and do not really know what it is like for her to have to go through life with all of these problems. It bothers her, she said, when people do not understand her condition, and she resents the fact that they may think she is fine based upon her appearance alone. Yet she also does not want people to know that she has a disability and to pity her. Although she had a rather hostile edge to her, Mrs. Frizzle's ability to acknowledge her vulnerability made her more likeable. But I was careful not to let my sympathy cloud my objectivity. As an expert, I was an advocate of the facts and not the patient.

When asked how she spends a typical day, Mrs. Frizzle said that it takes her about 2 hours to get ready in the morning: "I do everything slowly," she said, "and I have to do one thing at a time." She said that she was able to do rudimentary types of activities (e.g., feed her cat, make tea). She would take walks, although not as frequently or as far as she did prior to the surgery. She used to Rollerblade often, during the day and at night, and sometimes for great distances. Since the surgery, she has been completely unable to do this and many other physical activities she used to do with ease. She is unable to clean her apartment by herself and has someone come in to help (partially paid for by a local charity). She recently moved to a new location and many of her belongings remained in the moving crates because she did not have the energy to organize her apartment. Mrs. Frizzle said that she spent a lot of her time going to doctors' appointments and to therapists: She received trigger point injections and craniosacral therapy. These treatments helped ameliorate some of the pain in the back of her head, neck, and shoulder area but did not eliminate it. She said that often after an injection she feels bad and gets very dizzy, and there have been occasions when she has left the doctor's office and fallen down. She no longer writes like she used to, which was a very important part of her life and livelihood. In fact, she had been working on a novel for over 10 years but has not worked on it since the surgery. "Writing was everything to me," she said, "now it's like someone cut my heart out." She does not read as often either: The nystagmus makes it difficult, and her eyes hurt. Mrs. Frizzle presently has to nap during the day, and often she naps until dinnertime. She may then cook dinner and go to bed after that or perhaps watch television. "It depends on the day I've had . . . it's never the same—almost every day is filled with something related to my injury."

In discussing the possibility of brain damage as a result of the surgery, Mrs. Frizzle said that it was her understanding that her treating psychologist and the psychologist who did the first testing both felt as if her brain was affected because of her apparent word-finding difficulties and memory problems. She said that she does not remember what the neurologists have told her about possible brain damage, but it was her understanding that the surgeon "went into the arachnoid layer where CSF is stored." She later said that one of her ENTs believes that "scar tissue" has formed in the meninges and might be causing some of her pain. Mrs. Frizzle said that she has been told by some of her treaters that her dizziness, visual problems, and resulting disequilibrium are because of "the disconnection from her eyes and ears to the brain" as a result of the CSF leak. Whether or not these theories are true, it was clear that Mrs. Frizzle possessed more than a minimum knowledge about her condition, and she took an active role in her treatment and efforts toward recovery.

Mrs. Frizzle acknowledged that some of her condition may be emotional and not just physical. When asked about any apparent changes in personality, she indicated that others have told her that she is different from how she used to be. She used to be easygoing, but now she loses her temper easily and is less patient (although this has reportedly improved secondary to the nattokinase she is taking). She uses profanity more than before; she cited specific examples of her use of profanity in the doctor's office and the hospital where the surgery took place. She reports that she cries more easily and that "tears just come out on their own." When asked what her treating psychologist (who knew her before the surgery) would say, Mrs. Frizzle replied, "She would say I am not the same person that she treated back in 1984 while I was going through a divorce. I've always had my physical strength and was able to get on with my life." Mrs. Frizzle said that dizziness is the "most destructive" of all the symptoms: "It derails me," she said. One of the most difficult things about the dizziness is its unpredictability: "I never know when I am going to get a dizzy spell," she said. She added that she is more fearful now than she used to be and does not travel to areas of the city to which she used to travel; she is also very anxious when crossing streets. When asked about any suspiciousness/paranoia, Mrs. Frizzle became tearful and acknowledged that this was something new for her. "I feel like everybody is ganging up on me," she said. She relayed an experience in which she had misperceived something (seemingly sexual) an engineer in her building had told her; she was so embarrassed by her response that she reportedly did not leave her apartment for almost 2 weeks.

Behavioral Observations

As noted, Mrs. Frizzle arrived a half-hour early for the clinical interview, which took place on the first day. She said that she prefers to arrive at her appointments early because she does not know what to expect in terms of the traffic or her ability to maintain balance when crossing the street. She arrived an hour before the scheduled time on the second day, stating that she did not get the message about the change in her appointment time. Initially, she appeared somewhat upset, but was easily reassured that the appointment would begin shortly. She was not happy about having to come back for a third day, but she appeared calmer on that day. She was appropriately dressed on all occasions and listened to headphones while reading in the waiting room. She ambulated without noticeable gait disturbance; however, she tended to "hug the walls" when she walked, stating that she often bumps into them, especially when she is rounding a corner. Of note is the fact that when she rose from a seated position, she did so in a very slow and cautious manner; nevertheless, the dizziness would strike, and it often took her a few moments to gain her balance. On a few occasions, it appeared as if she were going to fall over, and she had to be supported briefly until she regained her balance. Overall, she came across as rather hysterical or "nonphysiological" in her presentation, but her disequilibrium occurred so consistently over the 3 days of testing as to be believable.

Mrs. Frizzle was fully alert, oriented, and cooperative on all 3 days. Her speech was normal relative to rate, rhythm, and prosody, and her thought processes were coherent, logical, and goal directed. Throughout the interview, she tended to be a bit tangential in her speech, getting off topic at various points in time. She was aware of this tendency and was able to correct herself in most instances. She was cognizant of the reason for testing and was able to articulate what led to the referral. She evidenced an appropriate range of affect throughout the evaluation, at times becoming frustrated and angry (when talking about how her life had changed since her injury). On other occasions, she became teary and appeared sad. During the administration of one test of executive function (Wisconsin Card Sorting Test; WCST), she became very frustrated; yet she was able to persist and complete the test with consistent effort. During sensory–perceptual testing, she became very dizzy after three trials of single visual stimulation; the task was discontinued following two trials of double simultaneous stimulation. Also of note was her sensitivity to light: She was about to put her sunglasses on during the testing, but the lighting was reduced to a lower level of illumination that seemed more tolerable to her. Overall, Mrs. Frizzle was cooperative and motivated throughout the testing. On occasion, she seemed to get fatigued, but she expressed an interest in continuing with the evaluation with the hopes of completing it in one or two sessions.

TEST RESULTS

Validity and Test Interpretation Considerations

In order to assess level of effort, motivation, and potential response bias on cognitive testing, performance on measures sensitive to malingering, erratic performance patterns, and invalid response patterns was assessed. Mrs. Frizzle's scores on the Victoria Symptom Validity Test (VSVT) (24/20) and the Test of Memory Malingering (TOMM) (46/50/45) were valid, suggesting no signs of suboptimal effort or an attempt to feign memory deficits. She reported feeling as if she may have transposed some of the numbers of the hard items on the VSVT because of the nytagmus. Her score on the Rey 15-item Memory Test recall (14) and recognition (15) trials were also both within normal limits. Her score on the forced-choice component of the California Verbal Learning Test–2 (CVLT-2) (16) was perfect, similarly indicating a valid response style. Her score on the Validity Indicator Profile (VIP) Verbal subtest was valid; the nonverbal score was invalid and reflective of a careless response style. This result does not suggest that she consciously put forth poor effort on this subtest; some individuals respond in this manner when they are distracted or fatigued or when they are hampered by intense and competing internal stimuli. Overall, Mrs. Frizzle was observed to put forth adequate effort throughout the testing.

The MMPI-2 Fake Bad Scale (FBS) score was 28; this is a scale that is often used to evaluate exaggeration of physical complaints, especially in compensation-seeking adults. Elevations of this magnitude suggest a high rate of endorsement of physical symptoms, leading some to opine that the symptoms are endorsed for purely secondary gain. On the other hand, patients with somatoform disorders as well as those with personality changes secondary to bona-fide medical–neurological conditions also score high on this scale. Moreover, feeling as if his or her symptoms are not believable to others may lead the person to over-endorse his or her complaints to "prove" to others how dramatically his or her life has changed as a result of the illness/injury. Also of note is Mrs. Frizzle's high degree of endorsement of "critical items," again reflecting a moderate amount of distress, manifesting primarily in symptoms of anxiety, depression, and somatic complaints. She related that after completing the MMPI-2, she began to feel angry and frustrated about her current circumstances and about how the surgery has negatively affected her life.

Summary

Results of the present, most comprehensive, neuropsychological evaluation to date reveal generally intact performance in most cognitive domains assessed (see Table 4.1). Indeed, Mrs. Frizzle scored at, or very close to, her estimated premorbid ability levels on the majority of the tasks administered. Any cognitive deficits that were apparent are considered mild or subtle in nature. However, even small decrements in cognitive functions can cause major disruptions to someone such as Mrs. Frizzle, who was clearly operating at an above-average to superior level before the surgery. Primary and relative difficulties were revealed on tasks measuring working memory and memory-retrieval skills, nonverbal abstract reasoning, visual–spatial abilities, organization and planning, and fine psychomotor speed, particularly with the left hand. Qualitatively, there was evidence of a number of difficulties, most notably problems on tasks requiring visual–spatial abstract reasoning and the reproduction of complex figures; in fact, her reproductions appeared very "organic-like." It is important to point out that the testing was done in a very quiet, structured environment where Mrs. Frizzle was able to direct her attention to the tasks at hand without external distractions. Problems may emerge for her in unstructured, distracting environments or when her psychological–emotional state causes an internal disruption to her capacity to think logically and in an organized manner.

TABLE 4.1. Neuropsychological Test Results for Mrs. Fizzle

Test	Standard scores
Victoria Symptom Validity Test	
Easy	24/24 (100%)
Latency	1.02 seconds
Hard	18/24 (75%)
Latency	2.01 seconds
Test of Memory Malingering	
Trial 1	46/50
Trial 2	50/50
Trial 3	45/50
North American Adult Reading Test	Estimated Premorbid Full Scale IQ = 121
Wechsler Adult Intelligence Scale–3rd Edition	
Full Scale IQ	119
Verbal IQ	115
Performance IQ	121
Verbal Comprehension Index	114
Perceptual Organization Index	109
Working Memory Index	108
Processing Speed Index	117
Vocabulary	12
Similarities	12
Arithmetic	12
Digit Span	13
Information	13
Comprehension	NA
Letter–Number	9
Picture Completion	15
Digit Symbol Coding	14
Block Design	11
Matrix Reasoning	12
Symbol Search	12
Wechsler Memory Scale–Third Edition	
Logical Memory I	SS = 12
Logical Memory II	SS = 13
Logical Memory LS	SS = 12
Face Recognition I	SS = 17
Face Recognition II	SS = 13
California Verbal Learning Test–Second Edition	
Trials 1–5 Total	$T = 48$
Trial 1	$Z = -0.5$
Trial 5	$Z = -1.0$
Short-Delay Free Recall	$Z = -1.0$
Short-Delay Cued Recall	$Z = -1.0$
Long-Delay Free Recall	$Z = -1.0$

(continued)

TABLE 4.1. *(continued)*

Test	Standard scores
California Verbal Learning Test–Second Edition *(cont.)*	
Long-Delay Cued Recall	$Z = -1.0$
Recognition	$Z = 0$ (16 hits)
Brief Visuospatial Memory Test–Revised	
Trial 1	$T = 40$
Trial 2	$T = 47$
Trial 3	$T = 37$
Total	$T = 40$
Learning	$T = 51$
Delay	$T = 45$
Hits	> 16%ile
False positives	11–16%ile
Rey Complex Figure Test	
Immediate Recall	$T = 29$
Delayed Recall	$T = 31$
Recognition	$T = 43$
Paced Auditory Serial Addition Test	
Trial 1	$Z = -1.36$
Trial 2	$Z = -0.38$
Trial 3	$Z = 0.26$
Trial 4	$Z = 0.54$
Trail Making Test	
A	$T = 45$
B	$T = 55$
Category Test	$T = 37$
Wisconsin Card Sorting Test	
Categories Completed	> 16%ile
Total Errors	25%ile
Perseverative Responses	14%ile
Perseverative Errors	16%ile
Failure to Maintain Set	> 16%ile
Learning to Learn	> 16%ile
Boston Naming Test	$Z = -3.2$
Finger Tapping Test	
Dominant	$T = 29$
Nondominant	$T = 32$
Grooved Pegboard	
Dominant	$T = 30$
Nondominant	$T = 33$

(continued)

TABLE 4.1. *(continued)*

Test	Standard scores	
	T-scores	
Minnesota Multiphasic Personality Inventory–2	? = 0	Hs = 92
	L = 52	D = 75
	F = 68	Hy = 94
	K = 52	Pd = 53
		Mf = 42
		Pa = 59
		Pt = 62
		Sc = 72
		Ma = 56
		Si = 41
Geriatric Depression Scale	23/30	Moderate to severe

Mrs. Frizzle's present IQ scores are highly consistent with these two tests conducted previously, and they suggest that her general intellectual abilities are essentially unimpaired and very close to her estimated premorbid skills. She showed the expected practice effects, having taken this test (or a similar version) twice previously. The subtest scores were essentially equivalent across evaluations (although the scores from the second evaluation were not included in the report), and she has improved in her overall attention/concentration abilities, at least compared to the initial testing. Yet the present test results reveal somewhat greater cognitive difficulties than were evident in the second evaluation; there is also more evidence of some problems compared to the first evaluation.

Based upon all the available information (e.g., record review, clinical interview, and test results), it is difficult to ascertain the exact etiology of Mrs. Frizzle's reported cognitive deficits. Indeed, her present psychological–emotional condition, in combination with the prominent physical symptoms and preoccupation with such symptoms, seemed to exert a significant influence on her capacity to perform certain cognitive functions. On the other hand, the qualitative difficulties she reported as well as the evident changes in her emotional condition (e.g., lability, tendency to "fly off the handle") suggest that there may be an organic component to some of her symptoms and complaints. She has a number of symptoms (e.g., vertigo, dizziness, anosmia, nystagmus) that appear to have central nervous system (CNS) causes or correlates. The possibility exists that she may have sustained some subtle frontal lobe damage as a result of the "intracranial contents being violated" (e.g., dural tear, subsequent CSF leak, development of aseptic meningitis).

Whatever the exact cause of Mrs. Frizzle's symptoms and complaints, be it psychological, organic, or some combination of the two, it was my opinion that there was certainly "something neuropsychologically wrong" with her brain that was not evident prior to the sinus surgery. What is even more evident to me is the fact that she has shown deterioration in functioning over time, so much so that there appears to be no conceivable way that she could ever return to her premorbid level and resume the kind of lifestyle to which she was accustomed over 5 years ago. In my opinion, part of her report of, and preoccupation with, her physical symptoms was secondary to the fact that there may be those who doubt the validity of her condition and the veracity of her complaints. Indeed, she harbors considerable anger and resentment toward those who are not sympathetic to her condition, let alone those whom she perceives to be at fault. Thus, her unconscious magnification or tendency toward somatization under stress may be a product of a need to prove to others how impaired she is and how much her life has been affected by the effects of the surgery. This is not to be misconstrued as representing a conscious or volitional attempt to feign or exaggerate for the purpose of financial reward.

DSM-IV differential diagnoses include:

Axis I	294.9	Cognitive disorder not otherwise specified
	296.22	Major depressive disorder, single episode, moderate, chronic
	300.02	Generalized anxiety disorder
	316	Mental disorder affecting episodic vertigo, Ménière's disease
Rule out	310.1	Personality change due to dural tear, cerebrospinal fluid leak; aseptic meningitis
Axis II	V71.09	No diagnosis
Axis III		Cerebrospinal fluid leak, episodic vertigo, fibromyalgia, anosmia, and Ménière's disease
Axis IV		Problems with primary support group, occupational problems, problems related to interaction with the legal system
Axis V	GAF = 55	(Current)

RESPONSE FROM THE ATTORNEY

I sent a copy of the report to Mrs. Frizzle's attorney. He called me the day he received it, stating, "What is all this mumbo jumbo about Cognitive Disorder, NOS, Fake Bad Scale, and exaggeration? I referred her to you for an evaluation of her cognitive abilities and here you are talking about all this stuff. What am I going to do when the defense sees this report?" Clearly, I was not expecting such a response, but I handled it in the same way I might deal with a patient who was not happy with something I had written about him or her . . . in a nondefensive manner with an eye toward education. I reminded Mr. Peterman that I had previously informed him that a comprehensive neuropsychological examination also included components addressing motivation and effort and psychological and emotional functioning. Moreover, the crux of the case as he described it to me really seemed to be the psychological and emotional consequences of the sinus surgery. I suggested that we set up a time to meet so that I could go over the results with him in greater detail; I also suggested that it would be wise for both of us to meet with the consulting forensic psychiatrist who would have a lot to say about Mrs. Frizzle's psychological and emotional condition. The three of us met over lunch at a local restaurant (paid for by the attorney). It seemed as if the psychiatrist and I were double teaming Mr. Peterman, because he had a hard time understanding psychological terms and concepts. He should already have been familiar with at least some of the terms before he decided to retain mental health experts. Nonetheless, the psychiatrist and I were successful in educating Mr. Peterman and reducing his apparent anxiety. In the end, it seemed as if we were the ones formulating the case strategy on his behalf—a scenario I would not recommend to nonattorneys.

DEPOSITION

For many weeks prior to the deposition, Mr. Peterman was quite anxious. He would call me virtually every other day to discuss some aspect of the case, to make sure that my opinions would not change, and to emphasize the psychological and emotional consequences of the case, not the issue of brain damage. Each time, I would reassure him and tell him that my opinions are accurately reflected in my report. He was a very thorough attorney, but his repeated phone calls began to irritate me; also, I knew that he might be upset when he received an invoice at the end of the case billing him for the time spent on the telephone! Yet, because this was the first time he had worked with a neuropsychologist, I wanted to leave a favorable impression with him. But, business is business. No doubt, he would be billing his client for the time spent talking to his experts and consultants.

I was deposed on the case about 6 months after I had evaluated Mrs. Frizzle and after the depositions of the two treating psychologists and the neurologist treaters. In preparing to be deposed, I had anticipated that the defense would have consulted with another neuropsychologist to assist them in their questions and approach. Going in to a deposition with this expectation "raises the bar" for me, so to speak, as I anticipate some fairly high-level questions that can likely only be thought of by another neuropsychologist. In this case, there was no disclosed defense neuropsychologist expert, and I was not asked to release the raw data to anyone, let alone defense counsel. I found this quite unusual, as I am asked to release the raw data to opposing counsel almost 80% of the time. Of course, I politely refuse, indicating that such information can only be released to another qualified professional. But, in this case, I was not asked to release the data to anyone.

After having the court reporter swear me in, the defense attorney started the deposition with the following question: "Dr. Heilbronner, how much money do you make serving as an expert witness?" Okay, I thought, so this is how we are going to proceed. We're going to dispense with the usual qualifying questions, when I became involved in the case, etc., and go right to their approach to the case . . . to discredit the plaintiff's experts as being biased and motivated by financial incentives. I responded, "Over what period of time are you asking about?" He said, "How about over the past 2 years?" I answered his question in a nondefensive manner and estimated to the best degree possible. Responding honestly and not becoming perturbed by these kinds of invasive questions is the best way to proceed: It leaves the impression that you are an able participant in the forensic arena. Indeed, their intent seemed to be to get me riled up at the outset of the deposition. Years ago, I may have been a bit bothered by such questions, especially when they came at the beginning of a deposition. Experience has taught me to relax, answer the questions to the best of my ability, and to serve as an advocate of the facts.

It seemed as if we spent most of the first hour responding to questions that related to my experience as an expert: What percent of the time am I retained by the defense versus the plaintiff? Are my fees the same for a clinical case as they are for a forensic case? How much have I billed Mr. Peterman, to date? Eventually, we got into Mrs. Frizzle's case. By then, it was clear sailing. I had spent 2 full days with her, had evaluated all the records, and knew the opinions of the treaters inside and out. The defense attorneys made efforts to characterize Mrs. Frizzle as a malingerer, which I effectively addressed. They also emphasized her presurgical psychological history, and in an attempt to make her seem like some kind of "basket case" even before this event transpired, asked questions such as "Doctor, isn't it true that Mrs. Frizzle has a premorbid psychological history?" "Isn't it true that she participated in psychological counseling for many years prior to her surgery?" "Isn't it also true, Doctor, that she has not really held a full-time job in the 5 years preceding the surgery?" I answered all of the questions honestly and politely corrected the attorney when he appeared to be misstating the facts in evidence.

OUTCOME OF THE CASE

Like many attorneys, Mr. Peterman did not call to inform me of the outcome of the case, even though he had promised to do so after the deposition had concluded. As far as he was concerned, my job was done and I had served my purpose for him and his client. But I had a real need to know how my testimony had impacted upon the process. I am not invested in the idea that my testimony or involvement is pivotal in determining the outcome of any case in which I am involved. However, this case held a special place for me for many reasons, the least of which was the fact that Mr. Peterman had invested a lot of time and money in the mental health aspects, which was the domain in which Mrs. Frizzle had suffered the greatest injury. I called Mr. Peterman about 1 month after the arbitration had concluded. He seemed happy to hear from me and told me in no uncertain terms that he had managed to secure a very satisfactory settlement for his client, thanks, in large part, to the testimony of his two mental health experts. He was not allowed to share with me the details of the settlement, but I was not particularly interested in the dollar amounts anyway. He had told me what I wanted to hear—that he valued the work I had done and felt that it was integral to obtaining a comfortable settlement for a person who had legitimately been damaged from medical negligence.

LESSONS LEARNED

This case did not occur that long ago, so I was not a novice in the forensic arena at the time I was involved. Nonetheless, I still learned a lot and might handle some aspects of the case a bit differently now. Here are some points to remember. Keep in mind that patients have often had previous experiences with other neuropsychologists that may not have been positive and that could color how they interact with you and how you are likely to perceive them, the opinions you derive from your examination, etc. Even though we are most often retained on cases where brain damage is an issue, it is not ethical to raise the issue of brain damage when it doesn't exist. Moreover, there may be other psychological and emotional issues that outweigh any apparent cognitive dysfunction. Clinical neuropsychologists are trained to be sensitive to, and keenly aware of, the psychological and emotional damages that are often involved in many medical malpractice cases. However, that formulation must be built upon thorough investigation of the issues via a sound clinical interview and the administration of reliable and valid psychological inventories. Finally, when you are testifying in court, always consider the possibility that someone (e.g., an attorney or another expert) may be watching you perform. In closing, I'd like to leave you with a final admonition for those of you venturing into forensic neuropsychology practice. In the wise words of the precinct sergeant from *Hill Street Blues* (for those of you old enough to remember that television program): "Be careful out there."

REFERENCE

American Psychological Association. (2002). Ethical principles of psychologists and code of conduct. *American Psychologist, 57,* 1060–1073.

5

Alleged Traumatic Brain Injury in a Spanish Speaker

LIDIA ARTIOLA I FORTUNY

My postdoctoral career as a clinical neuropsychologist started in a neuro-surgery unit at a university hospital in Great Britain, where I functioned both as a clinician and a researcher for a number of years. When I returned to the United States in the early 1980s, there had literally been an explosion in interest in neuropsychology. I started a private practice with no difficulty and soon began getting referrals from what, for me, were nontraditional sources: attorneys, judges, and caseworkers seeking neuropsychological opinions for other than strictly medical reasons. Pre-dictably, and given that I am a native speaker of Spanish and a polyglot, I began getting a lot of referrals of Spanish and other non-English-speaking individuals. For a number of years it was extremely frustrating to be asked to diagnose non-English speakers, particularly those with fewer than 8 years of formal education, without appropriate instruments. I eventually started a project to adapt English-language instruments that have high levels of acceptability within our profession into Spanish and to collect normative data on Spanish speakers. This undertaking culmi-nated in the publication of a Spanish-language battery (Artiola i Fortuny, Hermosillo, Heaton, & Pardee, 1999). The battery was normed with Spanish-speaking participants from southern Arizona, northern Mexico, and Madrid (Spain). It has rendered my assessment of Spanish speakers considerably easier, although much remains to be done in this area before the standards that exist in English-language instruments can be attained. At the present time, my forensic practice constitutes approximately one-half of my professional activities. Approximately 25% of the individuals I examine are clearly Spanish-language dominant. Frequently, these individuals have been examined previously by colleagues who are monolingual. Sometimes examinees with low levels of English fluency are tested in English; sometimes they are tested in Spanish through an interpreter. The quality of these evaluations varies widely, depending on the individual colleague's awareness of language and cultural issues and, it would seem, depending on their willingness to tolerate the odds that their work may be reviewed by a colleague who, in addition to being well trained in neuropsychology, is also fluent in the examinee's better language.

The examination I report in this chapter is one of many examples of my experiences in forensic practice with Spanish speakers. I attempt to provide a reasonably detailed account of the procedures I used in the course of this evaluation, given that availability of normed Spanish-language instruments is very limited compared to English. In addition, I try to provide some education on what I believe to be important aspects of the examination of non-English speakers that rarely present a problem during assessment of mainstream U.S. individuals.

"Mr. Corral" was referred by C.P., an attorney specializing in workers' compensation defense. During his initial telephone call, he explained that he wanted to refer Mr. Corral for independent neuropsychological examination. Mr. Corral had been employed for the previous 5 years as a skilled laborer by a cement company, and he had been promoted on a number of occasions. Mr. Corral was claiming total disability secondary to cognitive deficits and emotional complaints allegedly stemming from injuries sustained during an industrial injury 2 years earlier. Mr. Corral, whose first language was Spanish, had been examined by two board certified neuropsychologists, neither of whom claimed to possess fluency in Spanish. C.P. wanted to know if examinations conducted through interpreters could be considered valid and whether an examiner who had only partial fluency in the examinee's language could reach valid conclusions. Before deciding whether the referral was appropriate, I asked exactly how the previous evaluations had been conducted, whether the clinician communicated directly with the examinee, and, if so, what were the clinician's language qualifications. C.P. could only answer these questions partially because the reports in his possession were not clear. I also asked the attorney to give me a list of the instruments that had been used, explaining that it is important to be aware of the limitations imposed by nonstandard use of instruments, as well as the limitations imposed by the use of standard instruments on non-mainstream individuals. The list of instruments he gave me led me to believe that Mr. Corral likely had not been examined in a manner that could allow valid conclusions. Therefore, I felt that I might be of assistance in clarifying the situation, and I accepted the referral.

INDEPENDENT EXAMINATION OF JUAN CORRAL

Sources of Collateral Information

Medical records pertaining to the 2002 injury, reports and raw data of prior neuropsychological examinations, and Mr. Corral's deposition taken 1 month before the evaluation were reviewed and used to assist with collection of background information and to reach diagnostic opinions.

Review of Records

Mr. Corral was in his usual state of health until January 2, 2002. On that date, he was pouring cement in a pool area when he slipped and fell in the pool. The left side of his body hit the edge of the pool as he was falling. Depending on what records one reads, he was under water for anywhere between 30 seconds and 2 minutes. There appears to be agreement on the fact that he was pulled out of the pool by one of his co-workers, and that at that point he was awake and alert. Mr. Corral stated in an interview that during the event, he remembers invoking, out loud, a popular religious figure to come to his assistance. He reported a clear memory of the accident, including the ambulance ride to the hospital.

On admission to the medical center, he was reportedly fully awake and oriented. He complained of pain to his left thigh and foot as well as mild, diffuse pain elsewhere. He denied nausea or vomiting and had no shortness of breath. The initial clinical impression was "multiple contusions with blunt injury to the left chest and abdomen." He remained at the medical center for 2 days. A computed tomography (CT) scan conducted on the day of admission was interpreted as showing multiple punctate foci of increased signal intensity on the long TR pulsing sequences within the supratentorial white matter. The configuration was interpreted as most compatible with small vessel ischemic white matter disease, as opposed to injury-induced changes. A second CT scan conducted 2 days later, this time with contrast, revealed identical information. A magnetic resonance imaging (MRI) of the major arteries of the skull base was read as normal.

In May 2002, Mr. Corral was examined by Dr. B.W., a neurologist. Dr. B.W. noted that Mr. Corral had been referred because a blood clot was found on his MRI. Dr. B.W. also noted that Mr. Corral had struck the back of his head and "clearly suffered a closed head injury." Mr. Corral reported some weakness in his lower extremities, memory difficulties, poor appetite, difficulty sleeping, and nightmares. Dr. B.W. opined: "Clearly Mr. Corral has suffered a closed head injury. It does appear that he has some sequelae of closed head injury, namely memory difficulties and depression." Dr. B.W. recommended a neuropsychological examination by a board-certified neuropsychologist, Dr. A.H.

Prior Neuropsychological Evaluations and Treatment

Dr. A.H. (a monolingual, board-certified clinical neuropsychologist) examined Mr. Corral in June 2002. Dr. A.H. noted that English was Mr. Corral's second language, and that because of Mr. Corral's limited skills in English, the neuropsychological testing would be fairly circumscribed in scope. He was administered the following tests in English: Trail Making Test (Parts A and B), portions of the Wechsler Adult Intelligence Scale–Revised, Rey Auditory–Verbal Learning Test, Rey–Osterrieth Complex Figure Test, and Halstead Finger-Tapping Test. According to Dr. A.H., during the examination Mr. Corral did not understand English very well, and a number of the questions that were asked had to be interpreted by his wife. Dr. A.H. noted Mr. Corral's educational level to have been 8 years of schooling in Mexico. It is uncertain as to who provided this piece of information. Based on his examination, Dr. A.H. opined that "the [patient] is showing cognitive disturbances reflected by decreased concentration and attention and ability to shift his cognitive set that would be compatible with a postconcussional syndrome. He is also showing substantial difficulties with memory and speed of information processing. He appears depressed. There is probable evidence of a posttraumatic stress disorder present as well." Dr. A.H. felt that it would be worthwhile for a Spanish-speaking speech and language pathologist to work with Mr. Corral. He also felt that Mr. Corral should be referred to a Spanish-speaking psychotherapist. Dr. A.H. did not refer Mr. Corral to a

Spanish-speaking clinical neuropsychologist, even though there are several in his state.

In July 2003, Mr. Corral was seen for neuropsychological evaluation by Dr. M.G., a board-certified clinical neuropsychologist. Dr. M.G. speaks some Spanish and reported that he was able to communicate directly with Mr. Corral. He also said that Mr. Corral was bilingual. He used a bilingual technician to administer the tests. Dr. M.G. indicated that Mr. Corral had had 8 years of formal education in Mexico. He administered the Trail Making Test, Part A, and did not attempt Part B because it took Mr. Corral 89 seconds with two errors to complete the sample. No attempt was made to establish the examinee's level of literacy. Dr. M.G. administered the Rey Auditory–Verbal Learning Test in Spanish and noted that Mr. Corral's performance had worsened significantly for verbal learning and memory relative to Dr. A.H.'s (English-language) results. He also administered the Rey–Osterrieth Complex Figure Test and opined that Mr. Corral's performance was markedly impaired both in copying the figure and in remembering it. He concluded that Mr. Corral's overall neurocognitive functioning was worse than in January of the same year. He opined this was probably due to pain, depression, and anxiety, in addition to brain dysfunction due to effects of the accident. Dr. M.G. suggested that he should work with Mr. Corral to assist with his psychological problems, and he also recommended cognitive retraining. He appears to have treated Mr. Corral over a period of approximately 1 year.

At Dr. M.G.'s request, Mr. Corral was admitted in August 2003 to the R.H. Day Treatment Program. A report covering a 6-week period lists a very large number of limitations in this man, including decreased mobility, decreased visual acuity, headaches, dizziness, and a variety of "profoundly impaired" cognitive functions. It is not clear how these disabilities were assessed. It is also unclear how the clinicians went about communicating with Mr. Corral, with the exception of the physical therapist, who seems to have used an interpreter.

An R.H. Day Treatment Program report covering a second 6-week period continued to assess Mr. Corral as being "profoundly impaired" in a variety of areas, though again, it is unclear to me how these areas were assessed. Interestingly, moderate to severe expressive–receptive language deficits were assessed, but there is no explanation as to how this assessment was done. In that report, it also appears that an assessment done in Spanish of language-based deficits and cognitive function was conducted. However, there is no information as to who did the assessment, and no objective results were presented to buttress the opinions rendered. Of note also is that a speech–language pathology assessment was conducted, apparently through an interpreter.

An R.H. Day Program speech–language pathology report of November 2003 indicated that Mr. Corral had made significant progress in all short-term goals. Of note: There is no indication of the language in which the assessment was conducted. Approval for continued treatment was requested but denied by a neurologist, Dr. J.L., because, according to that clinician, "therapies of physical, occupational, and speech therapy do not secm to be helping."

A functional capacity evaluation of Mr. Corral was conducted in June 2004 by S.H., a rehabilitation psychologist. That evaluation was conducted through an interpreter, and there was a note indicating Mr. Corral's educational level to be 4 years, not 8 years, as previously reported. Based on review of records and examination, Dr. S.H. concluded that "Mr. Corral is permanently and totally disabled from sustained and gainful work activity. His highest level of occupational functioning is in a subsidized sheltered workshop environment."

Warning on Limits of Confidentiality

Before beginning the interview, I informed Mr. Corral that I am a clinical neuropsychologist and that I was hired to examine him by a defense attorney in order to gather information regarding his current neuropsychological status. I informed Mr. Corral that I would serve as an evaluator, not as a therapist. I explained that I would review his personal history with him, ask questions related to his emotional state, and that neuropsychological tests would be administered to him. Mr. Corral was also informed that I would prepare a lengthy report to the referring attorney and that the content of interviews, observations and results would not be confidential. He was informed that these limits of confidentiality are inherent to forensic evaluations. Mr. Corral appeared to have adequate understanding of the nature of the warning.

Background History

Juan Corral is a 42-year-old right-handed Mexican man born in a mid-sized town in the state of Nuevo León, Mexico. He has lived in the United States for the past 19 years. Mr. Corral reported completing 4 years of formal education in an urban Mexican elementary school. He said that he was the best student in his class in all subjects. He stopped going to school (as did his siblings) to help his family with living expenses. He spent some years working as a cement layer. His most recent occupation was as a foreman in a cement company.

Mr. Corral's father had died approximately 4 years earlier; he was an agricultural laborer. As far as Mr. Corral knows, his father never went to school. Mr. Corral's mother died when he was 6 years old; he did not know the cause of his mother's death or the length (if any) of her school attendance—only that she was a homemaker. Mr. Corral was essentially raised by his sister, who is 15 years his senior. He has five sisters and two brothers, all older; he does not remember his siblings' ages.

Mr. Corral had four children with his wife, one of whom passed away about 1 year ago, at age 18, evidently killed in a car accident when returning from a party. The surviving children are twin 15-year-old boys and a 13-year-old girl. Mr. Corral reports no family history of mental or neurological illness and denies any prior trauma to the head or any prior chronic illness. He never needed or received psychiatric or psychological treatment for any reason before 2002. He denies present alcohol consumption and admits to drinking socially before his accident. He denied ever using drugs, and he does not smoke.

Presenting Complaints

Mr. Corral's chief complaints were "pain in the brain, left leg, waist, and both heels." During interview he was unsure as to problems with attention and concentration, memory, language, and hearing. However, he endorsed numerous and severe memory complaints in response to a questionnaire. He was unsure as to whether his ability to move has changed since his injury. He stated that his personality has changed "a little."

Behavioral Observations

Mr. Corral presented as a very quiet gentleman with blunted affect and depressed mood. He responded to questions very vaguely and monosyllabically. When he did speak, his speech was normal in articulation and volume. Rate was reduced, and prosody could not be appropriately assessed. He tended to respond "I don't know" to my questions and repeatedly referred me to his wife, Petra, for answers. He did say he does not remember who his primary care physician is, but he later said that "Dr. M.G. prescribes nortriptyline, 40 mg, at night." He remembered that he sees Dr. M.G. every two to three months, that he talks with him, and that Dr. M.G. gives him memory tests "and all that." He did not initiate any type of conversation. He appeared to be able to sit comfortably for long periods of time.

During testing, Mr. Corral's level of cooperation and effort appeared adequate. He was quiet, responsive to conversational cues, but lacking spontaneity (verbal or motor). There was no evidence of frustration. All office questionnaires were read to Mr. Corral.

Procedures

Clinical interviews with Mr. Corral and his wife; Wechsler Adult Intelligence Scale–Revised (WAIS-R) (Performance subtests); Vocabulary subtest of the WAIS-R (Spanish Adaptation); Word Memory Test (WMT); Grip Strength Test; Finger Tapping Test; Spanish Neuropsychological Battery (Artiola i Fortuny et al., 1999), including Verbal Fluency, Auditory Memory, Visual Memory, Word List; Figure Memory; Story Memory; Stroop Color–Word Test.

The following tests were used to assist in determining Mr. Corral's dominant language: Boston Naming Test (Spanish, English); Token Test (Spanish, English); Verbal Fluency (Spanish, English). The raw test data were used for between-language comparisons.

I interviewed Mr. Corral and his wife. I am a native speaker of Spanish with tertiary education in both Spanish and English. Mr. Corral's level of education was estimated at 4 years. The evaluation was conducted in a quiet environment in my office. Tests were administered by D.M., a master's-level neuropsychology technician born and educated in Mexico, currently completing a PhD in psychology at a U.S. university. For the Spanish Neuropsychological Battery, published Spanish-language norms (Artiola i Fortuny, Heaton, & Hermosillo, 1998; Artiola i Fortuny et al., 1999) were used. Mr. Corral was compared to Anglo-Saxon standardization samples on Finger Tapping and Grip Strength, using the comprehensive norms for an Expanded Halstead–Neuropsychological Reitan Battery (Heaton, Grant, & Matthews, 1991). For the WAIS-R (Performance) he was compared to an Anglo-Saxon sample of similar demographic characteristics, using comprehensive norms for an Expanded Halstead–Reitan Neuropsychological Battery: A Supplement for the WAIS-R (Heaton, 1992). The Performance IQ reached with this procedure is used only to derive the T-score necessary to compare the examinee to the Anglo-Saxon standardization sample with similar demographic characteristics, not to actually assign an IQ estimate.

On the Spanish versions of the Boston Naming Test (adjusted for Spanish word frequency) and the WAIS-R (Vocabulary), Mr. Corral was compared to preliminary results of a normative study currently in progress. For the Token Test, norms from the Examen de Afasia Multilingüe (Rey & Sivan, 1991) were used.

Language Dominance

In an attempt to determine whether Mr. Corral was English or Spanish dominant, several tests were administered to him in both languages. In the Token Test of syntactic comprehension, Mr. Corral's adjusted score for the Spanish version was in the average range, relative to Spanish speakers with similar levels of education. In English, his raw score was less than half of his Spanish score. In the Boston Naming Test, Mr. Corral was able to name a total of 36 words out of a possible 60 in Spanish. In the English version, he was able to name a total of 16 words. Overall, even though both sets of results are poorer than expected, they are thought to indicate considerably better knowledge of the Spanish than the English language. He was able to generate a total of 25 words in 3 minutes, in response to a phonemic cue in Spanish; in English, he generated 10 words. The results were consistent with Mr. Corral's significantly better use of Spanish than English during conversation. He was, therefore, interviewed and tested in Spanish.

TEST RESULTS

Validity and Test Interpretation Considerations

A number of results suggested that we were not able to consistently elicit Mr. Corral's best efforts for success that are a prerequisite for accurately depicting a person's true cognitive capabilities. On the WMT, his scores were as follows:

    Immediate Recognition = 82.5% (fail)
    Delayed Recognition = 80.5% (fail)
    Consistency = 77.7% (fail)
    Multiple Choice = 45.0% (caution)
    Paired Associate Recall = 40.0% (warning)
    Free Recall = 17.5% (warning)
    Delayed Free Recall = 12.5%

In a recent study, the mean score of patients with moderate to severe brain injury was greater than 90% correct on each of the WMT effort measures. More importantly, Mr. Corral's results were worse than those of individuals with mild head injury, moderate to severe head injury, and severe head injury for both the symptom validity and the memory portions of the WMT. Failure on the WMT can be interpreted as evidence of response bias and brings the validity of a patient's test results into question. On the Dot Counting Test, he counted the grouped dots significantly more slowly than the ungrouped dots. This pattern of performance raises a significant red flag with regard to motivation, because it is usually associated with less than optimum effort in performing neuropsychological tests. Unfortunately, these results call into question the validity and representativeness of the rest of the test scores reported below.

Cognitive Test Results

Mr. Corral was oriented to place and situation, but not to time: He missed the exact date by 1 month. He was able to identify the president of the United States but was unable to identify his predecessor. He also correctly identified the president of Mexico but was unable to identify his predecessor. In response to a question concerning his knowledge of world or national news, he appeared generally aware of national news but was unable to elaborate on details. He was able to write his name and his address. A brief sentence written to dictation was educationally appropriate. He was able to count backward from 20 to 1, but he did so rather slowly, taking 37 seconds. He was unable to recite the Spanish alphabet accurately, making six errors, the first one after the letter *D*. He made two errors in the addition of serial 3's.

The present neuropsychological evaluation documents results generally in keeping with Mr. Corral's reported level of education. When compared to Spanish speakers of similar age and level of education, Mr. Corral scored at, or very close to, his estimated premorbid abilities on many of the tasks administered. He obtained *T*-scores in the average range in all areas except the word and color measures of the Stroop Color–Word Test, delayed recall of the Story Memory and Figure Memory tests, and learning score and immediate recall of the word list learning task (see Table 5.1). Of note, however, is that he had performed normally in similar tests during other evaluations. Recognition was in the normal range

TABLE 5.1. Test Scores for Juan Corral, January 2004

Measures	T-score	Measures	T-score
Figure Memory Trial 1	45	Grip Strength Right	12
Figure Memory Learning	38	Grip Strength Left	28
Figure Memory Delayed Recall	40	Finger Tapping Right	16
Figure Memory Discriminability	55	Finger Tapping Left	11
Story Memory Trial 1	40	Word List A Trial 1	50
Story Memory Delayed Recall	34	Word List A Total	33
Story Memory Learning	40	Word List B	47
Story Memory Discriminability	55	Word List A Short-Delay Free Recall	26
Verbal Fluency (PMR)	46	Word List A Short-Delay Cued Recall	36
Forward Digit Span	47	Word List A Long-Delay Free Recall	41
Backward Digit Span	62	Word List A Long-Delay Cued Recall	45
Forward Visual Span	52	Word List A Discriminability	38
Backward Visual Span	50	WAIS-R Picture Completion	45
Stroop Word	33	WAIS-R Picture Arrangement	45
Stroop Color	33	WAIS-R Block Design	36
Stroop Color–Word	38	WAIS-R Digit Symbol	44
Stroop Interference	41	WAIS-R Object Assembly	55
		WAIS-R Performance IQ	46

for all tests. Motor tests were performed very poorly, with some results as low as –3.5 standard deviations below the mean. However, he had performed normally in these tests in previous evaluations.

Mr. Corral's IQ could not be estimated in a valid manner because there are no Spanish-language IQ tests that include samples of individuals with fewer than 9 years of education. However, in order to compare his nonverbal abilities to those of Anglo-Saxon individuals with similar educational levels, he was administered the performance subtests of the WAIS-R. Relative to these individuals, Mr. Corral obtained a T-score of 46, which is in the normal and expected range.

Summary and Conclusions

1. Results on many tests were entirely in the expected range, given his age and stated level of formal education.

2. There were numerous inconsistencies between the present neuropsychological test results, the results obtained during the A.H. evaluation, and the results obtained during the M.G. evaluation. There were specific inconsistencies in Mr. Corral's performance of motor tasks when comparisons were made between results obtained from different evaluations.

3. A number of test results are so dismal as to be unbelievable. The findings are inconsistent with his level of functioning in day-to-day life. Indeed, he was unable to define even one word on a Spanish test of vocabulary; however, he was able to generate complex words on a fluency test. He was also able to understand a fair amount of written material in Spanish, and he certainly appeared to have no difficulty understanding fluent spoken Spanish. Additionally, he understood, discussed, and signed various Spanish administrative forms handed to him by this office.

4. During the present examination, Mr. Corral claimed to have no knowledge of certain basic facts regarding his accident and aspects of his current life, frequently deferring to his wife. In fact, his responses were so vague that I had to rely on Ms. Corral for a history. Yet, during his deposition, he was able to provide detailed information regarding events preceding the accident. In completing a questionnaire, he endorsed a very large number of memory complaints (including problems remembering both recent and remote events), yet his spontaneous complaints were only related to pain.

5. Mr. Corral's symptom validity results suggested that he was not putting his "best foot forward" on the cognitive measures.

To summarize: Mr. Corral was involved in a significant industrial accident in 2002. This accident clearly was accompanied by some physical discomfort and by a large number of complaints, which have changed and increased over time. Some of his treaters had deemed him to be totally disabled, and it appears that he himself may have come to believe this dismal conclusion. It is likely that he has had a maladaptive reaction to the injury, which has led to depression and personality changes. He also may have had some symptoms of posttraumatic stress early in the postinjury period. He lost a daughter shortly after his own accident, and he seems to have been profoundly affected by this loss. He has numerous and varied somatic complaints, the origins of which are not clear. Anger and frustration regarding his claim may be a significant contributing factor to the reported behavioral changes. Unfortunately, present and past results indicate that Mr. Corral may not have put forth his best effort during the evaluations, rendering the results invalid for the purpose of reaching conclusions regarding his cognitive status. If his complaints persist beyond the expected time of resolution of his litigation, psychiatric assessment and treatment should be considered.

Feedback to Referring Counsel

During a feedback session with C.P., I explained the results obtained by Mr. Corral and my interpretation as elaborated in the previous section. I also explained in detail the concerns I had regarding the previous neuro-psychological conclusions. I pointed out that Mr. Corral's level of education was 4 years and not 8, as had been indicated by some clinicians. Mr. Corral may have said that he went to school until age 8 (which would, indeed, give him about 4 years of formal education), and somewhere along the line this may have been misunderstood and passed along inadvertently. I explained to the attorney that our field knows a lot less about individuals with low levels of education (fewer than 8 years) than it does about individuals with higher levels of education (8 or more years). Neuropsychology has developed primarily in English-speaking countries, where it is quite difficult to find significant numbers of individuals with fewer than 8 years of education (Artiola i Fortuny, 2004). Hence, many English-speaking neuropsychologists in the United States have little, if any, experience with extremely low levels of formal schooling. When an individual with fewer than 8 years of formal education is assessed, caution must be exercised in order to ascertain that the problems experienced in test performance are not due to low level of education. Without appropriate age- and education-corrected norms, the interpretation of neuropsychological test results is impossible, or nearly so. Calling a patient brain damaged when, in fact, results may be a simple reflection of poor education is likely to have serious repercussions. I provided the attorney with references that address the effects of low levels of education on neuropsychological results and the effects of culture on the neuropsychological examination (e.g., Artiola i Fortuny & Mullaney, 1997, 1998; Artiola i Fortuny, 2004; Chávez & Oetting, 1995; Cole & Scribner, 1977; Cole, 1999; Nell, 2000; Luria, 1979; Rogoff & Chavajay, 1995).

I explained to C.P. that a number of clinicians who assessed Mr. Corral had apparently failed to take into account his extreme low level of education—or they may have been simply unaware of it. Consequently, they concluded that brain damage existed when, in fact, the explanation for the poor test results may lay elsewhere. Many of Mr. Corral's poor results were simply due to his extremely low level of education. When he was compared to a group of individuals with similar demographic characteristics, many of his results were in the expected range—even in spite of evidence of poor effort on his part.

Outcome of the Case

Approximately 5 months after completion of my report, I was called before the Industrial Commission for a hearing. C.P. did not call me ahead of time so that we could prepare for the hearing. He opened my testimony by asking me to recite my qualifications. My direct testimony on Mr. Corral was consistent with the written report. C.P. also asked me to give my opinion on validity issues that may arise when monolingual English-speaking clinicians perform neuropsychological evaluations of individuals who speak languages other than English. I explained the potential problems inherent in this practice and pointed out that, in addition to fine points of test validity, even gross errors in collecting simple factual information may occur (as seems to have been the case here) and can lead to erroneous interpretation of data. I also spent some time pointing out the special interpretive problems posed by individuals with very low levels of education.

During cross-examination, opposing counsel seemed more interested in annoying or destabilizing me than in my professional qualifications, the facts of the case, or my opinions. His questions focused on the details of my origins (birthplace, linguistic background). He attempted to establish that I spoke "Spanish" and not "Mexican, the language of Mr. Corral." This ploy, incidentally, has been utilized on a few occasions with no success. A clinician accused of speaking a brand of Spanish "different" from that of the examinee has to come armed with full knowledge of the limited range of variation of this geographically scattered language. Educating the trier-of-fact on the normative mechanisms that have been in place for several centuries in the Spanish language goes a long way in defusing an overly zealous opposing counsel's attempt to discredit. This particular attorney seemed upset that I had criticized the use by his witness of an interpreter to examine the claimant. I explained that it was my opinion that his witness was an otherwise well-qualified board-certified neuropsychologist, and that it was the failure to communicate directly with the examinee that had caused serious errors that could have been avoided. I did not criticize the qualifications of my colleague in any way, but I did indicate that whenever there is a barrier (linguistic or otherwise) between an examinee and a clinician, there exists a potential for (sometimes embarrassing) error, and that it is best to avoid this risk whenever possible. The attorney who hired me informed me 1 month later that the judge allowed Mr. Corral a limited number of sessions of psychological therapy with the Spanish-speaking therapist. He was found fit to return to work, with a 5% limitation of the whole person due to physical injuries.[1]

What Did I Learn?

The most satisfying aspect of forensic assessment is the opportunity to educate the legal profession and the trier-of-fact on the contribution that neuropsychology is capable of making. Although the case of Mr. Corral occurred recently, the diagnostic issues are essentially identical to those I have had the opportunity to address during the past two decades. Indeed, our field has undergone tremendous transformation; our databases of normative information have increased significantly as has our knowledge of the variables that affect test results. Similarly, we have become much more sophisticated in detecting insufficient effort. These advances have rendered the task of neuropsychological diagnosis more precise. Although assessment of non-mainstream individuals remains a challenging endeavor, I have learned that many recent advances can be applied to these individuals and improve our ability to make valid statements, provided that we keep up to date with the literature. Cases such as Mr. Corral's have motivated me and others to attempt to bring a solution to the problem, at least for Spanish speakers, by writing about it and by standardizing and norming instruments that can be used to assess these individuals in a manner that approaches the assessment of English speakers.

REFERENCES

Artiola i Fortuny, L. (2004). Perspectives in cross-cultural neuropsychology: Language, low education, and illiteracy. In J. Ricker (Ed.), *Differential diagnosis in adult neuropsychological illiteracy assessment* (pp. 66–107). New York: Springer.

---

[1]Under the statutes of workers' compensation, disability may be divided into three periods:

1. Temporary total disability is the period in which the injured person is totally unable to work. During this time he or she receives medical treatment.
2. Temporary partial disability is the period when recovery has reached the stage of improvement so that the person may begin some kind of gainful employment.
3. Permanent disability applies to permanent damage or to loss of use of some part of the body after the stage of maximum improvement from medical treatment has been reached and the condition is stationary.

Artiola i Fortuny, L., Heaton, R. K., & Hermosillo, D. (1998). Neuropsychological comparisons of Spanish speaking participants from the U.S.–Mexico Border Region vs. Spain. *Journal of the International Neuropsychological Society, 4*, 363–379.

Artiola i Fortuny, L., Hermosillo, D., Heaton, R. K., & Pardee, R. E. (1999). *Manual de normas y procedimientos para la Batería Neuropsicológica en Español* (Manual of norms and procedures for the Spanish Neuropsychological Battery). Tucson, AZ: *m* Press.

Artiola i Fortuny, L., & Mullaney, H. A. (1997). Neuropsychology with Spanish-speakers: Language use and proficiency issues for test development. *Journal of Clinical and Experimental Neuropsychology, 19*, 615–623.

Artiola i Fortuny, L., & Mullaney, H. A. (1998). Assessing patients whose language you do not know: Can the absurd be ethical? *The Clinical Neuropsychologist, 12*, 113–126.

Chávez, E. L., & Oetting, E. R. (1995). A critical incident model for considering issues in cross-cultural research: Failures in cultural sensitivity. *International Journal of the Addictions, 30*(7), 863–874.

Cole, M. (1999). Culture-free versus culture-based measures of cognition. In R. Sternberg (Ed.), *The nature of cognition* (pp. 645–664). Cambridge, MA: MIT Press.

Cole, M., & Scribner, S. (1977). Crosscultural studies of memory and cognition. In R. V. Kail, Jr., & J. W. Hagen (Eds.), *Perspectives on the development of memory and cognition* (pp. 239–271). Hillsdale, NJ: Erlbaum.

Heaton, R. K. (1992). *Comprehensive norms for an expanded Halstead–Reitan Battery: A Supplement for the WAIS-R*. Odessa, FL: Psychological Assessment Resources.

Heaton, R. K., Grant, I., & Matthews, C. G. (1991). *Comprehensive norms for an expanded Halstead–Reitan Battery*. Odessa, FL: Psychological Assessment Resources.

Luria, A. R. (1979). *The making of mind*. Cambridge, MA: Harvard University Press.

Nell, V. (2000). *Cross-cultural neuropsychological assessment: Theory and practice*. Mahwah, NJ: Erlbaum.

Rey, G. J., & Sivan, A. B. (1991). *Examen de Afasia Multilingüe* [Multilingual Aphasia Examination]. Iowa City, IA: AJA Associates.

Rogoff, B., & Chavajay, P. (1995). What's become of research on the cultural basis of cognitive development? *American Psychologist, 50*, 859–877.

6

Brain Injury When Chronic Pain Is a Prominent Diagnosis

Michael F. Martelli

My involvement in forensic practice developed as a natural consequence of providing assessment and treatment services in a physical medicine and rehabilitation setting. A majority of rehabilitation clients present with traumatic physical and neurological injuries and acquired and developmental physical and neurological disorders and impairments. Clinical service typically includes evaluation of impairment and disability and provision of rehabilitative recommendations and treatments. This process inevitably leads to encounters with such forensic contexts as Social Security Disability application, personal injury litigation, workers' compensation claims, disability insurance policy application, other health care insurance policy coverage, determination of competence to handle finances, and other important life functions or decisions.

The forensic context was uninvited; indeed it was thrust upon me, and I found it to be strikingly opposite to the more altruistic and benevolent interactions in rehabilitation. However, it is uniquely challenging. The forensic context usually affords longer periods of time with examinees, greater access to information that is not usually available, and greater external verification of inferences. Not even in graduate school was my methodology, procedures, and inferences more critically scrutinized. I believed, and still believe, that this critical examination fosters growth and development of neuropsychological skills and science. Disentangling the multiple contributors to cognitive dysfunction and to impairment and disability is a diagnostic challenge that requires careful scrutiny—and forensic work guarantees that this process will be critically scrutinized. Forensic work has helped me to define a model for the scientific practice of neuropsychology that applies more generally.

REFERRAL AND CONTEXT

The following case occurred several years ago, but it is one I find particularly interesting. It is illustrative of how neuropsychological test data are not always the primary assessment tool, and it represents what I like to think was a healthy general skepticism in the adversarial arena. Most of all, this case highlights a sensitive skeptic's efforts to resist "creeping adversarialism" and pursue more objective examinee understanding.

Having grown up in a blue-collar neighborhood in Pittsburgh, I maintain a somewhat healthy level of skepticism regarding all self-report to psychologists, perception of our tests and their strength, motivation of persons taking these tests, and the often overly exuberant endorsement of less than impressively powerful predictions without consideration of limitations. This skepticism extends to my sensitization to pressures that reinforce simplistic dichotomous inferences and nonobjectivity in the now prominent medical–legal arena—perhaps the last remaining frontier for a lucrative neuropsychological practice.

The referral for this case developed in an unusual manner. It was late in the afternoon on a Friday and I was trying to get out of the office before dark for the first time in a very busy week. Then the phone rang. A notably articulate and pleasantly toned gentleman introduced himself. He was the lead defense attorney in a personal injury lawsuit that was quickly approaching trial. An extension had been denied, and an independent examination was needed in relatively short order.

This firm was familiar to me for its specialization in defense work. Moreover, it had a reputation for relying on an array of expert witnesses who demonstrated considerable predisposition to favorably biased findings. In other words, this firm preferred experts who had reputations for freely engaging in the world's oldest profession. I had some confirmation of this reputation through providing rehabilitation services to a couple of previous clients who were involved in personal injury lawsuits. One of the cases included a very bright young man who had sustained a severe traumatic brain injury (TBI) that required excavation of about one quarter of his right hemisphere and produced prominent executive deficits. The defense neuropsychologist opined that he was essentially unimpaired because of an average IQ score. The accident reconstruction expert reported insufficient impact in the accident to produce the bodily injuries sustained, speculating that they may have happened prior to the tractor-trailer running over the compact car. The other case's details were similarly alarming.

This referral was not something I expected to be interested in; I was clinically overworked and overinvolved in other projects. In fact, I had the first opening in my schedule for a few years, wanted to finally take some vacation, and as a salaried employee, earned nothing extra doing forensic work. Finally, having been strongly influenced by Ted Blau's "Forensic Psychology Rules of the Road" (Blau, 1984, 1992), and having adapted an early version of a summary of guidelines for navigating the adversarial arena (included in Tables 6.1 and 6.2), nonacceptance of this case seemed almost certain.

"Well, what brings you to call me"? I uttered curiously. He indicated that his firm was interested in procuring an independent neuropsychological examination from a practitioner with specialized treatment experience working with persons with mild to moderate TBI and postinjury adjustment. He indicated that they were interested in employing a highly qualified expert with good credibility to perform an objective evaluation, and they wanted an objective opinion from a rehabilitation professional to contrast with what they perceived as blatantly skewed opinions from the treating neuropsychologists who had performed previous evaluations. I still didn't expect to have time, but the case started to sound less unappealing; so I agreed to juggle my schedule for an appointment Monday morning.

The attorney arrived for the meeting with an associate. He explained that the plaintiff had sustained an apparent mild TBI but was claiming persistent severe impairment 3 years later. They further explained that the plaintiff had been examined and followed by two nationally prominent neuropsychologists who were diplomates with impressive training credentials, well published, involved in national organizations and the training of postdoctoral fellows, and engaged in a lot of medical–legal work. The neuropsychologists, both of whom performed more defense-

TABLE 6.1. Recommendations for Promoting Objectivity in Expert Testifying Witnesses

1. Guard against inherent biases favoring the retaining side/party. Strive for objectivity by resisting attorney enticement into joining the adversarial and partisan attorney–client team.

2. Strive for objectivity by resisting pressure to provide differentially favorable findings to the retaining side.

3. Balance cases from plaintiff and defense attorneys and resist partisan specialization in an adversarial legal system.

4. Respect role boundaries and do not mix the conflicting roles of treating doctor, expert, and trial consultant.

5. Spend sufficient time directly evaluating the examinee and the examinee population for whom expert testimony is given.

6. Avoid cutting of corners; be thorough; insist on adequate time; and rely on standardized, validated, well-normed, and well-accepted procedures and tests. Use only specific, appropriate norms; take into account symptom base rates; and consider all competing explanatory factors for symptoms.

7. Review all available information before arriving at opinions; always include and consider contradictory facts and evidence and never arrive at opinions that are inconsistent with the plaintiff's records, test data, and behavioral presentation.

8. Guard against excessive "black-and-white" findings; recognize the limitations of scientific, medical, and neuropsychological opinion, and that few findings are black or white or attributable to a single event (e.g., Occam's razor).

9. Guard against motivational threats to assessment validity. Always assess response bias and always attempt to facilitate response validity.

10. Perform critical self-examination (e.g., Sweet & Moulthrop's [1999] questions) in every medical–legal case. Keep running statistics and strive for balance in ratios relating to favorability of findings to retaining party, defense versus plaintiff referrals, and black/white versus mixed findings.

11. Pursue objectivity by maintaining vigilant guard and actively, critically, and tranparently addressing and reporting possible bias and potential limitations in (a) competence and expertise, (b) evaluation measures and procedures, and (c) inferences and interpretations.

12. Dispute opinion of other experts only in pursuit of objectivity, in the context of complete and accurate representation of the other experts' findings, inferences, and conclusions.

13. Identify personal values and biases, anticipate possible effects in medical–legal work, and monitor every case accordingly.

14. Develop an ethical behavior habit. In addition to #10, keep ethical standards, case books and reports, and a collection of articles in a handy place for frequent review. Consult colleagues frequently about ongoing potential ethical issues. Periodically perform critical comparative review of past defense versus plaintiff-referred cases. Strive for objectivity and a reputation as such.

15. Make efforts to develop and employ formal mechanisms for monitoring objectivity, the validity of diagnostic and prognostic statements against external criteria, and receipt of objective feedback from peers.

16. Promote increased awareness (e.g., give talks, write, teach, engage in dialogue) within the forensic professions of issues relating to ethics and scientific objectivity (e.g., promoting use of professional ethical standards by courts in assessing admissibility of evidence; Shuman & Greenberg, 1998).

Note. Based on Martelli, Bush, and Zasler (2003); American Psychological Association (2002); Sweet and Moulthrop (1998); Blau (1992); Brodsky (1991); and the Committee on Ethical Guidelines for Forensic Psychologists (1991).

related work, were well known for virtually never agreeing with each other on anything. In this case, they both provided treatment, collaborated on the case, and opined severe persistent neurobehavioral impairment.

I could feel the momentum changing as interest steadily increased and hopes for my vacation faded. Subsequent to a review of my curriculum vitae (CV), a summary conversation about the scope of the examination vis-à-vis the research literature and this examiner's experience regarding the long-term effects of milder TBI, reassurance that the other neuropsychologists' national prominence would not influence my objectivity, and their acceptance of my assertion to perform the same assessment independent of the referral source, I agreed, albeit with some reluctance.

BACKGROUND INFORMATION

Postinjury neuropsychological, psychological, and medical records were received and reviewed, followed later by preinjury medical, school, and employment records. R.G., a right-handed Middle Eastern male in his mid-30s, was the plaintiff in the personal injury lawsuit. Briefly, his medical, educational, occupational, and social history includes immigration to the United States in his late teens after completion of 1 year of college in Europe in order to complete a master's degree in health technology. He is trilingual and was employed in a private health clinic and as a part-time teaching instructor at the local university medical school. He completed a PhD in health administration while working. R.G. was married in the United States shortly after graduating with his master's degree, and he now has three children between the ages of 1 and 4.

R.G. was injured in an accident 3 years earlier when he was struck in the head by an 8-foot-long, 100-pound fence post being carried by another shopper in a home improvement store. Records indicated that he was struck in the back of his head with the post and fell to the floor. Contrasting witness reports suggested that he was struck in the right temporal or occipital region of his head, fell to the floor striking his back, and may have struck the floor with the left posterior region of his head. The blow resulted in a loss of consciousness estimated at between 10 and 30 minutes. He was transported to the nearby emergency room at a major university hospital trauma center, where he was awake but noted to be briefly unresponsive. R.G. experienced an estimated 3-hour posttraumatic amnesic period from the blow to his head, an initial Glasgow Coma Scale (GCS) score of 14, a back injury that produced acute pain diagnosed as strain/sprain, and headache and nausea. Computed tomography (CT) scans of the head and back were read as unremarkable. ER records indicate that R.G. was clear and fully oriented at 3 hours postinjury. He was discharged from the ER later in the day, complaining of headache and resolving mild blurred vision with prescriptions for ibuprofen and Phenergan.

R.G. experienced a complicated recovery course. An attorney was retained a couple of weeks after the accident. In the first month postinjury, records indicated that he complained of persistent head, neck, and back pain, nausea, diplopia, difficulties with concentration and memory, decreased hearing acuity, and increased irritability. He returned part-time to his job as a doctoral-level health care technician 3 weeks postinjury, incrementally increasing work hours to 4 full days per week after a couple of months. This schedule was reduced to 3 days per week after consultation with a physical medicine and rehabilitation doctor, secondary to complaints of constant and fairly severe head, neck, and low back pain that was significantly irritated by driving or prolonged sitting, disturbed sleep, irritability, and decreased concentration and memory.

One month postinjury, he was evaluated by a neuropsychologist with whom he was familiar from brief previous collegial contact. Findings included:

- A pattern of diffuse neuropsychological impairment characterized by decrements in multiple areas of thinking efficiency (attention/ concentration, processing speed, complex thinking, memory, organization, problem solving) and upper extremity strength, speed, and dexterity.
- Self-report of moderately severe persistent and widespread pain with dizziness and sleep disturbance (no standardized measures of pain complaint were administered).
- Significant emotional distress (e.g., Beck Depression Inventory score indicative of clinical depression) estimated to possibly amplify cognitive impairments.
- A just-above cutoff score on the Portland Digit Recognition Test (PDRT), attributed to emotional distress (although no neuropsychological test scores were deemed reduced by emotional distress).

- Recommendation against psychotherapy, as this might make R.G. "even more anxious."
- Recommendation for magnetic resonance imaging (MRI) and electroencephalogram (EEG).
- No discussion of the raw data, which suggested inconsistencies that may have reflected poor motivation (e.g., intact Paced Auditory Serial Attention Task [PASAT] vs. impaired performances on Wechsler Memory Scale—Revised [WMS-R] Mental Control and Digit Recall subtests).
- No discussion regarding what, if any, current medications (Ultram, hydrocodone, Ambien) were employed before and during testing, or the possible effect of pain or medications on test results, or potential effects of involvement in litigation.

Three months postinjury, with persistent head, neck, and back pain, dizziness and emerging angry outbursts, R.G. was diagnosed with major depression, and he began outpatient psychiatric and physical therapy treatment. After an insurance change, he was referred to another neuropsychologist and underwent repeated neuropsychological evaluations at 12, 20, and 32 months postinjury. These revealed a pattern of persistence in all previously noted areas of neuropsychological deficiency, along with persistent emotional distress and significant pain-related distress, and only token suggestion of the possible influence of emotional, pain, and motivational effects on test results.

A review of R.G.'s neuropsychological records was notable for the following:

- Failure to improve in purported postconcussive symptoms.
- Questionable effort suggested on many neuropsychological tests.
- Little to no discussion of possible negative impact on test findings of medication effects, pain-related distress (reportedly high on all test dates, including extremely high current pain ratings at time of testing), or pain tolerance; English as a second language and/or disinterest in testing; and minimal isolated mention of emotional distress, emotional motivations, and borderline scores on mostly less sensitive symptom magnification and effort/motivation tests (e.g., Rey 15-item Memory test).
- Interpretation of consistency of poor overall test scores as evidence of valid test results and organic brain injury.
- Absence of previously recommended MRI or EEG.

Outpatient multidisciplinary chronic pain management services, including psychological services, were begun 2½ years postinjury, coincident with diagnosis of lumbar radiculopathy and performance of a discectomy. On medical advisement, R.G. withdrew from his regular job position and developed a home-based health technologist placement service (vs. practice) while maintaining his one-afternoon-a-week position as a clinical instructor.

A multidisciplinary work capacity evaluation performed just prior to this examiner's evaluation listed insufficient work tolerance for preinjury occupation, "symptom magnification" without abnormal illness behavior, and depression and anger estimated to be "likely disruptive" to rehabilitation efforts.

INTERVIEW

R.G. presented as an attractive, neatly groomed, polite, humble, unassuming, and endearing individual with a pleasing voice that suggested at least some need for approval. Formal explanation informing him about the nature, scope, and unique features of independent examinations were noted to produce visible signs of anxiety. However, he was subsequently relieved by reassurances that I insisted on efforts at objectivity and was dedicated to performing the same examination, had his attorney referred him and provided his informed consent.

During the interview, R.G. displayed intermittent anxious and dysphonic affect and readily and sometimes dramatically displayed grimacing, sighs, and stretching of facial muscles as expressions of pain, consistent with his decision to withhold his pain medication in order to perform "as I really am." This announcement served to herald his intention to highlight his pain-related symptoms. During testing, he would sometimes deny being in great pain when he looked in relatively great distress, but at other times would behave more melodramatically about what seemed to be relatively less overall physiological arousal and distress.

R.G.'s examination was conducted under special circumstances in order to minimize the potentially distracting effect of chronic pain and associated symptoms, to emphasize the most effective interview (which continued throughout testing in an interactive and intuitive manner), and to foster sufficient rapport (Hart, Martelli, & Zasler, 2000; Hart, Wade, & Martelli, 2003; Martelli, Zasler, Nicolson, & Hart, 2001). A heating pad, a comfortable chair, lumbar support, flexible use and placement of a roll table, frequent position changes and breaks (including use of the interview as a break) with attention to facial expressions and distress signals, adjusted lighting, slow pace, and even use of the examinee's musical relaxation tape were all employed.

This approach was based on a combination of factors: (1) review of the relevant literature regarding effects of pain on cognitive functioning (see Table 6.2); (2) the fact that the examinee already had been tested four times previously (and I did not know at the time that he was assessed an additional time just prior to my examination); (3) clear observation of pain distraction along with interview and test data indicating somatic hypervigilance; (4) the examinee's indication that pain interfered with performance on all previous examinations; (5) my observation that impromptu interview during testing is often more effective in reducing guardedness and more fruitful, given benefit of ongoing test observations and opportunity for subsequent clarifications; and (6) my experience that useful and extended interviews are too often neglected in forensic neuropsychological examinations yet often provide the most revealing information.

The exam included extensive interviewing, approximately 15 hours of total face-to-face contact for interview and testing over a 4-day period, a 30-minute telephone interview of his wife during a break from her work, and a review of a 10-inch stack of medical records. The unusual 4-day format for examination, which was indicated after part of the interview on the first session, was readily agreed to by R.G., although approval from the referring attorney required several phone calls. A similar request was made and agreed to regarding the phone interview of R.G.'s wife.

Interview and test observation data were especially rich and significant, and these were cultivated by a flexible interviewing style. Interviewing was assisted through use of my usual recording method: a small, silent, wireless keyboard held in my lap, on which I typed in a well-practiced and fairly unobtrusive manner that allowed frequent verbatim recording while looking at the examinee.

R.G. reported persistent complaints in all previously reported areas, with highly consistent independent corroboration by his wife on structured questionnaire and interview:

TABLE 6.2. Recommendations for Assessing and Minimizing the Confounding Effects of Chronic Pain during Neurocognitive Examinations

1. Chronic pain and associated symptoms must be considered a source of performance variance in neuropsychological testing and performance.

2. Consideration should be given to postponing neuropsychological assessment in cases where pain and related symptomatology (especially sleep disturbance) have not yet received specific and appropriately aggressive treatment focus.

3. Altered test conditions should be considered to promote optimal performance and minimize discomfort and emotional distress (e.g., comfortable seating/positioning, use of accustomed esthetics, cushions, heating/ice pads, optimized ergonomics, frequent breaks, frequent standing or position changes, modified lighting, etc.).

4. Arrange for assessment by a chronic pain specialist in cases where there is (1) pain-related complaint that interferes with everyday functioning and performance, (2) suggestion of poor pain adaptation, or (3) a neurologically atypical cognitive profile.

5. Although assessing the presence and severity (Verbal or Visual scales; observation) of pain periodically during testing for correlation with performance is important, assessing the cumulative effects of coping with pain and associated symptoms appears to play a more important role. Supplementing the interview with administration of symptom checklists that assess associated complaints of chronic pain (e.g., fatigue, sleep disturbance) by the patient with independent ratings by corroborators, may be helpful. The repeated administration of a sustained, attention-demanding, timed test at the end of a session may help identify or corroborate possible fatigue-related deficits.

6. Standard measures of mood and emotional–personality functioning, as well as measures specifying assessment of response to pain, should always be employed. Significant emotional distress, negative beliefs about pain and illness, and lifestyle interference that seems inconsistent or disproportionate should increase the level of caution in attributing performance decrements to brain dysfunction versus other causes.

7. Assessment of any response bias (pain as well as other complaints) should be conducted to identify exaggeration and to estimate effects of chronic pain on ability to sustain optimal performance as well as avoidance. Inventories that address primary and secondary gains and motivation, as well as primary and secondary losses, should be employed.

8. Pain medications represent another possible moderator variable, and caution must be exercised in interpreting test results for persons who rely upon them for pain management. Simply instructing clients to desist from using medications during testing is not an adequate solution, because the effects of unmodulated chronic pain may be worse for some aspects of cognitive functioning than induced opiate analgesia (Lorenz, Beck, & Bromm, 1997).

Note. Based on Martelli, Zasler, Bender, and Nicholson (2004).

- Decrements in sustained/simultaneous attention, focused attention and recent memory, comprehension, speed of information processing and reasoning, recent memory, expression, efficiency of information processing.
- Headache and neck ache, sensation changes, sensitivity to noise and light, nausea and decreases in energy, balance, sexual interest, and milder problems with blurred vision, tinnitus, dizziness, coordination, speed and strength, and sleep and appetite.
- Marked difficulties with anxiety and irritability and moderate difficulties with depression, moodiness, impatience, restlessness, frustration/stress tolerance, self-confidence, and motivation/interest.
- Marked reductions in sports/recreation activities and moderate difficulties with anger management, getting along with wife and family and others, management of household chores, sexual functioning, worry about health, and reduced social activities.

R.G.'s description of his greatest postinjury complaints was telling. He offered that "I can't play with my children" due to (head, neck, back) pain, while fighting tears and shuddering. He complained that since the injury, he was "not enjoying life . . . everything is a struggle . . . sleeping with my wife . . . I don't like getting up . . . not able to work in my profession without pain . . . feel so exhausted." Regarding pain, he explicitly indicated, "This is my major problem, number one."

R.G.'s pain included lower back and left leg pain and headaches. Back and leg pain were described similarly as constant numbness with increasing burning and tingling with increased activity or prolonged sitting. This pain, which had remitted somewhat, was described as worsening subsequent to a lumbar discectomy. He also reported headaches that are associated with a reduction in focused attention and concentration and that increase with cognitive demand, stress, back pain, and other triggers. He additionally reported that pain disrupts his sleep several times every night, and it often disrupts his wife's sleep; he awakens when he turns and "never" gets a night of refreshing sleep. In response to query about general effects of pain and associated symptoms (e.g., sleep disturbance, medication effects, fear of pain), he offered that "it always" affects his concentration, making him "foggy . . . slow" and more notably with tasks requiring greater concentration and speed. Regarding previous neuropsychological assessments, he reported significant pain-related concentration difficulty on all of them.

Regarding any pain interventions, R.G. noted that pain medications (despite disliked side effects) and lying down helped with pain tolerance, but that these interfered with ongoing activities and were often not available as an option (e.g., at work, where lying down and taking stronger psychoactive medications was not permitted). Additionally, he reported a characterological dislike for medications and sensitivity to their effects, indicating displeasure at having to take medications that only partly helped symptoms and produced side effects he didn't like. He further indicated that taking medications conflicted with his religious beliefs. He noted that although his pain had shown some slow gradual improvement, he was very disappointed that surgery had only worsened it. Importantly, although R.G. reported memory problems, and all previous assessments confirmed this, his description of such lapses were much more consistent with concentration problems. That is, the examples he provided indicated variable memory dysfunction that tended to be largely correlated with increased pain, stress, distress, fatigue, and sleep and mood disturbances.

In terms of his relationship with his wife, he reported self-doubt and significant resentment that the injury had reduced his capacities, including his ability to provide for, prove his worth to, and earn the respect of his wife. His response to query about sex included the report that pain prevented sexual relations, although he denied sexual dysfunction. This discussion was notably followed by an abrupt transition to ambivalently expressed anger about his accident.

When pointedly questioned about his residual anger toward the person who had caused his accident, R.G. erupted emotionally and hollered out loudly, with stuttered anger and tears, that "he didn't call the hospital or my home . . . [the store] did not even call to see if I was all right . . . I know I wouldn't do that to my enemies . . . I am a f—ing human being, not a dog [with abruptly increased animation, anger, tears, trembling]." This outburst contrasted greatly with his uniformly pleasant, polite, and controlled presentation, and his wife's report that he never cursed. Further inquiry revealed that "they did nothing . . . I got the bills [from the hospital] . . . and I paid them, I am still making payments on the bills. . . . I have no insurance . . . only their insurance company called worried about me suing. . . . I would never treat someone like that." Regarding his handling of these unpleasant memories and anger, R.G. noted: "I don't want to think about it. . . . I don't know why they would do that . . . the guy carrying the post . . . if it was me, I would have gone to the hospital. . . . But they just let . . . he just left. . . . From what I was told in his deposition, he saw me collapse and . . . ”

In a subsequent phone interview with his wife, she noted that both she and her husband suspected that discrimination against R.G. for being Middle Eastern was a factor. She reported that fear and anger and a desire to obtain medical treatment compelled her to contact an attorney. In response to a subsequent query about a hunch ("How long has R.G. had sexual performance problems?"), she partially gasped out "I can't believe he told you that. He hasn't told anyone. . . .” He is so embarrassed. . . . It happened right after the injury and has never really returned. . . . He is afraid to try . . . afraid to talk about it or tell his doctors." Her further report about an infection related to a postsurgical scar was interrupted by her own questions about just what, and how, her husband had revealed this information. This questioning was redirected to elicit the report that preinjury, R.G. had frequently talked about plans for the future, including areas of professional growth and family expansion. He was a "go-getter," sociable and "bubbly" and happy, but all that has disappeared and been replaced with silence, fear, depression, a sense of inner emptiness, poor coping and problem solving, and generalized reductions in energy and motivation.

BEHAVIORAL OBSERVATIONS AND TEST RESULTS

Neuropsychological test selection in R.G.'s case was complicated by attempts to avoid repetition of tests employed on the four previous examinations. It was necessary to balance the use of the most reliable, valid, and well-normed instruments with attention to practice effects. Given no dearth of previous test data, I chose to use a few different, less known, and/or older test versions and subtest combinations. Because I administer all of my own tests, test selection was flexible and adjusted in response to ongoing test performances and patterns.

A summary of tests administered and findings is presented in Table 6.3.

R.G.'s test performance, including effort/motivation to perform well on testing, was variable, punctuated by intermittent grimaces and other nonverbal expressions of discomfort and distress that sometimes appeared less than fully credible. This behavior was a prompt for testing of limits and creative adaptation of some administration procedures.

TABLE 6.3. Summary of Neuropsychological Tests Administered and Findings

Tests administered

- Adapted Neurobehavioral Symptom Checklist (completed by examinee and wife); Behavior Change Inventory (examinee and wife); Katz Adjustment Scale (wife)
- North American Adult Reading Test
- Category Test, Trail Making Test, Tactual Performance Test (TPT), and Grooved Pegboard
- Computerized Assessment of Response Bias (CARB), Word Memory Test (WMT), Rey 15-item Memory Test
- Millon Inventory of Personality Styles
- Minnesota Multiphasic Personality Inventory–2 (MMPI-2)
- Multidimensional Pain Inventory (MPI), Kinesiophobia Scale, Hendler Low Back Pain Screening Test
- Paced Auditory Serial Addition Test–Revised (PASAT-R)
- Rey Auditory–Verbal Learning Test (RAVLT)
- Rey–Osterrieth Complex Figure Test (Meyers version)
- Ruff Figural Fluency Test
- State–Trait Anxiety Inventory and State–Trait Anger Expression Inventory
- Wechsler Adult Intelligence Scale–Revised (WAIS-R), Verbal subtests
- Wide Range Achievement Test–Revised (WRAT-R)
- Williams Inhibition Test
- Zung Depression Inventory

Test findings

Attention/concentration

- Simpler concentration and vigilance tasks: low average to borderline impaired, except for suspiciously poor Digit Span.
- Visual–motor scanning and sequencing tasks: very slow and inefficient, suggesting significant impairment if performed effortfully or without distraction.
- Complex, demanding, speeded information-processing task PASAT-R: at least mildly impaired range score was very consistent with previous evaluations; unusual pattern of stable scores across easier to harder trials.

Overlearned verbal skills

- Most areas assessed: average to low-average performances; consistent with previous assessments.
- Generative verbal fluency: mild to moderate impairment; slightly improved compared to previous assessments.
- Despite consistent scores, qualitative inconsistencies noted on spelling across administrations; some familiar words spelled correctly on one occasion and unusually on another.

Verbal reasoning

- Lower than expected performance, quite consistent with previous evaluations.
- Serious questions about motivation and effort level, as well as possible effects of English as a second language and generalized pain and adjustment-related distress.

(continued)

TABLE 6.3. *(continued)*

Memory functions

- General verbal memory performances: moderate to severe impairment, consistent with previous evaluations; recognition not relatively better than recall.
- Visual nonverbal memory: relative strengths noted only in a complex figure recognition for which this examinee has had more than one prior testing exposure; atypical, suspicious pattern of recall.

Sensory and motor skills

- Moderate impairment roughly comparable to previous evaluations.

Nonverbal reasoning and problem solving

- Category Test (nonverbal reasoning, logical analysis, and problem solving): mild to moderately impaired, similar to 1 month postinjury.
- TPT (tactile performance, tactile–spatial learning, and problem solving): moderate to severely impaired; much more impaired/slower compared to previous administration.

Symptom validity measures (dedicated)

- WMT: suspiciously poor (more similar to "simulators" than to severe brain-injured patients).
- CARB: suspiciously poor.
- 15-Item Test: 10

Clearly, disruptive pain behavior seemed to interfere with his attention during testing (e.g., scores up to twice as impaired on similar tasks when he appeared to be in pain). Moreover, his performance appeared somewhat variable, depending on instructions. For example, R.G.'s best (above average) and clearly most demonstrably effortful performance (e.g., fixed his gaze on the words, actively anticipated next words, and did not attend to any physical discomfort) was on a reading test (North American Adult Reading Test) that was introduced both as insensitive to decline after brain injury and as a comparative estimate of preinjury ability. He obtained an estimated premorbid IQ of 119, despite having English as a second language. In contrast, his score on a parallel task not introduced as such (Wide Range Achievement Test–Revised), fell in the below-average range, punctuated by greater vigilance to physical discomfort (e.g., grimaces, facial and neck muscle stretching, eye squinting) and greater demonstrated difficulty reading words with less apparent dedication to optimal performance. When queried about English, R.G. attested to exposure to numerous TV and educational programs as a child, insisting that he had acquired "everything" Americans do, explicitly suggesting that any observed impairments were due to the injury and not to cultural factors.

R.G.'s Digit Span performance was suspiciously poor; testing limits, by introducing a highly effective chunking enhancement strategy, did not produce the expected improvement. On a verbal categorical reasoning test (Similarities subtest), readministration on a subsequent testing occasion revealed a similar score but discrepant responses to the items. His mildly to moderately impaired performance on the Tactual Performance Test, although appearing credible, was poorer than on two previous occasions with different examiners.

The poor memory profile patterns on the Rey Auditory–Verbal Learning Test (including a prominent recency effect atypical of true brain injury) and the Rey–Osterrieth Complex Figure Test were consistent with his performance on a previous examination, but did not improve despite previous exposure, and revealed only slightly better recognition than recall. Trail Making Test B performance was slow in that the examinee seemed to scan past the numbers and proceed more slowly than on comparable tasks. His performance on a complex, speeded serial addition task, the Paced Auditory Serial Attention Test, did not show the expected decline with increased difficulty. On the Williams Inhibition Test (1992), a fairly simple nonverbal reasoning, cognitive flexibility, self-control task designed for severely impaired persons, he showed poor performance (vs. only mild impairment on the much more difficult Category Test) that only improved to borderline after a second administration.

Overall, R.G.'s atypical and poorer than expected performance patterns on select neuropsychological tasks contrasted negatively with most of his behaviors during the interview. Furthermore, many of his performances appeared quite inconsistent for an individual sustaining less than a severe brain injury who was performing as a clinical instructor and comanaging a home-based business. Finally, R.G.'s scores on two dedicated measures of symptom validity (CARB, WMT) suggested at least mildly suboptimal effort consistent with borderline scores on similar, but more obvious, measures of effort on previous assessments. Undoubtedly, qualitative and subjective indicators converged in suggesting suboptimal effort and/or effort to perform suboptimally. Further indicators suggest that pain-related internal distraction, sleep deprivation, frustration, a desire to dramatically present symptoms, emotional distress, and/or other motivational factors contributed as significant sources of variance in test performance scores.

With regard to his emotional status, R.G.'s responses on objective personality and emotional status measures demonstrated validity configurations consistent with a pattern of highlighting of symptoms, a plea for help, and/or a "distress" profile. However, the clinical profiles were interpretable and externally consistent across measures and with the interview and historical data. Integration of interview and historical information with objective measures indicated a significant amount of generalized emotional distress that appeared fairly diffuse. A summary of relevant emotional findings includes the following interpretations:

- Attempts to strongly characterize and even amplify cognitive, emotional, and physical symptoms and subjective distress.
- Somatic and cognitive symptom hypervigilance, hyperarousal, and somatization tendencies.
- Poor current internal coping resources for managing emotional distress, especially with regard to angry/resentful emotions, pain, and coping with perceived changes in functional status.
- Minimization of emotional conflicts (incompatible with coping with postinjury pain and life disruption) and low tolerance for emotional and physical distress. A characterological (premorbid) low pain tolerance was suggested by interview (e.g., reported disruptive pain when previously cut his finger) and strongly characterized on all personality, somatic symptom, emotional status, and disability measures (e.g., rated worst pain as 15 on a 10-point scale; MPI classification as "dysfunctional pain coper"; MMPI-2 somatization traits; Millon Inventory of Personality Styles; Work Capacity evaluation report; Kinesiophobia Scale score—all suggesting pain-phobic responses).
- Significant and poignant unresolved anger, resentment, and perceived victimization regarding the persons responsible for his injury and pain, failed surgery, changes in cognitive efficiencies, and other multiple associated life interferences and disruptions that have occurred postinjury.
- Cultural influences specifically relating to expectations of correcting injustice by imposing retribution, lest he perceive himself as having failed his own expectations regarding his religious beliefs (i.e., interview indications, with collaboration from MMPI-2 critical items: "When people do me wrong, I feel I should pay them back if I can, just for the principle of the thing"; " I feel as if I have been punished without cause"; "I brood a great deal").

- Perceptions of helplessness, hopelessness, and stress that grossly exceed internal resources for coping; feeling exhausted and overwhelmed, compounded by extremely low ego strength.
- Evidence that posttraumatic emotional distress is (1) significantly impacting current adaptation to postinjury impairments, (2) exacerbating symptoms, and (3) exerting an inhibitory effect on long-term adaptation and recovery.

Interestingly, a review of R.G.'s revelations during the interview indicated a startling contrast with his neuropsychological test performances. Whereas the test performances were often suspicious, he seemed unquestionably open to revealing many aspects of almost all of his many distresses. In fact, at the end of the examination, he complimented me, indicating that he thought I was the only psychologist who understood him and that he "couldn't wait" to get a copy of the report from his attorney.

IMPRESSIONS

The results of R.G.'s previous and current neuropsychological assessment represent a database that imposes serious limitations with regard to any inferences about the degree and severity of residual neuropsychological impairment or associated cerebral dysfunction. By history, R.G. sustained a traumatic brain injury, which could perhaps best be categorized as "complicated mild." However, the recovery pattern was *not* characterized by expected improvement but rather by a persistence of deficits and protracted disability. In addition, a considerable amount of questionable motivation compromised the validity of the test findings. Hence, I had little confidence that the test results accurately reflected his true neuropsychological abilities at that time.

Delight is a good adjective for describing the lead defense attorney's reaction upon preliminary verbal report of these results. However, in keeping with the considerations of a skeptic pursuing balance and attempting to perform the same evaluation independent of the referral source, and in efforts to challenge and subject every finding to critical scrutiny, I resisted the easy solution of joining the defense attorney team as an adversary who could simply make an assertion of dichotomous malingering to offset the other slanted evaluation findings of severe impairment. Instead, I pursued a conceptualization that hopefully integrated all information obtained in the examination for the best understanding of this examinee—regardless of the partisan interests of the referral source.

Despite ample evidence of exaggeration on testing, there were too many findings that were incompatible with a simple unidimensional diagnosis of malingering. For instance, R.G. actually minimized some apparently genuine and significant problems, including sexual dysfunction and distress over postsurgical disfigurement. Striking was his minimization of problems with sexual performance in contrast to his wife's regarding it as a very important impairment. This is opposite of the pattern usually seen with TBI malingerers (e.g., Sbordone, Seyranian, & Ruff, 2000).

The most important data source for this examination, and the most revealing information to date, was the interview. Creativity in conducting it notwithstanding, the interview findings were quite revealing, and much of the information was both inconsistent with a simplistic malingering diagnosis and indicative of a constellation of vulnerability factors that seemed to predispose him to poor postinjury adaptation.

Importantly, review of the records suggested a significant iatrogenic component to R.G.'s symptoms and disability. In some ways, they read like an introductory guide to manufacturing disability and poor postinjury outcome. Missing was early and appropriate differential diagnosis and early and aggressive treatment that would have helped to resolve his problems and prevent persistent symptoms. Instead, R.G. initially received a kind of neuropsychological "Law of the Instrument" evaluation, which paid exclusive attention to brain injury while mostly neglecting prominent symptoms of posttraumatic head, neck, and back pain, significant emotional distress, sleep deprivation, medication effects, and motivational factors. Notable was the early failure to (1) recognize multiple poor prognostic risk factors, or (2) appreciate the critical importance of early intervention in primary pain and emotional distress symptom areas. Worse, he received an almost unfathomably misguided recommendation "against" psychotherapy, when it should have been intensively provided very early on.

Diagnoses from R.G.'s neuropsychological treaters' earlier examinations attributed to brain injury symptoms often much more compatible with chronic pain, associated concomitants (e.g., sleep disturbance, somatic vigilance, pain medications, fatigue), and emotional distress. Undoubtedly, early postinjury experiences usually set the stage for future expectancies and postinjury adaptation. There is an abundant literature demonstrating the importance of early intervention in minimizing disability for both brain injury and chronic pain patients. In my opinion, misdiagnosis, underdiagnosis, and late intervention strongly contributed to R.G.'s poor postinjury adaptation and persistent symptoms. Specifically, the initial misdiagnoses shaped a pattern of misattribution, failed improvements, and disability expectation.

When treatment finally did proceed more intensively, it came very late and in piecemeal fashion. Even psychiatric and chronic pain providers appeared to suffer from the initially established momentum of misattribution of symptoms to brain injury, rather than seeing the more comprehensive clinical picture of chronic pain, adjustment disorder, residual anger, low motivation, medication effects, sleep deprivation, and biopsychosocial and coping variables, not to mention cultural factors. The failure of a psychologist specializing in the treatment of chronic pain to detect or intervene with R.G.'s inhibited anger and resentment is telling and reflects a consensual validation of a misattribution that removed hope for improvement.

The underappreciation of R.G.'s pain was critical. It was apparent to me during the interview that pain was his primary and most disabling acute symptom, even from early postinjury. Pain and its concomitants (e.g., sleep disturbance, somatic preoccupation, fear of pain, fatigue) can have a more disabling effect across a wider range of neurocognitive functions than brain injury or many other types of injuries (Nicholson & Martelli, 2004). Further, the available evidence strongly supports the conclusion that chronic pain, especially head and neck pain, independent of TBI, can and often does produce impairment of cognitive functioning. This conclusion is supported by multiple lines of evidence from studies of acute and chronic pain in humans and animals, and from experimental, clinical, and neurophysiological studies (Martelli, Zasler, Bender, & Nicholson, 2004) that indicate negative effects, especially on attentional capacity, processing speed, memory, and executive functions. Finally, resolution of postconcussive disorders frequently seems to hinge on resolution of, or improved coping with, posttraumatic pain. Further complicating the late treatment of R.G.'s pain is evidence that he has a low premorbid pain tolerance, low general premorbid tolerance for conflicts and distress, significant problems coping with pain and other injury sequelae, and significant generalized emotional dysfunction.

Another important and apparently neglected factor in R.G.'s assessment and treatment records related to cultural differences. Clearly, there is a dearth of norms for specific English as a Second Language populations. The importance of considering this limitation, along with how cultural factors can affect test findings and interpretation, is prescribed by

American Psychological Association (2002) Ethical Standard 9.06. In R.G.'s case, there were several important considerations. In Middle Eastern cultures, where dualism is not assumed, there is less separation of physical (and cognitive) and emotional pain. During the interview, R.G. seemed to blend his report of physical, cognitive, and emotional distress, and this style required repeated questions and clarifications. Imaging of R.G.'s initial back injury revealed no structural defects. However, only 2½ years later, he was diagnosed with lumbar radiculopathy and underwent surgery. This medical event eliminated malingering as an explanation for back pain but strongly indicated that chronic pain (and its associated and cumulative effects) is an infinitely better explanation for his pattern of mostly unchanging deficits. Indeed, the clear indication of chronic pain begs for consideration of psychophysiological explanations (e.g., inhibited intense anger) of his ongoing disability.

R.G.'s significant persistent rumination and resentment about his injury also seemed amplified by his perception of cultural and religious discrimination. His injury caused him to violate his traditional religious beliefs against the use of medication, and even surgery did not relieve pain. Further, in describing his expectations about the person and the store correcting the injustice and his need for retribution, he clearly indicated belief that this was a cultural and religious sanction ("God willing"). Finally, the treatment he received after the accident seemed to represent to him a kind of rejection by the country into which he was trying so hard to assimilate and against which still had trouble expressing anger.

With regard to his emotional status, R.G.'s multiple postinjury stresses were previously delineated. Anxiety—as an immediate, lasting, and poorly treated postinjury reaction—produces a cognitive bias that selectively favors the processing of dangers and threats. Unremitted, it is associated with hypervigilance to symptoms and a psychophysiological hyperreactivity that increases signs of distress, aggravates symptomatology, and maintains symptoms beyond the normal recovery period. Persistent pain and fear of pain were significant triggers for R.G.'s anxiety and other emotional distress.

Clearly, blame, anger, resentment, and perceived victimization seemed to be intertwined with R.G.'s anxiety, causing psychophysiological hyperreactivity. Inhibited aggression is known to produce some of the most severe psychophysiological disturbances. Anger/blame/victimization, all of which are negative prognostic indicators, can be expected to wreak havoc on postconcussional symptoms, extending them long after neuropsychological recovery, especially in the context of anxiety-based attributional biases (e.g., catastrophizing about pain, medication effects, loss of control, uncertainty about the future, additional losses), psychosocial stress, and so on. In fact, the best explanation available to me is that the deterioration in R.G.'s back was a product of a patho-psychophysiological process resulting from his intense but inhibited anger and resentment. It seemed that the holding in of anger and its ambivalent, unmodulated, and displaced expression, together with subsequent guilt and fear, exhausted him even more than fighting off the distraction from chronic pain, depression, and anxiety.

Concentration problems that probably contribute significantly or primarily to all of R.G.'s cognitive complaints, and some test findings, appear to result foremost from chronic pain, exhaustion and fatigue, depression, anxiety, fear of failure and inadequacy, and, perhaps most importantly, unrequited anger and residual resentment. R.G. would not improve clinically until he achieved some resolution regarding his anger and the need to cope with chronic pain.

DEPOSITION

During a scheduled meeting, the defense attorneys were interested in systematically reviewing every particular demonstration of suspicious performance on the dedicated effort measures and atypical or invalid response patterns. They requested specific references and articles to justify all assertions. They seemed to be much less interested in the findings regarding pain or emotional distress and, in fact, questioned why these areas were addressed at all, given that they were convinced the plaintiff was just a "malingerer." They argued that "even if pain and emotional distress are genuine," if I presented those findings in deposition against the opposing side's findings of severe impairment from brain injury, it would only balance things out to perhaps moderate brain injury impairment. Although I did not "buy" this argument, they nonetheless seemed satisfied to be armed with a lot of detailed ammunition to argue that the plaintiff was "malingering."

The deposition was scheduled by the plaintiff's attorney 1 week later in my office. A brief predeposition meeting with the defense attorney duo replayed the previous meeting. The deposition, in contrast, seemed like the previous meeting in reverse. The plaintiff's attorney was accompanied by a well-known plaintiff's personal injury trial consultant. I was asked to review the findings and initially asked how my examination produced different findings from the two eminent neuropsychologists who, at that time, had much more impressive credentials. I explained that I had specialized experience in both pain and brain injury, did my own testing, spent much more face-to-face time with the examinee, and did a much more extensive interview. I logically responded to questions aimed at challenging my interpretation of suboptimal performance and was apparently convincing enough that they changed tactics in favor of questions aimed at establishing that numerous symptoms and complaints were legitimate: "Dr. Martelli, is R.G. malingering pain? . . . Is he malingering sleep disturbance? . . . Is he malingering emotional distress?" Next they asked questions intended to relate these symptoms to R.G.'s injury. Apparently pleased that I had not labeled their client a complete malingerer and was attributing many symptoms to his injury, they simply asked for details delineating the effects of pain and emotional dysfunction on R.G.

On cross-examination, the questions represented efforts to more strongly characterize and generalize evidence of malingering, to label R.G. a malinger and cast doubt on all of his symptoms: "Dr. Martelli, isn't the WMT a malingering test? . . . Doesn't his score indicate malingering? . . . If he isn't telling the truth, isn't he lying? . . . If a person exaggerates on several things, then shouldn't he or she be doubted on everything?" They seemed frustrated by my explanation that exaggeration and true impairment are not mutually exclusive.

Discussions with the defense attorneys immediately before and after the deposition clearly highlighted some frustration with my not conceptualizing R.G. in terms of a mutually exclusive dichotomy. From their perspective, he either had severe impairment from a brain injury, or he was a malingerer—and since I did not think he had significant brain-injury-related problems, he must be a malingerer. They expressed disbelief that I didn't share their anger at R.G. The associate even commented that he thought I was weakening their case.

Unexpectedly, upon coming out of my office after the deposition, I noticed that R.G. was in the waiting room. He and his attorneys met briefly, after which he appeared in the door of my office. He indicated that he desperately wanted to "get better" but had lost hope. He asserted that he had reread my report several times and showed it to his wife. He said that he felt even more strongly that I was the only professional who had understood him and that after a discussion with his wife, he had some renewed hope for improvement. He thanked me and said he hoped to see me again.

CASE OUTCOME

Although I avoided a potential source of bias by not becoming too friendly with the referring attorneys, I was less successful in suppressing my interest in learning the outcome of the case. I got a phone message about 1 week after the deposition. The case had settled and the scheduled court date was cancelled. I couldn't resist calling to learn the details. The lead attorney reported unexpected surprise and pleasure that R.G. had instructed his attorneys to settle the case and remove the claim for permanent brain damage, drastically reducing his demand for coverage of past medical bills and a nominal amount for future coverage. The attorney further commented that he continued to strongly disagree with my unwillingness to call him a malingerer but conceded that "sometimes you just can't predict. . . . " Notably, I never heard from anyone in that law firm again. I also did not hear from R.G.

CONCLUSIONS

R.G.'s lawsuit should have been focused on pain, its associated symptoms, and emotional dysfunction. Had it focused on these areas, and had it afforded him early and aggressive treatment for sustained injuries that he could not afford himself, much of his distress and disability could likely have been prevented. Rather, it appears that much of his disability was learned—and his neuropsychologists were the teachers.

At the core of all bioethical principles, and virtually every ethics code issued by every health care profession, is the avoidance of harm. In R.G.'s case, the improper diagnosis and misattribution of probable chronic pain symptoms to brain injury harmed him by not availing him of the early intervention necessary to help prevent chronic pain. Consistent with recent revisions and current ethical principles in medicine and psychology (Nicholson, 2005; Martelli, 2005; Martelli et al., 2004; Martelli, Bush, & Zasler, 2003), available options for brain injury specialists who do not have specialized training and experience in pain management include (1) referral to a professional with specialty competence; (2) consultation with such specialists when referrals cannot be made; or (3) acquisition of knowledge, supervision, and training as indicated. When professionals provide assessment in which chronic pain is an issue, they have an ethical obligation to obtain the necessary training, skills, and experience to conduct such an examination (e.g., using appropriate techniques), or to openly state the limitation in their expertise and the tentativeness in their opinions and conclusions.

LESSONS LEARNED

This case occurred early in my career and early in my involvement in forensic work. It actually happened at a time when the prevailing zeitgeist was seemingly more concerned about false negatives, or not detecting brain-injury-related sequelae, than false positives, or misattributing symptoms to a brain injury that had not occurred. This was a predisposition I also shared, to some extent. Clearly, critically examining the work of others helped me to sensitize myself to the pitfall of misattributing symptoms to brain injury that actually emanated from other causes. It has helped refine and improve my own clinical practice. It has spurred me to conduct ongoing literature reviews about the other sources of variation in neuropsychological performance and test scores, which has culminated in writing that I hope has contributed a few useful sources to the scientific literature. In this particular case, it was the presence of pain that had a particular influence.

Interestingly, posttraumatic pain is a frequent concomitant of traumatic brain injuries. However, the assessment and treatment of persons with pain are complicated and challenging processes. Pain is a complex, multidimensional subjective experience with no clear or objective measures. Chronic pain and its concomitants (e.g., sleep disturbance, somatic preoccupation, fear of pain, fatigue) can have a more disabling effect across a wider range of functions than brain or many other types of injuries (Nicholson & Martelli, 2004). Especially relevant in the case of concomitant brain injury is the conclusion from multiple lines of evidence indicating that pain can, and often does, produce impairment in cognitive functioning. Further, resolution of post concussive disorders frequently seems to hinge on resolution of posttraumatic pain (Martelli et al., 2004). These factors create a differential diagnostic dilemma that can only be remedied by familiarity with many important issues and the current knowledge base in the specialty field of pain management.

The standards for specialty knowledge and training for assessing effects of pain parallel those for brain injury. Weekend workshops, casual and outdated familiarity with the methods and knowledge base, or utilization of a few pain-related tests is clearly insufficient. At the present time, we are experiencing an increasingly restrictive health care environment.

Reimbursement from clinical services is precipitously diminishing, managed care resources are dwindling, and the opinions and recommendations of neuropsychological and other practitioners are being subjugated to decisions from financial gatekeepers. In contrast, there is considerable enticement and reinforcement, from the subtle to the overt, for much higher reimbursement for forensic sources. This reinforcement, which by its nature operates as effectively below the level of conscious awareness, also applies to the rendering of opinions that fits with the characteristic preference of the legal system for black/white, either/or opinions. Complying with this preference is more likely to garner future referrals than more complex and conceptual diagnostic conclusions and inferences.

In this present chapter I have provided a couple of tools that represent the learning that was spurred, in large part, by the case presented here. These tools include some of my own attempts to refine my practice and resist reinforcement from potential sources of nonobjective influence. Table 6.2 includes recommendations that may help disentangle pain as a confound in the interpretation of neuropsychological test performance. Table 6.1 includes a summary of specific recommendations I have found useful for promoting objectivity in my forensic practice. These are offered in the hope of sharing some of the lessons I have learned.

REFERENCES

American Psychological Association (2002). Ethical principles of psychologists and code of conduct. *American Psychologist, 57,* 1060–1073.

Blau, T. (1984). *The psychologist as expert witness.* New York: Wiley.

Blau, T. (1992). *The psychologist as expert witness.* Workshop presented at the annual meeting of the National Academy of Neuropsychology, Reno, NV.

Brodsky, S. L. (1991). *Testifying in court: Guidelines and maxims for the expert witness.* Washington, DC: American Psychological Association.

Committee on Ethical Guidelines for Forensic Psychologists. (1991). Specialty guidelines for forensic psychologists. *Law and Human Behavior, 15*(6), 655–665.

Hart, R. P., Martelli, M. F., & Zasler, N. D. (2000). Chronic pain and neuropsychological functioning. *Neuropsychology Review, 10*(3), 131–149.

Hart, R. P., Wade, J. B., & Martelli, M. F. (2003). Cognitive impairment in patients with chronic pain: The significance of stress. *Current Pain and Headache Reports, 7,* 116–126.

Lorenz, J., Beck, H., & Bromm, B. (1997). Cognitive performance, mood and experimental pain before and during morphine-induced analgesia in patients with chronic non-malignant pain. *Pain, 73*, 369–375.

Martelli, M. F. (2005). Ethical challenges in the neuropsychology of pain: Part 1. In S. S. Bush (Ed.), *A casebook of ethical challenges in neuropsychology* (pp. 113–123). New York: Swets & Zeitlinger.

Martelli, M. F., Bush, S. S., & Zasler, N. D. (2003). Identifying and avoiding ethical misconduct in medicolegal contexts. *International Journal of Forensic Psychology, 1*, 26–44. Accessed June 20, 2003, from ijfp.psyc.uow.edu.au/IJFPArticlesIssue1/Martelli.pdf.

Martelli, M. F., Zasler, N. D., Bender, M. C., & Nicholson, K. (2004). Psychological, neuropsychological, and medical considerations in the assessment and management of pain. *Journal of Head Trauma Rehabilitation, 19*, 10–28.

Martelli, M. F., Zasler, N. D., Nicholson, K., & Hart, R. P. (2001). Masquerades of brain injury: Part I. Chronic pain and traumatic brain injury. *Journal of Controversial Medical Claims, 8*(2), 1–8.

Nicholson, K. (2005). Ethical challenges in the neuropsychology of pain: Part 2. In S. S. Bush (Ed.), *A casebook of ethical challenges in neuropsychology* (pp. 124–130). New York: Swets & Zeitlinger.

Nicholson, K., & Martelli, M. F. (2004). The problem of pain. *Journal of Head Trauma Rehabilitation, 19*(1), 2–9.

Sbordone, R. J., Seyranian, G. D., & Ruff, R. M. (2000). The use of significant others to enhance the detection of malingerers from traumatically brain injured patients. *Archives of Clinical Neuropsychology, 15*(6), 465–477.

Shuman, D. W., & Greenberg, S. A. (1998, Winter). The role of ethical norms in the admissability of expert testimony. *The Judge's Journal*, pp. 11–17.

Sweet, J. J., & Moulthrop, M. A. (1998). Self-examination questions as a means of identifying bias in adversarial assessments. *Journal of Forensic Neuropsychology, 1*, 73–88.

Williams Inhibition Test. (1992). Philadelphia: Cool Springs Software.

7

A Rising Star Too Quickly Fades
Mismanagement of Sport-Related Concussion

MARK R. LOVELL
JAMIE E. PARDINI

In looking back over the past two decades, it appears that my (M.R.L.) increasing involvement in forensic practice has actually occurred insidiously, without my conscious selection of this type of work as a career path. In retrospect, it now seems that my increasing involvement with athletes within a forensic context has been an outgrowth of two primary factors. First, work with athletes has assumed an ever-increasing proportion of my clinical practice, therefore increasing the chances that my involvement with particular athletes might develop into a forensic case even if it did not start out that way. For example, not infrequently, a neuropsychological evaluation that was originally completed ostensibly to assist in making return to play decisions after injury ends up after the fact (often years later) being part of a legal proceeding. This most often occurs when an athlete alleges that he or she was returned prematurely to the playing field, thus jeopardizing his or her career. Second, lawsuits regarding alleged brain injury in athletes (especially professional athletes) have become increasingly commonplace in recent years. This is particularly true regarding mild traumatic brain injury or concussion, where there is relatively sparse "objective" information (e.g., neuroimaging data) that can either confirm or negate a claim that an athlete was treated improperly by a particular physician or team.

Over the past twenty years, I have come to realize that, in a very real sense, *all* evaluations that I undertake with athletes represent potential forensic cases due to the litigious nature of our society and the high potential for re-injury following athletes' return to play. Indeed, I have spent many an anxious Sunday as a spectator watching a professional athlete take the playing field after a neuropsychological evaluation only days before. What if he or she is re-injured? Am I liable for being part of the return to play decision? Yet, in the final analysis, I feel that my involvement in the forensic aspects of sports neuropsychology has undoubtedly made me a more careful clinician in all aspects of my practice.

CASE DESCRIPTION

When "Becky Sikorski" presented to me (M.R.L.) for an independent neuropsychological evaluation, she had just completed her fifth season as a professional athlete in a nonhelmeted sport. Fortunately, she had been able to earn a living through participation in the team, as well as through a variety of smaller endorsement deals. Because of her athletic accomplishments (which included being the most valuable player [MVP] on a world championship team during her second and third years), spunky attitude, and trademark hairstyle, she was well known in the United States and Europe.

The purpose of my evaluation with Becky was to determine if she had experienced cognitive and physical losses related to a suspected mismanagement of a recent series of concussive injuries. The athlete and her agent were suing the management of her team for "forcing" her into "medically unsound behaviors" by "threatening" her with contract violations and loss of future playing time toward the end of her fourth year and throughout the fifth year of her career.

Because Becky had traveled overseas for this evaluation and had other professional commitments during her stay in our country, I had to manage the evaluation time carefully: My access to her, in person, was limited by the 3-day duration of her visit. I began by discussing the limits of confidentiality as well as the typical rules and procedures of a forensic neuropsychological evaluation. I reminded Becky that because the evaluation was ordered for legal purposes, the official "client" in the evaluation was actually the attorney (although Becky was the one being tested), and that any information I gathered as part of the evaluation could be used by her attorney in court proceedings. Thus typical confidentiality rules between a neuropsychologist and patient were not applicable. I also informed her that I would not be able to provide her with feedback regarding her performance on tests or my conclusions due to the forensic nature of this case; that instead, I would send the report to and discuss my findings with her attorney, who could then disclose the test results to her if he wished. Once I had completed this informed consent procedure, I began the interview by having Becky tell me her story in her own words.

BACKGROUND INFORMATION

Approximately three-quarters of the way through her fourth season on the team, Becky found herself facing off with a player from the opposite team in an attempt to secure the ball. Although she has no recollection of the skirmish, or even of the game up until that point in time, she has since watched game films and talked to other women on her team about the play. Apparently, Becky jumped up for the ball at the same time as the other team's player, and the two struck heads and fell to the ground. The opposing player did not lose consciousness and was able to control her fall by bracing with her hands and feet. From her description of the game film, it appears that Becky lost consciousness when the two players butted heads in mid-air, then fell to the ground. Unable to brace herself, she seemingly incurred a second impact that involved striking the back left region of her head on the ground. The sound of her head hitting the ground was audible to the crowd, and a collective gasp can be heard on the game film.

According to Becky's review of the game tape, she was unconscious for approximately 2 minutes. Once she fell, paramedics arrived at her side immediately, and she was quickly "spine boarded" and taken to the regional hospital's emergency room. Becky stated that a friend from college, who had been watching the game, accompanied her on the ambulance ride and throughout her stay at the hospital. Becky reportedly was quite confused when she awoke and seemed to have no recall of having played in the game at all; in fact, she did not recall any events of that whole day. She was able to remember going out to dinner with friends the night before the injury. When emergency room physicians asked her basic orientation questions, she was able to state the month and year, but not the date; she knew her name and her friend's name, but did not seem sure of where she was (either the name of the hospital or the city). Becky's neurological examination in the ambulance revealed unequally reactive pupils, though a neurological examination approximately 3 hours later was within normal limits. In addition, a computed tomography (CT) scan of the brain was unremarkable.

Though neuroimaging and neurological exam were unremarkable at the hospital, Becky was kept overnight for observation because of her significant confusion, duration of amnesia, and the fact that she was participating in an "away" game and would not have proper observation in a hotel room. Becky was released approximately 24 hours after her admission. The repeated neurological exam prior to discharge was again unremarkable. In addition, her period of retrograde amnesia had shrunk to approximately 4 hours prior to injury; thus she remembered activities earlier in the day, though she never recalled the events of the game or the trip to the game with her team. In terms of posttraumatic or anterograde amnesia, she experienced a solid 70 minutes of memory loss, with an additional 50 minutes of "spotty" anterograde amnesia. Her disorientation and confusion, according to hospital records and her friend's report, had cleared approximately 90 minutes postinjury.

At discharge, Becky was instructed to rest, with no significant physical activity for 1 week, and to work out and train in a noncontact fashion for 1 week. If everything went well during those 2 weeks, she could then return to play. Becky strictly followed these instructions. Her coach and the owner of her team called her twice a week during her 2 weeks of rest and noncontact activity. They asked how she was feeling and expressed their desire to get her back out to play, because the team appeared to be having a difficult time without her in a crucial position. She complained to them of headaches, fatigue, and intermittent dizziness, and they reassured her that she just needed to "get back on the horse," that she was likely not feeling well because she had not been very active or competitive. Becky knew that she felt poorly, but on the other hand, she knew that she always felt fatigued when she was inactive.

At the end of her mandatory 2-week noncontact period, Becky felt much better, had fewer headaches, and only felt dizzy when she rose in the morning. Although she had been cleared for working out after 1 week, Becky stated that she did not work out very often during the noncontact period. She reported that on the first day of week 2, she took a jog around her neighborhood, but had to stop after approximately one-half mile because she developed a sharp headache, dizziness, and mild nausea. Becky walked the rest of the way that day and reported to me that she felt "very nervous" about her condition. Although she reported to her coach, manager, and athletic trainer that she had been able to jog and lift weights during the second week, she reported to me that she continued to rest after she had the troubling experience with jogging. She believed that if she just rested for the remainder of her time off, she would be ready to go back to play when she was scheduled to do so. She wanted to go back to play so as not to disappoint her teammates and the rest of the organization.

The day Becky was scheduled to return to practice and play with the team, she arrived at the gym feeling uncertain. She pulled her coach and athletic trainer aside and stated that she still "didn't feel right." The athletic trainer had her perform stretching, jogging, and drills with the team. Approximately 1 hour into practice, Becky walked to a bench and sat down. Her head was pounding, she felt dizzy, and she had "dry heaves," though she never vomited. Many of her teammates appeared concerned, as did the athletic trainer, who sent her to the locker room to lie down. Her coach later visited her in the locker room and reminded her that it was "very important" that she play in this week's game against the team's chief rival, and to continue to play, because there were very important international matches coming up. He expressed sympathy for her struggle but knew she was a "tough girl"—and, after all, it was "just a concussion."

Becky played and practiced with the team for the next several weeks with no improvement in symptoms. She continued to develop headaches, dizziness, and nausea after most practices, and she sometimes sat out general drills in order to recover for more position-specific drills during practice. Although she continued to play reasonably well, and her play contributed to a winning record for the remainder of the season, she did not perform at her previous level, and she, the coach, the trainer, and management noted that she appeared to have less endurance. Unfortunately for all parties involved, the second-string player was a young rookie who could not perform as well as the concussed Becky could. She completed the season with little improvement in her symptoms; she hoped that she would fully recover in the off-season.

Now that she was no longer concentrating on athletic competition, Becky began to focus on the financial and contractual aspects of her current and pending endorsement opportunities, as well as on buying a house and taking a few college courses, hoping to one day finish her bachelor's degree in finance. Her headaches and dizziness persisted at mild levels when she worked out at her gym for approximately 1–2 hours per day. She admits that she "took it easy" on herself, working out much less vigorously because of her symptoms. However, more troubling symptoms began to emerge. Now that the demands of her daily activities had changed, she began to really notice problems with attention/concentration and short-term memory. She felt overwhelmed when she was required to "think about more than one thing at a time," and emotionally she felt more irritable and quick tempered.

When I asked her to think back to determine if these symptoms were actually "new" symptoms that had emerged in the off-season, she stated that they indeed were not, though she noticed the symptoms more because of the lifestyle and work changes that the off-season brought. In hindsight, she reflected, even her husband had noticed her quick temper and distractibility. When I later asked her husband about her symptoms in an overseas phone conversation, he stated that he noticed her changes in emotion and attention, but attributed it all to having a tough season and problems with her coach and management. Her husband was a professional athlete as well, and he felt she was likely "over" the concussion and just having other problems.

When the team reunited to begin training for her fifth season as a professional athlete, Becky was hopeful that she was ready to play. Although she still had mild problems with the symptoms she had previously described, their frequency and intensity had abated over the 4 months of the off-season. In fact, she stated, there were many days (sometimes more days than not) in each week when she felt "completely back to normal," even while working out. However, there remained other days where a hard workout or stressful situation would cause her symptoms to reemerge, and she would "crash" for a few days.

Becky successfully completed a week of low-impact low-demand conditioning without any symptom-related difficulties and was really beginning to feel "on top of [her] game." However, for the rest of the season, she struggled with headaches, dizziness, and nausea after most of her intense workouts or games. Again, she sought counsel and expressed concern with the coach and athletic trainer, believing that there was something wrong with her. Both encouraged her to keep playing through her symptoms because "there must not be too much wrong" with her, given her continued good performance on the team. Becky did, in fact, continue to play well, though she certainly was not going to be in the running for MVP, as she had been twice before. When she was feeling her worst, her coach and manager often warned her that if she did not play for a specified number of game minutes or practices, she would lose playing time in the future, even after she was healed. This possibility was unnerving to Becky, because she was already concerned about the potential long-term financial ramifications of not playing.

Becky's enjoyment in playing and being with the team began to wane. Because of her difficulty with symptoms, inability to play up to her personal standards, and the cognitive (attention/concentration, short-term memory) and emotional (irritability) problems associated with her injury, Becky experienced the onset of a depression. She reported ambivalence, sadness, increased crying, decreased appetite, insomnia, and a gradual loss of interest and pleasure in activities and people who once brought her joy. She called in sick often and appeared to withdraw from her teammates. Her ambivalence was evident in her playing behaviors. When she felt the worst, she withdrew and did not fully participate, and when she felt a little better she would push herself very hard in order to secure her place on the team. On the days when she did push herself, she felt terrible afterward and experienced an exacerbation of symptoms for at least 2 days, sometimes so severe that she stayed in bed until the next practice.

When the season ended, Becky approached her coach and management to obtain a referral for a specialist, in order to determine why her symptoms were not improving. She was referred to the team physician, who stated that a mild concussion should not cause her continued difficulty. At her next meeting with management, Becky was told that the team would be releasing her within the next 2 weeks, and that she needed to "rest up" in order to approach and try out for other teams in the preseason. When Becky questioned the team's ability to terminate a contract with yet another year promised, the team manager informed her that she was being terminated due to her violation of the contract through failure to participate in team-mandated activities.

My task was to determine if Becky demonstrated neurocognitive deficits associated with her initial injury and its subsequent likely mismanagement. Becky had never received baseline cognitive testing, though her academic history suggested that her performance should be at least in the average range. She described herself as an "average" student in high school and college, generally earning a "B" average in her coursework. She reported no history of learning or attentional disorders. Also, Becky reported scoring 1000 on the Scholastic Aptitude Test (SAT).

NEUROPSYCHOLOGICAL TESTING AND RESULTS

The following day, I administered a neuropsychological test battery that consisted of a combination of paper and pencil and computerized tests. Table 7.1 reports the battery used, as well as the standard scores for Becky's performance on each measure.

Though Becky performed within expected levels on many of the cognitive tests, she demonstrated areas of likely attenuated cognitive functioning. First, she exhibited somewhat of a flattened learning curve on verbal list-learning tasks. Throughout the Rey Auditory–Verbal Learning Test (RAVLT), she seemed to have difficulty keeping track of the words she had said to me, and she was therefore somewhat repetitive when recalling the words. There was certainly evidence of retroactive interference, because she had great difficulty with List B and the Short-Delay recall portion of the test. However, she was able to recall all but one of the words she originally encoded on the long delay portion of the test. In addition, she demonstrated low-average performance on the ImPACT Computerized Test Battery verbal memory composite, with closer examination of individual test scores revealing difficulty with initial encoding.

Becky also demonstrated difficulty with tasks requiring processing speed. Her performance on the Symbol Digit Modalities Test (SDMT), though accurate, fell more than one standard deviation below the average for her age group. In addition, her performance on the Processing Speed Composite of ImPACT fell in the low-average range, which is certainly believed to be below premorbid expectations.

She exhibited performances that were within expected levels on visual memory tasks, attention tasks, and simple speed tasks. In addition, her performance was within normal limits on tasks requiring cognitive flexibility, set maintenance, and the ability to respond to changing task demands.

Regarding her symptom presentation, Becky endorsed (both in the clinical interview and on the Post-Concussion Symptom Scale) several symptoms consistent with postconcussion syndrome. Specifically, she endorsed mild problems with irritability, moderate difficulty with headaches, nausea, dizziness, attention/concentration, short-term memory, irritability, and feeling mentally "foggy," and severe problems with insomnia (falling asleep and staying asleep), sadness, nervousness/anxiety, and emotionality (total symptom score = 48). On the Beck Depression Inventory–II (BDI-II), she endorsed significant levels of sadness, pessimism, loss of pleasure, perception of being punished, loss of interest,

TABLE 7.1. Becky's Neuropsychological Test Results

Test administered	Raw score	Standard score
Rey Auditory–Verbal Learning Test		
List A Learning Trial 1	8	$z = 0.5$
List A Learning Trial 2	9	$z = -0.4$
List A Learning Trial 3	9	$z = -1.1$
List A Learning Trial 4	10	$z = -0.85$
List A Learning Trial 5	10	$z = -1.05$
List B	5	$z = -0.79$
Immediate Recall of List A	7	$z = -1.68$
Delayed Recall of List A	9	$z = -0.78$
List A Recognition	15	$z = 0.94$
Brief Visuospatial Memory Test–Revised		
Learning Trial 1	8	$T = 54$
Learning Trial 2	10	$T = 51$
Learning Trial 3	10	$T = 44$
Total Recall	28	$T = 50$
Delayed Recall	10	$T = 47$
Symbol Digit Modalities Test		
Total Correct	46	$z = -1.15$
Trail Making Test		
A	20	$T = 51$
B	84	$T = 32$
ImPACT Computerized Test Battery		
Verbal Memory Composite	84	15th %ile
Visual Memory Composite	87	71st %ile
Processing Speed Composite	31.45	15th %ile
Reaction Time Composite	0.52	67th %ile
Controlled Oral Word Association Test		
FAS	45	$z = 0.03$
Animals	20	$z = -0.35$
Auditory Consonant Trigrams		
9 seconds	14	$z = 0.88$
18 seconds	12	$z = 0.22$
Wechsler Adult Intelligence Scale–III Digit Span Subtest		
Total Score	20	$AS = 12$
Forward Span	7	
Backward Span	6	
Wisconsin Card Sorting Test		
Categories Completed	6	Within normal limits
Failures to Maintain Set	0	Within normal limits
Post-Concussion Symptom Scale		
Total Score	48	Moderate to severe
Beck Depression Inventory–II		
Total Score	34	Severe

indecisiveness, loss of energy, and insomnia. She also reported mild to moderate levels of worthlessness, decreased appetite, concentration problems, and self-criticism.

Before Becky left my office, I reminded her that she would not receive feedback from me regarding her test results, though her attorney would likely discuss these with her once he received my report. However, as is typical for me, I made some suggestions about how she could better manage her postconcussion symptoms from this day forward. It was recommended that she avoid significant levels of physical and cognitive exertion until her symptoms began to resolve (if not completely, at least plateaued at mild and tolerable levels). She was not to perform any activity that exacerbated the symptoms. Becky was advised to avoid any activity that would place her at risk for additional head injury, including practices and games, until she was symptom free at rest and exertion and cleared by a medical professional to return to contact sport.

If she managed her symptoms appropriately, resting on days when she was more symptomatic, I believed that she would be able to effectively carry out activities of daily living, including being an active participant in the management and negotiation of her business affairs. As with physical exertion, however, I suggested she take frequent breaks or even reschedule appointments when she was significantly symptomatic and required to perform tasks requiring high degrees of concentration. I advised her to consider delaying enrollment in other college courses until she was feeling better, physically and emotionally.

Regarding her depression, I suggested that Becky see a psychologist or psychiatrist so that she could begin to address her response to the accumulating losses she had experienced. Clearly, she felt alone in trying to handle financial losses, reduced athletic performance, losses in relationships with her coach, athletic trainer, and some team members, as well as feelings that her husband was not being fully supportive of her as she recovered from the injury. I believed that she could benefit from psychotherapy, pharmacotherapy, or both.

CLINICAL INTERPRETATION

Overall, it was my opinion, with a high degree of medical certainty, that Becky was experiencing postconcussion syndrome that was the direct product of her concussion. I also felt that the concussion and its symptoms did not resolve in a timely fashion because the initial injury was not properly managed. Becky should not have returned to physically exertive activity, especially high-risk contact activity, while she was still experiencing significant symptoms of the concussion.

I also felt that the difficulties observed on neuropsychological testing were the result of the injury and resultant postconcussion syndrome, as well as the depression that was secondary to this injury. It would be difficult, if not impossible, to determine the independent contribution of the injury and the depression. However, because it was my opinion that both her postconcussion syndrome and the depression were products of the mismanaged injury, I did not see this outcome as being problematic, at least from a legal perspective (though I leave it up to the attorneys to worry about these issues).

CASE OUTCOME

Deposition

Approximately 6 months after my evaluation, I participated in a deposition concerning the findings of Becky's case. Although out-of-court settlements were attempted, Becky's case ended up going to trial. Plaintiff's council was seeking payment for Becky for the remaining year of her contract, citing that she was unlawfully declared in violation of contract and was, in fact, being punished for her injury. Her attorneys also charged that she had lost a significant amount of income from endorsements because of the mismanagement of her injury, which had caused her to be "out of play" longer than necessary. I was again called to testify on behalf of Becky, and the results of my examination were challenged in the cross-examination. During the deposition, the main adversarial focus of the defense attorney was an attempt to dissociate Becky's depression from her injury, implicating her depressive symptoms as being the underlying cause of her cognitive complaints.

Upon direct examination by Becky's attorney, an initial description of mild traumatic brain injury (concussion) was presented and scientific literature was cited that demonstrated neurometabolic changes following injury. In addition, recent published literature from the National Football League (NFL) and a number of collegiate studies were cited as evidence that concussion can and does lead to persistent symptoms in some individuals. Finally, Becky's neuropsychological test results were presented as evidence of her injuries. Cross-examination centered initially on an attempt to exclude my testimony, based on the fact that I am not a physician. However, this effort was unsuccessful; the acceptance of my work by a number of professional teams was seen as evidence of my expertise in the area of mild traumatic brain injury. Next, the defense attorney focused on the overlap of Becky's symptoms with a number of psychiatric disorders such as depression. In addition, it was suggested that there were potential secondary gain issues that may have been fueling Becky's report of persistent symptoms. This issue was put forth to me in the form of the following question: "Mr. Lovell, isn't it possible that people who have a large amount of money at stake may exaggerate or make up symptoms?" After reminding the attorney that I was a doctor, I countered this argument by stating that there was absolutely no evidence on testing or during my interview that Becky was exaggerating her symptoms.

Trial Testimony

A similar scenario to the deposition ensued during the trial. The defense attorney's argument that Becky's symptoms were related to an "emotional disorder" rather than to a mild traumatic brain injury was based largely on the nonspecific nature of her postconcussion symptoms. In fact, during the trial, the defense had the *Diagnostic and Statistical Manual of Mental Disorders, Fourth Edition* (DSM-IV; American Psychiatric Association, 1994) marked as an exhibit and made a point of listing (in court) a number of symptoms from the mood disorder diagnostic criteria. Specifically, her diminished cognitive abilities, fatigue, irritability, and insomnia were attributed to depression rather than to concussion. On the contrary, Becky's attorney argued that her concussion was the proximate cause of her symptoms and was therefore the basis for her symptoms and resulting loss of income. In court, Becky's attorney countered the defense argument by listing symptoms from the DSM-IV postconcussional disorder criteria.

The defense also introduced the testimony of an older local neurologist who stated that there was no evidence of a brain injury in this young woman and that her deficits were "functional" in nature. He further stated that her neurological examination was normal, that she had no positive findings on her CT scan and therefore had no objective evidence to support her claim. Upon cross-examination by Becky's attorney, the superficial foundation of the neurologist's opinion was exposed by asking him direct questions regarding recent published literature on concussion in athletes.

As was the case during my deposition, my courtroom testimony was aimed at providing objective evidence that Becky was indeed injured. Using a brain model as well as a brief video of a concussed NFL athlete, a description of the neurometabolic nature of concussion was presented to the court. Becky's test results were presented in graphic form (large charts) that compared her test scores to norms for other females in her age group. Finally, the issue of potential additional brain injury if she were to continue to compete was discussed.

At the completion of the trial, Becky was awarded the financial compensation that would be due to her based upon her contract with the team. She was not, however, awarded for the "loss of income" that potentially occurred due to loss of endorsements. The defense attorney's argument against compensation for Becky's lost endorsements was based on the uncertain nature of these contracts and the fact that these contracts were, in fact, not guaranteed. In other words, there was no way of knowing whether Becky would have been able to maintain her contract or maintain additional contracts in the future, regardless of her athletic performance.

After the trial, Becky never again returned to athletic competition; however, I have heard she is quite a successful coach of an amateur team in her country, as well as a broadcast announcer when the games are televised.

LESSONS LEARNED

I learned one particularly valuable lesson from this case. First, the somewhat subjective nature of Becky's postconcussive complaints resulted in a "muddying of the waters" with regard to the establishment of liability. This "muddying" relates to the fact that traditional "objective" neurodiagnostic procedures are almost always "normal" following concussion. Therefore, in the absence of any anatomical evidence of injury, it is the role of the neuropsychologist to convince the judge, jury, or arbitration panel that the plaintiff did, in fact, experience an injury. In our litigious culture where frivolous law suits are common, it is relatively easy for a defense attorney to suggest that the plaintiff is either malingering or has "psychological" issues that are leading to his or her symptoms. This position is often supported in court by the testimony of a neurologist, neurosurgeon, or other physician who testify that there is nothing "objectively wrong" with the plaintiff.

Ironically, the sports concussion literature has recently created a counter to this argument, because there is now clear documentation of cognitive deficits in even mildly concussed athletes following injury. The acceptance of the validity of injury-related cognitive deficits in athletes is now being increasingly utilized to bolster claims of cognitive deficits in concussed nonathletes injured in motor vehicle accidents, assaults, and falls. The reasoning here is that if athletes (who often have non-guaranteed contracts and therefore significant incentive to play) can develop persistent neurobehavioral difficulties following injury, it is completely reasonable to accept these deficits in nonathletes. This argument is often bolstered in court by the testimony of a neuropsychologist who has a relationship with a local or regional sports team, thus increasing the interest of the jury and lending credibility to the argument. In our "sports-crazy" culture, the reality is that an affiliation with a professional or collegiate team does promote an acceptance of the credibility of the testimony of the expert.

REFERENCE

American Psychiatric Association. (1994). *Diagnostic and statistical manual of mental disorders* (4th ed.). Washington, DC: Author.

8

Feigned Cognitive Symptoms in Alleged Toxic Exposure

Like Father, Like Son

KYLE BRAUER BOONE

I first become involved in forensic neuropsychological cases 20 years ago, while a postdoctoral fellow in the Department of Neuropsychology at UCLA. I discovered that I enjoyed the forensic (i.e., "detective") nature required by these assessments. I also perceived that it was in a forensic setting that neuropsychology really "shines." That is, the results of our objective, verifiable testing makes us of particular value to the courts, and especially in cases involving feigned cognitive symptoms, neuropsychological data are more objective and accurate than findings from any other discipline.

When I embarked on a career in neuropsychology, I had not "planned" to pursue a research focus in the area of symptom fabrication. However, as I found myself repeatedly sitting across from patients such as those described below, I was struck by the limited tools we had at our disposal to objectively document symptom fabrication. I often strongly "felt" that patients were faking, but as a psychologist committed to rigorous assessment procedures, I knew it was important to be able to operationalize and objectify what it was about a particular patient's behavior that set off my "alarms." Closely observing what the patients did and said helped to develop a sense as to which types of test paradigms would be effective in detecting dissimulation.

After years of conducting neuropsychological assessments, test administration can become rather "humdrum" as one tediously "ticks off" how many tests are left to be administered. However, when assessing someone who is feigning, the testing process itself becomes fascinating as one observes the patient's approach to symptom fabrication.

CASE 1: 77-YEAR-OLD FATHER

"Mr. Alfred Brown," a 77-year-old mechanic/maintenance worker, sued his former employer for injuries claimed to have occurred from continuous exposure to toxic chemicals during his 43-year employment with the company. The lawsuit was initiated 11 years after he retired, and Mr. Brown claimed, as recorded in his deposition, respiratory problems and sleeplessness of at least 10 years' duration, which he attributed to the toxic exposure. However, the breathing difficulties only reportedly occurred when he rode his bicycle for 30 minutes or more and when he laid down. Mr. Brown indicated that it would take him 30 minutes to fall asleep but he would awaken 3–4 hours later and remain awake. Of interest, he never complained of these problems during his periodic physical examinations during the years at work or for the first 11 years postretirement, and on exam 8 years after his retirement he had specifically denied the presence of respiratory problems or insomnia.

Over the ensuing months of the litigation process, Mr. Brown began to complain of cognitive difficulties, and he was seen for neuropsychological evaluation by the plaintiff's expert. It was concluded from this testing that Mr. Brown had slight to moderate impairment in cognitive skills in the context of average to low-average IQ scores (Verbal IQ = 83, Performance IQ = 93, Full Scale IQ = 86). However, no tests were administered to assess whether or not he was performing with his best effort on neuropsychological testing. In addition, no consideration was given to the impact of his low educational level (10th grade) on the test scores, and no medical history was obtained, which would have allowed exploration of alternative etiological factors for any observed cognitive decrements. Low-average scores were judged to reflect "mild impairment" when these would likely be consistent with estimated premorbid levels of function. Of relevance, Mr. Brown was fully independent in activities of daily living (including traveling) and demonstrated no attention or memory problems when answering deposition questions.

My neuropsychological evaluation of the plaintiff occurred 3 months after the initial neuropsychological exam. At the time of my assessment, I had been forwarded the previous neuropsychological report as well as the plaintiff's deposition and various medical records from treating physicians. I was aware that Mr. Brown had exhibited evidence of faking a hearing impairment during audiological assessment 2 months prior to my exam. He had produced normal neurological exams, although brain magnetic resonance imaging (MRI) had revealed possible cortical atrophy and white matter hyperintensities. In addition, he had been diagnosed with coronary artery disease and borderline hypertension; he had a history of chest pain, heart palpitations, and elevated cholesterol; and he was prescribed Cardizem and Mevacor. He also was described as having mild hypothyroidism. His medical history was further noteworthy for prostate surgery, two hernia repairs, and surgery to his right eye to correct damage from a work-related injury 10 years prior to retirement.

Prior to my exam, either or both of two possibilities seemed likely:

1. That Mr. Brown was faking his symptoms as suggested by (a) the fact that he had apparently faked hearing impairment shortly before my evaluation; (b) he was currently claiming physical symptoms of at least 10 years' duration, although he had denied any such symptoms 5 years ago; and (c) he appeared to be "adding" symptoms (i.e., cognitive) as the lawsuit progressed.
2. That Mr. Brown might indeed have below-average cognitive skills but that these could be consistent with his low educational level and/or the result of white matter hyperintensities, as shown on the brain MRI, and the effects of cerebrovascular disease.

Neuropsychological Examination

Clinical Interview

The cognitive symptoms that Mr. Brown attributed to exposure to workplace chemicals included decreased memory and inability to "do anything anymore." When asked to provide an example of a memory lapse, he stated that he would forget the names of people but then would recall them 30 minutes later. When asked to provide an example of things he could not do anymore, he said that he was unable to write checks because his "writing is terrible." The only physical symptom he reported was long-standing heart palpitations. When asked if he thought the palpitations might be related to his employment history, he commented, "It could have something to do with it." Of interest, he did not spontaneously report the various other symptoms that had been claimed in medical records. Regarding emotional functioning, he stated that the cognitive losses frustrated him and that he "probably" was depressed.

Mr. Brown stated that his history was negative for head trauma, brain infections, stroke, seizures, diabetes, alcohol or drug abuse, or birth or developmental abnormalities. His only language was English. He had attended school through the 10th grade, obtaining "pretty good" grades; he denied any history of learning disability or difficulty learning to read, although he acknowledged that he "never had enough patience" for reading. He had held employment as a maintenance mechanic for 43 years.

Mr. Brown was raised by an adoptive family and had no information about his biological parents. He was married twice, and his second wife died at the time of his retirement. He had one son from the first marriage, with whom he had had no contact for the past 10 years. His two younger sons lived locally and had never married. All three sons had completed high school; the oldest was a machinist, the middle son "took care of properties," and the youngest son did "odd jobs" and worked "on and off" for the same company as the patient.

Mr. Brown reported that in a typical day he worked in his yard, went to his son's house for lunch, and then returned home. He also indicated that he would go for daily walks with his dog and with a neighbor.

Behavioral Observations

Mr. Brown was a right-handed, Caucasian male who arrived on time and was accompanied to the testing session by his youngest son (Case 2). He was observed to be well groomed and casually but appropriately attired. Speech characteristics were unremarkable; he was talkative and initiated conversation, and responded quickly to interview questions. Thought processes were well organized and relevant. No examples of memory impairment were observed during the testing session (e.g., asking questions already asked and answered). Mr. Brown did not exhibit any significant hearing impairment; he did not ask that test instructions be repeated, and his responses were appropriate to test instructions, indicating that he had heard and understood them. In terms of psychological characteristics, he generally appeared unconcerned and indifferent, and/or noninsightful, when performing poorly on tasks. For example, despite committing 7 errors out of a possible 12 on a simple counting task, he spontaneously commented, "Am I doing good? I hope so!" He did not appear to be overtly depressed and actually appeared somewhat euthymic; no signs of severe psychiatric disturbance were observed (e.g., hallucinations, delusions).

Mr. Brown began the session by insisting "I'm telling you the truth!", but various aspects of his test responses suggested that he was, in fact, not applying his best effort on the cognitive tasks, and that he was attempting to portray himself as more cognitively impaired than is actually the case.

Test Results

Mr. Brown failed five out of five measures specifically administered to discreetly assess motivation and cooperation with the testing procedures. Specifically, on the Warrington Recognition Memory Test—Words, he obtained a score of 21 out of 50 (and he also required almost 10 minutes to complete the recognition trial, a markedly slow performance). Research using this test has indicated that a cutoff of 29 successfully identifies malingerers (Millis, 1992). Similarly, he obtained a score of 2 out of 15 on the Rey 15-item Memory Test (free recall = "I II," recognition = 0), a score well below the cutoff for suspect effort (Boone, Salazar, Lu, Warner-Chacon, & Razani, 2002). On the Dot Counting Test, he made 7 errors out of a possible 12, and did not reduce his counting time when presented with grouped dots; his overall E score was 53, a performance that substantially exceeds the standard cutoff of 17 for identification of noncredible performance (Boone, Lu, & Herzberg, 2002a). On the Rey Word Recognition Test, he only recognized as many words as he recalled on trial 1 of the Rey Auditory–Verbal Learning Test (RAVLT) (i.e., three words), a performance suggestive of suboptimal effort (Lezak, 1983). Finally, on the b Test, he made 46 commission errors and 191 omission errors, and he required more than 18 minutes to complete the test, for a total E score of 1,195, which markedly exceeds the cutoff of 160 used to identify suspect performance (Boone, Lu, & Herzberg, 2002b).

Mr. Brown also showed a noncredible pattern of performance on some standard cognitive tests sensitive to feigned performance. Specifically, he obtained a score of 5 on Reliable Digit Span (Greiffenstein, Baker, & Gola, 1994). In addition, his copy of the Rey–Osterrieth Complex Figure was impaired (20/36), and, of note, he failed to reproduce a very obvious detail (i.e., the bottom right-hand portion of the rectangle)— a rather unlikely performance. On the 3-minute delayed recall trial, he indicated that he could recall none of the figure, and when presented with a recognition task that included the target figure and six foils, he chose an incorrect option, again a nonplausible performance. On measures of overlearned information, such as reciting the letters of the alphabet or counting backward from 10, Mr. Brown made numerous errors (on alphabet recitation he omitted *F*, and *R* through *W*; counting backward, he placed *17* between *16* and *15* and omitted *13, 11, 10, 6,* and *1*; and he required lengthy periods of time to complete the tasks (16 seconds and 36 seconds, respectively). However, inexplicably, on another measure of remote memory/fund of general information (Information = 25th percentile), he performed normally.

Mr. Brown stated that he was unable to read the items of the Minnesota Multiphasic Personality Inventory–2 (MMPI-2) and declined to complete the test using an audio format. He suggested that his son read him the items, but this was viewed as unacceptable from a test validity standpoint; thus, administration was aborted.

Inconsistency between Test Scores across Testing Sessions

Three months prior to the current testing, Mr. Brown had obtained a Digit Span score within the low-average range (16th percentile) and a Picture Completion score within the average range (37th percentile). However, on current testing, Digit Span was impaired (1st percentile) and Picture Completion was borderline impaired (5th percentile). True brain injury leads to stable cognitive losses that can be replicated on subsequent testing session; brain injury is not associated with cognitive scores that markedly fluctuate across testing sessions. If a change in functioning occurs, it would be characterized by an improvement in scores on the subsequent testing session due to a test practice effect. There is no brain injury mechanism associated with remote exposure to toxins ending at least 10 years prior to testing that would explain a large drop in attention and visual-perceptual skills from normal to borderline or impaired across two testing sessions conducted only 3 months apart.

Inconsistency between Test Scores and Activities
of Daily Living

Mr. Brown's test scores did not match how he actually functioned in his daily life activities. Specifically, the test scores, if taken at face value, would indicate that he had a profound memory impairment and markedly impaired attentional skills. However, individuals with marked memory and attentional impairments show fairly consistent and prominent memory and attentional failure in all their behaviors. For example, they frequently restate information they have already provided because they have forgotten what they said previously. They continuously re-ask questions because they do not recall having asked the questions and receiving the answers. The attentional difficulties take the form of continuously losing track of what they are doing and what they are saying, and having to be continually reoriented to the task at hand. Mr. Brown did not demonstrate any of these behavioral patterns during the interview. In addition, if he had a true profound impairment in memory, he would require board-and-care placement or other 24-hour supervision, because the memory impairment would preclude him being able to care for himself (e.g., he would not remember any recent information aside from the previous 3–5 minutes of his life). Mr. Brown, in fact, lived alone and handled household responsibilities independently (e.g., cleaning, laundry, yard work), and he was able to travel; a person cannot engage in these activities independently with a profound memory impairment. Also of note, he claimed an inability to read (and therefore could not complete the MMPI-2), yet in his deposition he had admitted reading newspaper articles about toxic chemicals in his place of employment.

CASE 2: 45-YEAR-OLD SON

Mr. Brown's 45-year-old son, "David Brown," had been employed for 2 years by his father's employer when he was 21–23, at which point he was laid off; he then returned to work as a custodian, fabrication helper, stock clerk, and mail clerk when he was 28, ending when he was 38 when he was again laid off. He had worked part time for a retail department store in the ensuing years. Like his father, he filed suit against his former employer alleging that continuous exposure to toxic chemicals had resulted in injury to his brain, respiratory system, and internal organs.

D. Brown was previously seen for neuropsychological evaluation by the same plaintiff's neuropsychological expert who had evaluated his father. It was concluded from this testing that he had slight to moderate impairment in cognitive skills. Again, no tests were administered to assess whether or not he was performing with his best effort on neuro-psychological testing. A previous psychiatric evaluation by a defense psy-chiatrist had concluded that the patient was malingering, in that his "dementia-level" scores on mental status testing were not consistent with his activities of daily living (e.g., living independently, reading, going to plays and movies).

Records provided to me indicated that D. Brown had required some special education coursework during high school (at least, in math), had received poor work evaluations, and been noted to have some diffi-culties in memory and word-retrieval 10 years previous to this exam, when he had been hospitalized for depression.

Prior to my exam, either or both of two possibilities seemed likely:

1. That D. Brown was faking his symptoms, as suggested by the results of the psychiatric evaluation. Also, the fact that the father, who was also a party to the son's lawsuit, had been found to be feigning cognitive symptoms on neuropsychological evaluation raised an expectation that the same behaviors might be mani-fested by the son.
2. That D. Brown might have below-average skills, but that these would be reflective of baseline function as evidenced by poor per-formance in school and poor subsequent work performance.

Neuropsychological Examination

Clinical Interview

The only cognitive symptom reported by D. Brown was reduced memory. When asked to provide an example of a memory lapse, he stated that he would lay keys down and forget where he put them (who doesn't?). In terms of physical symptoms, he stated that he experienced headaches three times per day (each lasting a "few seconds"!). In addition, he said that he experienced stomachaches and cramping, which sometimes occurred two times per day but other days not at all. He also claimed to experience chest pains "once in a while," occasional pains in his shoulder and neck, and shakiness and jitteriness. When asked if he experienced any emotional symptoms, D. Brown reported that he did not sleep well and that he "never used to have this problem."

D. Brown stated that his history was negative for head trauma, brain infections, stroke, seizures, diabetes, alcohol or drug abuse, birth or developmental abnormalities, or cardiac problems. Surgeries included appendectomy and tonsillectomy, and he was hospitalized for gastrointestinal bleeding in his mid-30s. The patient was currently being evaluated for hypertension. Whereas he had denied a psychiatric history, the records indicated that he had been psychiatrically hospitalized 10 years previous to this evaluation due to headache and depression related to the death of his mother and being "yelled at" by a work supervisor. D. Brown underwent previous neuropsychological testing at that time and was reported to show declines in short-term memory and word-retrieval.

D. Brown's only language was English. He had completed high school with "B" and "C" grades, and he denied any history of learning disability or attention-deficit disorder, but reported that he had attended special classes for math coursework, at least.

Behavioral Observations

D. Brown was an ambidextrous, Caucasian male who arrived on time and was accompanied to the testing session by an older brother. He was observed to be well groomed and casually but appropriately attired. Speech characteristics were unremarkable, and his thought processes were well organized and relevant. No examples of memory impairment were observed during the testing session (e.g., re-asking questions already asked and answered), although of note, he claimed that he did not recall undergoing neuropsychological evaluation 6 months previously—a rather unbelievable assertion. In terms of psychological characteristics, D. Brown generally appeared unconcerned and indifferent when performing poorly on tasks. No signs of severe psychiatric disturbance were observed (e.g., hallucinations, delusions). Regarding his interpersonal demeanor, D. Brown interacted in a mildly petulant manner, and he disclosed information very slowly and only with prodding. He stated that he was experiencing a headache during the interview but did not show any overt signs of pain or discomfort (e.g., grimacing, holding or rubbing his head or neck, repositioning himself).

Various aspects of his test responses, as discussed below, suggested that he was not applying his best effort on the cognitive tasks, and that he was attempting to portray himself as more cognitively impaired than is actually the case. It is also of note that he was not truthful when providing a psychiatric history (e.g., he denied any previous psychiatric disorder but had been hospitalized for depression 10 years earlier), raising questions regarding the forthrightness of his presentation, in general.

Test Results

D. Brown failed three of five measures specifically administered to discreetly assess motivation and cooperation in the testing procedures. Specifically, on the b Test, he made 5 "d" commission errors and 46 omission errors, and obtained a total E score of 183, which exceeds the cutoff of 160 used to identify suspect performance (Boone, Lu, & Herzberg, 2002b). On the Dot Counting Test, he committed three errors, and one error involved miscounting seven dots as eight, a performance virtually pathognomonic for feigning (E score = 11; Boone, Lu, & Herzberg, 2002a). He achieved a total score of 19 (10 recalled, 9 recognized) on the Rey 15-item Memory Test, which falls below the cutoff of 20 used to identify suspect effort (Boone, Salazar, et al., 2002). In contrast, he obtained a score of 41 on the Warrington Recognition Memory Test—Words, which exceeds the cutoff of 29 (Millis, 1992); however, his performance was atypical due to slow completion time (> 6 minutes to execute the recognition trial). He also scored within normal limits on the Rey Word Recognition Test (8, with 1 false positive).

D. Brown also showed a noncredible pattern of performance on some standard cognitive tests sensitive to feigned performance. For example, his copy of the Rey–Osterrieth Complex Figure Test, although within normal limits (33/36), was noteworthy for omission of detail #11 (i.e., the face)—a highly unusual occurrence, in this examiner's experience.

Borderline to impaired scores were obtained on the Trail Making Test, Parts A (45 seconds) and B (he indicated that he did not know how to proceed past item "H," and the test was discontinued at 98 seconds); recall of the Rey figure ("I don't remember any of it"); verbal fluency (FAS = 16); RAVLT (7 words learned, 5 words after interference, 4 words on delay, 10 words recognized); Wechsler Memory Scale—Revised (WMS-R) Logical Memory (I = 3rd percentile, II = 4th percentile); and WMS-R Visual Reproduction (I = 5th percentile; II = 1st percentile [nothing recalled]). In contrast, scores on the Information and Picture Completion subtests were within the average range (25th percentile and 50th percentiles, respectively), and speed on the Finger Tapping Test was average to low-average (right = 48.6, 15–20th percentile; left = 45, 25–30th percentile).

D. Brown did not complete enough items on the MMPI-2 (300 in 2 hours) to produce a scorable protocol.

Inconsistency between Test Scores across Testing Sessions

On cognitive testing 1 year and 6 months prior to the current testing, D. Brown had performed normally on the Trail Making Test A, obtaining scores of 27 seconds and 35 seconds, respectively. Similarly, on previous testing, recall of paragraph details was low-average to borderline, whereas word list learning was low-average to average, in contrast to the borderline to impaired scores observed on current testing. Of particular note, 6 months prior to current testing he had performed within the average range in immediate and delayed recall of Visual Reproduction figures (54th and 61st percentiles, respectively). Finally, scores on the Finger Tapping Test also deteriorated over the 6-month interval, with left-hand performance declining by 20% (previous exam: right = 53, 45–50th percentile, left = 57, 90–95th percentile).

Actual brain insult leads to relatively stable cognitive deficits. If a change in cognitive scores occurs over time, it should reflect improvement due either to recovery or to a practice effect. There would be no brain injury mechanism to explain a marked drop from normal performance at 7 years posttoxin exposure to borderline to impaired scores at 8 years posttoxin exposure.

Inconsistency between Test Scores and Activities of Daily Living

Test scores did not match how D. Brown actually functioned in his daily life activities. Specifically, his test scores, if taken at face value, would indicate that he had a marked memory impairment, especially for visual information. Individuals with such impairment become lost when navigating, and may forget if they have turned off the stove or locked doors. However, D. Brown was able to live alone successfully, and he spent his time going to movies and plays (which depend on intact visual memory) and reading magazines, newspapers, books, and biographies.

Subsequently, the results from cognitive testing were issued in report format to the defense attorney, who indicated that the findings matched his suspicions. The court requested evaluations by an agreed-upon medical examiner, who judged that the patients did not have any neurocognitive dysfunction secondary to exposure to workplace chemicals. The plaintiffs did not receive any compensation for the alleged neuropsychological dysfunction.

LESSONS LEARNED

These cases helped me to learn that evidence of noncredible cognitive performance is detected from numerous parameters, not just whether a patient fails one or two effort tests. In the case of the father, he failed six of six formal indices and showed illogical inconsistencies in test scores across test sessions, and between test scores/behavior and how he actually functioned in daily life activities (e.g., couldn't read MMPI for me, but read newspaper articles describing chemical exposure in his workplace). The medical records also exposed inconsistency in symptom report, with Mr. A. Brown claiming symptoms that he had denied prior to the initiation of the lawsuit, as well as evidence that he had been suspected of fabricating hearing impairment. Similarly, the son failed three of five effort indicators, and also showed nonsensical discrepancies between test scores across testing evaluations and between test scores and how he actually functioned in daily life activities.

These two cases also demonstrated to me that individuals, even first-degree relatives from the same environment who are feigning cognitive deficits from the same alleged etiology, approach symptom fabrication somewhat differently. The father was fairly indiscriminate, feigning symptoms on virtually every task administered, whereas the son was more selective and, in fact, passed most recognition memory tasks, including a forced-choice paradigm. D. Brown demonstrated the need for administration of several effort indicators; if only the Warrington Recognition Memory Test—Words, standard administration of the Rey 15-item Memory Test (i.e., without recognition trial), and/or Rey Word Recognition Test had been used, his symptom fabrication would not have been detected. Finally, Case 1 reassured me that our effort measures are likely to be robust in detecting suspect effort even in elderly individuals with low educational level.

The question arises as to whether these patients had any true cognitive or psychological disturbance. Given the father's history of cardio-vascular disease and white matter hyperintensities, he was at risk for mild cognitive decline (Boone et al., 1992), separate from any toxic exposure. Similarly, the son had reportedly had special education placement, suggesting at least some developmental cognitive weaknesses. A work evaluation from the first year he began employment with the company stated that "he must improve on his ability to carry out his work assignments." In addition, 10 years previously, D. Brown had undergone neuropsychological evaluation in the context of a psychiatric hospitalization, and he was found to have deficits in memory and word retrieval at that time. However, the fact that both patients were faking on testing indicated that they themselves did not believe they had any significant cognitive deficits; if they truly believed in their cognitive complaints, there would have been little motive to feign impairments (e.g., if a person is convinced that he or she has a broken leg, he or she does not need to fake pain and mobility problems during the orthopedic exam).

MMPI-2 data were not available, so it is unknown to what extent these patients were depressed, although this condition would not account for the very poor effort they exerted on measures to rule out symptom feigning. Research has shown that depression does not lead to elevated false positive rates on effort tests (Lee et al., 2000). In addition, in the case of the father it might be questioned whether false positive identifications are increased in advanced age, but again this contingency does not appear to be the case; although modest correlations are found between some effort tests and age, older patients do not actually fall below cutoffs to detect noncredible performance (Boone, Salazar, et al., 2002; Boone, Lu, & Herzberg, 2002a, 2002b). The father also reported that he only attended school until the 10th grade and did not like to read, although he denied a history of learning disability; the son had required at least some special education placement. However, even if they did have learning disabilities, such disabilities do not cause patients to fall below cutoffs on such effort tests as the Rey 15-item Memory Test, Dot Counting Test, or b Test (Boone, Salazar, et al., 2002; Boone, Lu, & Herzberg, 2002a, 2002b).

The neuropsychologist's mandate is to objectively measure and document cognitive function across multiple domains. However, if a patient is not applying adequate effort, this goal is no longer achievable, and the mission then shifts to carefully and thoroughly documenting evidence of noncredible performance.

REFERENCES

Boone, K. B., Lu, P., & Herzberg, D. (2002a). *The Dot Counting Test.* Los Angeles: Western Psychological Services.

Boone, K. B., Lu, P., & Herzberg, D. (2002b). *The b Test.* Los Angeles: Western Psychological Services

Boone, K. B., Miller, B. L., Lesser, I. M., Mehringer, C. M., Hill-Gutierrez, E., Goldberg, M. A., & Berman, N. G. (1992). Neuropsychological correlates of white-matter lesions in healthy elderly subjects. *Archives of Neurology, 49*, 549–554.

Boone, K. B., Salazar, X., Lu, P., Warner-Chacon, K., & Razani, J. (2002). The Rey 15–Item Recognition Trial: A technique to enhance sensitivity of the Rey 15–Item Memorization Test. *Journal of Clinical and Experimental Neuropsychology, 24*, 561–573.

Greiffenstein, M. F., Baker, R., & Gola, T. (1994). Validation of malingered amnesia measures with a large clinical sample. *Psychological Assessment, 6*, 218–224.

Lee, A., Boone, K. B., Lesser, I., Wohl, M., Wilkins, S., & Parks, C. (2000). Performance of older depressed patients on two cognitive malingering tests: False positive rates for the Rey 15–Item Memorization and Dot Counting Tests. *The Clinical Neuropsychologist, 14*, 303–308.

Lezak, M. D. (1983). *Neuropsychological assessment* (2nd ed.). New York: Oxford University Press.

Millis, S. (1992). The Recognition Memory Test in the detection of malingered and exaggerated memory deficits. *The Clinical Neuropsychologist, 6*, 406–414.

9

An Unexpected Excursion

Sexual Consent Capacity in a Nursing Home Patient with Alzheimer's Disease

DANIEL C. MARSON
JUSTIN S. HUTHWAITE

I (D.C.M.) received a legal education and practiced and taught law for 4 years before returning to graduate school and becoming a clinical psychologist with specializations in geropsychology and neuropsychology. My legal education and training have informed my activities as a neuropsychologist in a variety of ways, including my approach to psychological report writing, my grantsmanship (grant writing has a number of similarities to writing a legal brief), my choice of research interests (i.e., competency and medical–legal issues in neurocognitive disorders), and ultimately my day-to-day mindset as I practice neuropsychology. Not surprisingly, I have always been attracted to forensic neuropsychological practice because it represents a natural convergence of my dual professional training. There are definite advantages to understanding the epistemology and to "speaking the language" when working with attorneys. My forensic expert activities have ranged from standard personal injury cases to mass tort litigation to capital murder defenses. However, my primary area of forensic activity and interest has involved issues of civil competency: conducting contemporaneous or retrospective evaluations of financial capacity, medical decision-making capacity, and testamentary capacity (Dymek, Atchison, Harrell, & Marson, 2001; Marson, Huthwaite, & Hebert, 2004; Marson et al., 2000; Marson, Chatterjee, Ingram, & Harrell, 1996; Marson, Ingram, Cody, & Harrell, 1995). These cases, which have generally involved older adults as the protagonists, require a variety of professional skills, including a conceptual understanding of competency assessment issues, knowledge of the legal elements of different civil capacities, and the ability to integrate clinical, psychosocial, functional, and legal information (often over a defined retrospective time period) to arrive at a clinical judgment of capacity (Marson & Briggs, 2001; Marson et al., 2004).

THE REFERRAL AND RETENTION

I received the call at 6:25 P.M. on October 24, 2001, while working late in the office on a grant application. The caller identified himself as "Mr. Thomas Counsel," an attorney in Des Moines, Iowa, with whom I had no prior experience. Mr. Counsel indicated that he had received my name from "Ms. Brenda Eager," a young and skilled lawyer with whom I had worked on two other competency cases in the past.

Mr. Counsel stated that he was representing the family of "Ms. Stella Patient," a 76-year-old woman with dementia who was recently deceased. Mr. Counsel informed me that Ms. Patient's family had brought a civil lawsuit against "Sweet River Nursing Home" (SRNH), where she had been cared for between 1999 and 2001. Mr. Counsel explained that one evening in November 2000, Ms. Patient had left SRNH without permission in the company of an adult man. After Ms. Patient was discovered that evening to be missing, nursing home staff called the police and an investigation was started. It was determined by nursing home staff that the man involved was "Mr. Byron Lucky," the son of another SRNH nursing home resident, whom he had been visiting that day. Later that same evening, Ms. Patient and her male companion returned to the nursing home. Ms. Patient was immediately taken to a local hospital and emergency room, and Mr. Lucky was detained by the police. Medical workup that evening was positive for recent sexual intercourse, and subsequent DNA testing confirmed that Mr. Lucky was her sexual partner.

Mr. Counsel stated that the following day, SRNH contacted their consulting neuropsychologist and requested an evaluation to determine Ms. Patient's sexual consent capacity. The neuropsychologist reportedly saw Ms. Patient that same day and determined that she had sexual consent capacity at the time of the excursion from the nursing home the previous night. Mr. Counsel indicated that he and the plaintiffs had concerns about the accuracy and the basis of the SRNH neuropsychologist's judgment regarding capacity. He inquired if I would be willing to serve as a consultant and potentially as an expert witness in the case with regard to the specific issue of Ms. Patient's sexual consent capacity.

I was intrigued by the case because I had never been involved in a forensic matter involving an issue of sexual consent capacity in an individual with dementia, no less a now-deceased one! However, despite my initial interest, I outlined the protocol steps that would be necessary before I would become involved. I explained to Mr. Counsel that I would need to apply for and obtain approval to participate from my academic institution. I indicated that I would need to receive a letter of retention that would outline the capacity in which he wished me to serve on this case. I also discussed my professional fee and indicated that I would need a specified advance retainer before becoming involved in the case.

Mr. Counsel requested that I seek institutional approval and stated that he would prepare a letter of retention. He also requested that I send him a copy of my CV. Mr. Counsel indicated that upon receiving notice of my institution's approval as well as receipt of my CV, he would provide me with pertinent medical and legal records as well as my retainer fee.

After the phone call was concluded, I made a brief note of our conversation and then e-mailed a copy of my CV to the address he had provided me. I also completed an institutional form requesting permission to participate in external activities. Two days later I received by overnight mail a letter of retention from Mr. Counsel. I attached a copy of this letter to the institutional form and submitted it to my department chair. Several days later I was informed that institutional approval had been obtained, and I e-mailed this information to Mr. Counsel. Three days later I received a large box of records and an accompanying letter and retainer check from Mr. Counsel and his law firm.

THE RECORDS

The records received were voluminous and appeared to represent the complete (or nearly complete) records of the case. The file included records kept by SRNH, emergency room records from "Westside Hospital" in Des Moines, police records, a brief videotape of Ms. Patient completed by her family the day after her nocturnal excursion, various depositions by those involved in Ms. Patient's treatment or care as well as other plaintiff experts, and two neuropsychological reports. One of these neuropsychological reports contained the evaluation conducted by "Dr. Jacques Psychologist," the consulting neuropsychologist who worked on a contract basis with SRNH. The other neuropsychological report was prepared by "Dr. Alan Veteran" about a month after the incident. Mr. Veteran was a practicing clinical psychologist in Des Moines who had been retained by Mr. Counsel and the plaintiffs to evaluate Ms. Patient.

Nursing Home Records

Ms. Patient was admitted to SRNH on March 13, 1999. Initial evaluation by the nursing home psychiatrist, "Dr. Tim Psychiatrist," about a week after Ms. Patient moved into SRNH, indicated that she was a 74-year-old Caucasian female with 12 years of education and an occupational history of working as a secretary. In his examination, Dr. Psychiatrist noted that Ms. Patient was not oriented to day, month, or year. Dr. Psychiatrist indicated a diagnosis of probable Alzheimer's disease, of moderate severity, and stated that Ms. Patient could not function without supervision, was unable to care for herself, and required immediate 24-hour supervision.

According to family report, Ms. Patient had been experiencing gradual but progressive cognitive decline over the past 7 years. Her daughter reported that she had significant difficulties performing instrumental activities of daily living (IADLs), including driving, cooking, housekeeping, managing her personal finances, and managing her personal medications. Specifically, Ms. Patient had reportedly often forgotten to take her medications, had overdrawn her bank account on several occasions, had forgotten to turn off the stove on more than six occasions, had left numerous dirty dishes piled up in the sink, and was reported by neighbors to be driving erratically. Ms. Patient was also reported as being unable to provide a cohesive history.

Other family and agency reports corroborated this history. Ms. Patient was admitted to SRNH after demonstrating cognitive decline and diminished ability to live independently over a 7-year period. Her family noted that she was wearing the same clothes over the course of a few days, had a poorly kept apartment, was driving recklessly, consistently left the oven and stove top on, had difficulty managing her personal finances, had lost over 20 pounds unintentionally, and was forgetful about taking her medications. She was also noted to drink alcohol excessively, if not supervised.

Immediately prior to coming to SRNH, Ms. Patient had been placed in another nursing home in the Des Moines area, but returned to live with family for a brief period after wandering away from this nursing home and refusing to return to it. During the brief time with family members, Ms. Patient was noted to require significant help with activities of daily living (ADLs) and to have impaired decision-making ability and near total unawareness of safety issues. She was also noted to become agitated at times with family members. After 3 days, her family was no longer able to cope with her caregiving needs and successfully obtained placement at SRNH.

During her 2-year stay at SRNH, Ms. Patient's cognitive level fluctuated, with Mini-Mental State Examination (MMSE) scores ranging between 17 and 22 during the first year. Difficulties were regularly documented in her orientation to time, and her short-term memory was reportedly very poor. She did not experience any significant change in her medical status during her initial 2 years at SRNH. Physically, she was independent with ambulation but was aimless in her activity, tending to wander the halls continually during the day. Ms. Patient required supervision with her ADLs. Given her prior history of elopement, she, like other residents, wore a "wander-guard" ankle bracelet that was designed to trigger an alarm if she left the premises without proper authorization. As with all residents of SRNH, Ms. Patient was permitted to leave the nursing home premises only after staff were appropriately alerted and only when staff and family had given their approval.

During her time at SRNH, Ms. Patient was reported by staff as having "good days and bad days." She was pleasant and friendly, likely to engage in conversation with anyone with whom she came into contact. Because family and SRNH staff had noted that Ms. Patient frequently experienced sundowning (i.e., confusion in the late afternoons or evenings), family members' visits were conducted earlier in the day. Nursing notes from SRNH's records 5 months prior to the incident in question indicated that the patient had no recollection of the prior day's events. Family members noted that Ms. Patient varied day to day in her ability to recognize family members or recall their names.

Facts of the Case

With regard to the incident in question, SRNH records and staff reports indicated that on the evening of November 22, 2000, a man had approached Ms. Patient on the unit and struck up a conversation with her. The nurse responsible for Ms. Patient's care during the evening shift had reportedly assumed that this individual was a family member with whom the nurse was unfamiliar. About 15 minutes later, a second nurse, "Ms. Carmella Heinz," noted that Ms. Patient was continuing to talk with this male individual, whom Ms. Heinz identified as Mr. Byron Lucky, a son of another SRNH resident who frequently visited his ailing mother. Although Ms. Heinz was not the primary nurse responsible for Ms. Patient's care, she was familiar with Ms. Patient and her frequent socializing with visitors. Ms. Heinz went back to preparing medications for several of her patients.

Unbeknown to the staff, Ms. Patient's ankle bracelet had apparently been removed, and she was noted to be missing from SRNH 30 minutes later when a scheduled status check of patients was performed. The visitor log was reviewed and did not reflect any visitors who may have checked Ms. Patient out of the facility. An emergency meeting was held with all of the nursing staff, and it was confirmed that Ms. Patient was last seen with Mr. Lucky, although no one had witnessed them physically leaving the facility. Upon the conclusion of this brief meeting, "Mrs. Marie Head Nurse," the head nurse, immediately called Ms. Patient's daughter to inquire about any known visitors who may have taken Ms. Patient off the nursing home premises. The daughter stated that she was not aware of anyone, and after a quick check with family members, confirmed that no one had been to visit Ms. Patient over the past 4 hours. Ms. Head Nurse informed the daughter about the known facts of the situation and stated that she would be notifying the police immediately after hanging up the phone.

Mrs. Head Nurse immediately notified the police upon the conclusion of her conversation with Mrs. Patient's daughter. After obtaining the identity of Mr. Lucky, two officers were sent to Mr. Lucky's home, while other officers met with staff at SRNH. Police were informed by Mr. Lucky's wife that he was supposed to be attending a Shriners club meeting that evening. Later that evening (about 2 hours after the disappearance), Mr. Lucky and Ms. Patient returned to SRNH and to Ms. Patient's floor. Ms. Patient presented at this time in no apparent distress. Mr. Lucky was detained by police for questioning, while Ms. Patient was taken to Westside Hospital Emergency Room for investigation of possible sexual and/or physical assault. At SRNH, Mr. Lucky admitted to taking Ms. Patient out of the nursing home but denied any sexual activity, claiming that they had simply driven and talked.

Emergency Room Medical Records

Medical records indicated that Ms. Patient presented to Westside Hospital Emergency Room at 10:30 P.M. on November 22, 2000, for evaluation of possible sexual assault and rape. On presentation, she was reported by "Dr. E.R. Physician" to be confused, agitated, and vigorously objecting to a physical evaluation by the attending physician. Ms. Patient was noted to be unable to sign her name or to provide consent for treatment. Dr. E.R. Physician judged Ms. Patient to be "extremely demented" on presentation. Ms. Patient was reportedly unable to provide any coherent history of the events of the evening and explicitly denied any recollection of sexual activity or possible rape. Emergency medical evaluation revealed fresh abrasions in the vaginal region and clear evidence of recent sexual intercourse, including the presence of semen and motile sperm. Subsequent DNA testing linked the collected semen to Mr. Lucky.

Family Videotape

On the morning of November 23, 2000, the day following the events, Ms. Patient's son and daughter conducted a private videotaped interview with their mother in her private room at SRNH. This videotape included a brief assessment of the patient's cognitive functioning. The videotape demonstrated the patient to be oriented to person only, unsure of her son's identity and relationship to her (i.e., she identified her son as a cousin) and unable to recall an identified word after 5 minutes, despite several reminders throughout the brief evaluation. She did successfully identify her daughter. Ms. Patient denied having any recollection of the events that had transpired the previous evening, and laughed in a confused manner when asked if she had recently had sex. She denied ever having gone with a visitor outside of the nursing home and denied ever engaging in any sexual activities, although she reported having a "boyfriend."

Neuropsychological Evaluation 1: Defense Expert

Dr. Jacques Psychologist, a neuropsychologist previously contracted by SRNH to provide mental health consultation and treatment services to its residents, was contacted by the SRNH administrator in the afternoon of November 23, 2000, the day after the events. Dr. Psychologist was asked to conduct a mental status evaluation and specifically to evaluate Ms. Patient's capacity to consent to sexual relations. Dr. Psychologist met with Ms. Patient that same day. He reviewed Ms. Patient's nursing home records and conducted approximately an hour-long interview, which included mental status testing and an MMSE (Folstein, Folstein, & McHugh, 1975). Ms. Patient's score on the MMSE was 20/30 and notable for impaired orientation to year, season, city, county, and to her current residence in a nursing home. Ms. Patient was unable to report her correct age and had no free recall (0/3) for three items presented verbally to her after 3 minutes. Ms. Patient was also unable to perform some tests of working memory, including spelling a word backward and performing serial 7's. Ms. Patient had difficulty understanding this task and actually began counting forward by 7's. She had difficulty with most questions of reasoning/judgment on examination. Dr. Psychologist noted her thought processes to be mildly confused and her emotional state to be slightly irritable.

Dr. Psychologist also asked Ms. Patient about the sexual encounter of the previous evening. According to Dr. Psychologist's evaluation notes, psychological report, and deposition testimony, Ms. Patient spontaneously reported that she had met Mr. Lucky recently and wanted to have sex with him. Dr. Psychologist noted that she stated that she did not have any fear or regrets about her sexual involvement with him, and that her decision was voluntary and uncoerced. According to Dr. Psychologist, she also demonstrated an acceptable understanding of the risks of leaving the nursing home and of engaging in casual sex. Ms. Patient reportedly had no recollection as to how her wander-guard ankle bracelet had been removed.

Dr. Psychologist's Deposition

In his deposition, Dr. Psychologist was questioned regarding his finding that Ms. Patient had mild Alzheimer's disease. He indicated that, based on his review of SRNH medical records, Ms. Patient's cognitive functioning had improved after being placed on Aricept. He tended to disregard the multiple staff notations concerning Ms. Patient's substantially impaired memory, orientation, and judgment. Dr. Psychologist reported his belief that Ms. Patient had mild Alzheimer's disease but was nonetheless still able to consent to sexual intercourse. Deposition testimony reflected that he based his impression predominantly on her MMSE score and on her comments during his interview with her.

Neuropsychological Evaluation 2: Plaintiff's Expert

At the request of plaintiff's counsel, Dr. Alan Veteran conducted a comprehensive neuropsychological evaluation in December 2000, about a month following Dr. Psychologist's evaluation. During the interview, Dr. Veteran noted that Ms. Patient was unable to understand the purpose of the evaluation, even when it was carefully explained to her. Dr. Veteran also observed that Ms. Patient was unable to recall information seconds after it was presented and could not remember his name, despite his telling it to her numerous times throughout the evaluation. Ms. Patient reportedly misreported the year by 12 years, was not oriented to the month or the day of the month, and could not tell time on a watch. She reported that she lived with her daughter instead of in a nursing home. Ms. Patient also misreported the number of children she had and the name of her late husband. When she asked where her husband was, she commented, "I guess he's dead."

With respect to the incident at issue, Dr. Veteran indicated that Ms. Patient had no knowledge or recollection of the events whatsoever, including leaving the nursing home, getting into Mr. Lucky's vehicle, where they went, or the sexual relations that ensued.

As part of the evaluation, Dr. Veteran administered the Wechsler Memory Scale–III (WMS-III; Wechsler, 1997b) and the Wechsler Adult Intelligence Scale–III (WAIS-III; Wechsler, 1997a). On the WMS-III, Ms. Patient was unable to report her correct age, the current president of the United States or the one who proceeded him, the current year (she said 1974), the month, the day of the month, her location, or the city. Ms. Patient reportedly had 0% recall for Logical Memory I (immediate recall) and Logical Memory II (delayed story recall), and was unable to recall a single word pair across all four trials on the Verbal Paired Associates subtest. She had very poor recognition memory and a negative response bias on Faces I (3 of 48 faces). Testing on the WAIS-III resulted in a Verbal IQ of 70 (2nd percentile), which reflected a probable mild to moderate decline from a clinical estimate of premorbid verbal intellectual functioning.

In his report, Dr. Veteran concluded that at the time of the incident, Ms. Patient had severe dementia and lacked the competency to consent to anything, including treatment and sex. Dr. Veteran also noted that Ms. Patient's judgment was severely impaired and that she had little insight into her capacity. He further noted that as a result of her dementia, Ms. Patient would be unable to comprehend or remember what was happening to her and would likely respond to the requests or cues of anyone in her immediate setting. Dr. Veteran felt that Ms. Patient would be unable to assert her will in refusing to have sexual relations or even remember that she had engaged in sexual relations immediately afterwards.

VIEW OF THE CASE AND FORMULATION OF OPINIONS

Having reviewed the records in the case, I began to formulate my opinions regarding Ms. Patient's cognitive functioning, diagnostic status, dementia stage, and capacity to have sexual relations on November 22, 2000. I then planned to relay my view of the case and opinions to Mr. Counsel. It would then be his decision, and that of his clients, as to whether they wished to use me as an expert witness in the litigation.

Cognitive Functioning

There was incontrovertible evidence in the record supporting substantial cognitive impairment and dementia in Ms. Patient. Findings from Dr. Veteran's evaluation and from family, physician, and SRNH report reflected profound short-term memory impairment as well as impairments of working memory and abstraction and loss of verbal intellectual functioning. I was impressed by the reported 7-year history of progressive cognitive decline. Functional changes consistent with dementia included impaired capacity for a number of IADLs and ADLs, including management of her personal finances, management of her medications, cooking, housekeeping, driving, and basic self-care skills (e.g., her unintentional weight loss). The range of MMSE scores (17–22) was highly consistent with dementia.

Dementia Etiology

The record also provided strong support for a primary progressive dementia of the Alzheimer's disease (AD) type. Ms. Patient's 7-year history of cognitive decline was reportedly gradual and progressive, with no stepwise changes suggestive of a vascular or other neurological contribution. In his admission note for SRNH, Dr. Psychiatrist indicated a diagnosis of AD, and this diagnosis appeared to be well-established both before her admission to SRNH and also during her care there. Identification of dementia etiology and dementia stage (see below) are useful because they provide a conceptual and empirical framework for making retrospective capacity judgments.

Dementia Stage

Several sources of evidence suggested that Ms. Patient had entered into the moderate stage of AD at the time of the incident in question. The profound nature of her short-term memory loss (with recall duration of only seconds), her MMSE scores between 17 and 22, and the reported duration of cognitive decline (7 years) were suggestive of the early-moderate stage. Behavioral changes consistent with moderate AD included Ms. Patient's aimless wandering of the halls, her ongoing elopement risk, and her increasing inability to recognize close family members such as her son. Such recognition failures are not characteristic of patients with mild AD, but are seen in those in the moderate and severe stages of the illness.

Based on the information in the record, I completed a Clinical Dementia Rating (CDR; Morris, 1993) form for Ms. Patient. The CDR is designed to assist in staging patients with AD and related dementias. Ms. Patient's CDR was a 2.0 and her sum of boxes score was a 15. These findings supported an assignment of moderate stage AD-type dementia for Ms. Patient.

Capacity to Consent to Sexual Relations

My next task was to form an opinion concerning Ms. Patient's capacity to consent to sexual relations—the central issue of the case and my main charge. This was the issue upon which the two other psychologists involved in the case differed so dramatically.

It is important to recognize that a diagnosis of dementia, or findings of cognitive impairment, are themselves insufficient to support a judgment of incapacity to consent (Marson & Briggs, 2001). In my clinical experience I have assessed individuals with dementia who still possess the capacity to engage in important matters such as making a will or making medical treatment decisions. It is always necessary to evaluate the functional abilities constituent to the capacity in question, in conjunction with secondary diagnostic, cognitive, and other evidence, before arriving at a capacity judgment.

The general conceptual framework for assessing decisional capacity involves an examination of four different consent abilities (Appelbaum & Grisso, 1988; Grisso & Appelbaum, 1995; Marson et al., 1995; Roth, Meisel, & Lidz, 1977). These abilities and their underlying definitions are:

- The capacity to "evidence" a choice. This standard focuses on the presence or absence of a decision, not on the quality of the decision (Roth et al., 1977).
- The capacity to "appreciate" emotionally and cognitively the personal consequences of a choice. This standard emphasizes the patient's awareness of the consequences of a decision: its emotional impact, rational requirements, and present and future risks and consequences (Roth et al., 1977).
- The capacity to reason about a choice, or make a choice based on "rational" reasons. This standard tests the capacity to use logical processes to compare the benefits and risks of various decision options and weigh this information to reach a decision (Appelbaum & Grisso, 1988).
- The capacity to make a choice based on an "understanding" of the situation and alternatives. This standard requires memory for words, phrases, ideas, and sequences of information (Appelbaum & Grisso, 1988).

The next step was to apply this conceptual assessment framework to the context of consent to sexual relations in a nursing home setting. This translation resulted in the following requirements for a valid consent to sexual relations: Ms. Patient would need (1) to make an actual volitional decision to have sex or not; (2) appreciate the personal consequences of making such a decision (e.g., leave the nursing home without permission; accompany a man she did not know; undergo the risks of sexually transmitted disease with such a partner); (3) be capable of reasoning in a comparative way about the risks and benefits of having sex with an unknown gentleman; and (4) sufficiently understand the situation regarding a sexual relationship outside of the nursing home setting and different alternatives available to her.

After reviewing the record, it was my professional judgment that Ms. Patient probably lacked all four of the above abilities related to sexual consent capacity. First, it appeared highly questionable that a volitional act to have sex could have occurred. Given her profound short-term memory impairment, confusion, and general disorientation, Ms. Patient probably did not understand why she was leaving the nursing home with her new male companion (even if they had previously discussed having sex), and simply followed his cues throughout the course of the evening. Second, it is highly improbable that Ms. Patient appreciated the personal risks and consequences of her behavior that evening. Nursing home staff had already noted Ms. Patient's lack of safety awareness, and her departure with a male companion known to her for only a short time reflects a marked lack of insight and very poor judgment. Third, given her documented impairments in reasoning and her inability to retain any factual information, it is very unlikely that Ms. Patient would have been capable of engaging in any kind of reasoning process concerning the merits of sexual activity with Mr. Lucky. Finally, it was clear that Ms. Patient fundamentally lacked an understanding of her situation (including that she was a resident in a nursing home), risks of her proposed behavior, and alternative choices and courses of action with respect to romantic activity.

For all these reasons, it appeared clear to me that Ms. Patient lacked sexual consent capacity on the evening in question. Corroborating support in the record for this capacity judgment included the emergency room's recognition of Ms. Patient's inability to consent to treatment, and the findings of Dr. Veteran regarding the patient's decisional incapacity in December 2000.

Reconciliation of Dr. Psychologist's Capacity Findings

In formulating opinions in the case, a final issue concerned the evaluation and findings of Dr. Psychologist. As discussed above, Dr. Psychologist had evaluated Ms. Patient the day after the event and found that Ms. Patient possessed sexual consent capacity. In my judgment, Dr. Psychologist's opinion in the case lacked credibility for several reasons. First, Dr. Psychologist was the consulting neuropsychologist to SRNH, and also to a number of other nursing homes in Iowa that were owned by SRNH's parent company. A substantial portion of Dr. Psychologist's practice income appeared to derive from his consulting activities for SRNH and its "sister" nursing homes. Thus, Dr. Psychologist's objectivity and credibility in the case appeared potentially compromised by this professional relationship to SRNH.

Second, and more important, Dr. Psychologist's capacity findings and judgment in the case were strikingly inconsistent with the record evidence of her memory impairment. Specifically, the record made clear that Ms. Patient's short-term memory was profoundly impaired, with recall latencies of only seconds before new information was lost. This finding is consistent with Dr. E.R. Physician's observation that Ms. Patient had no recollection of the events earlier in the evening, and with Ms. Patient's inability to recall any information about these events when questioned directly by family members the following morning in her room at SRNH.

In contrast, Dr. Psychologist's report and deposition testimony suggested that a factually full and refreshingly frank discussion occurred between him and Ms. Patient on the topic of her sexual activity the previous day. Per Dr. Psychologist, Ms. Patient spontaneously reported that she had met Mr. Lucky recently and wanted to have sex with him ("I wanted to do it"), that she indicated "no fear or regrets" about her actions, that her decision was voluntary and uncoerced, and that she also demonstrated an understanding of the risks of leaving the nursing home and engaging in casual sex.

What does one make of this? The woman described by Dr. Psychologist is not the same woman who appears in the rest of the record. Assuming that this patient material reported by Dr. Psychologist was not simply manufactured, my professional judgment was that Ms. Patient's "discussion" of her sexual activities simply represented confabulations that were cued by leading questions from Dr. Psychologist. If Dr. Psychologist presented all of the relevant material in the form of leading questions, Ms. Patient could work with, and respond to, the questions within the confines of her working memory. Thus, in my judgment, the different statements and quotes attributed to Ms. Patient appeared to simply reflect her parroting back to Dr. Psychologist material that he himself had composed and presented in emotionally inviting leading questions to her. This explanation was the only way I could reconcile Dr. Psychologist's findings with that of the record as a whole.

COMMUNICATION OF OPINIONS TO PLAINTIFF'S COUNSEL

I set up a telephone conference call with Mr. Counsel in order to discuss the opinions in the case. After presenting my opinions, he asked a number of questions regarding my dementia staging and capacity opinions. He then asked whether I would be willing to testify to these opinions at deposition or trial as an expert witness in the case. I indicated that I would be willing to do so, but expressed a preference for limiting my travel if possible. He indicated that he would shortly be disclosing me to defense counsel as another expert witness that would be called at trial.

THE DEPOSITION

About 3 months later I received a notice for a deposition duces tecum (bring with you) by "John Defense-Attorney, Esq.," the attorney for SRNH. Mr. Defense Attorney and Mr. Counsel traveled out of state to Birmingham to conduct the deposition at my office. The deposition, which continued for 7 hours, began as most depositions do. Mr. Defense Attorney reviewed my professional credentials, including my legal background. He also reviewed my clinical and administrative responsibilities (i.e., roles as clinical neuropsychologist, director of neuropsychology within the Department of Neurology, associate director of the Alzheimer's Disease Research Center [ADRC], supervisor to postdoctoral fellows), my research focus on competency and capacity issues, and my prior experience as a forensic consultant and expert witness.

Mr. Defense-Attorney also reviewed the documents I had produced in response to the discovery requested within his notice of deposition. These included my CV; articles, treatises, and other evidentiary sources on which I had based my opinions; correspondence with counsel; fee statements and invoices for professional services; prior deposition and courtroom testimony; and medical and legal records reviewed in the present case. In addition to the document request, Mr. Defense-Attorney questioned me specifically about the professional fees I had earned thus far in the case and inquired about specific conversations that I had had with plaintiff's counsel in preparation for the deposition. Finally, he questioned me about my prior work and experience as an attorney.

Mr. Defense-Attorney eventually turned to my professional opinions in Ms. Patient's case. As discussed further below, he focused almost exclusively on my cognitive, diagnostic, and dementia staging opinions. He was particularly interested (and I believe concerned) about my conclusion that Ms. Patient was suffering from moderate (not mild) stage AD at the time of the events of November 22, 2004. As part of this discussion, I discussed the videotape of Ms. Patient made by her family the day following the events. I noted her substantial memory loss as well as her failure to recognize her own son who was carrying out the family interview, and indicated that these evidentiary findings were highly consistent with moderate AD as opposed to mild AD. I was challenged by defense counsel about the possibility that Ms. Patient might not have wanted to discuss her activities of the prior evening with her son while being video-taped. I testified that it was my impression that Ms. Patient's responses and behaviors on the videotape were not indicative of privacy concerns or of personal evasiveness, but rather reflected her profound amnesia and previously reported prosopagnosia: She was capable neither of recall-ing these very recent events nor of consistently recognizing her own son.

In addition to my discussion of the videotape, I reviewed the psycho-logical test findings of Dr. Psychologist and Dr. Veteran. I indicated that Dr. Veteran had performed more comprehensive testing with Ms. Patient than did Dr. Psychologist. I noted that Dr. Veteran interviewed Ms. Patient and assessed her cognitive functioning with the use of the WAIS-III and the WMS-III. I noted that Dr. Veteran's impressions of profound memory loss and advanced dementia were far more consistent with those of Dr. E.R. Physician and the record as whole than were those of Dr. Psy-chologist. I also pointed out that Dr. Psychologist's testing was primarily limited to the MMSE and that this brief measure is, at best, a crude esti-mate of cognitive functioning in comparison to more comprehensive neuropsychological testing. Discussion also centered on the MMSE score of 21/30 obtained by Dr. Psychologist and how that score corresponded to a dementia stage of moderate.

Toward the end of the deposition, Mr. Defense Counsel for the first time raised the issue of Ms. Patient's capacity status by obliquely asking "Would you agree with me that memory is not a good indicator of lack of capacity?" The line of reasoning pursued by counsel was based on litera-ture suggesting that executive functions, in general, were more potent predictors of decisional capacity status than short-term memory—with the unstated implication being that Ms. Patient's profound memory loss was therefore somewhat irrelevant to her sexual consent capacity status. I carefully refrained from accepting Mr. Defense Counsel's premise and argument in this regard. I noted that short-term memory function and the ability to encode new information were vitally related to decisional capacity in several respects. In particular, the consent ability of compre-hension/understanding is completely dependent on acquisition and retention of factual information relevant to the decisional context. In the case of Ms. Patient, I stated that I believed that her short-term memory loss was probably the preeminent cognitive factor related to her incapac-ity, because the extent of her memory loss made it impossible for Ms.

Patient to even create a factual context within which to reason through, form, and make decisions.

No further questions regarding competency generally, or Ms. Patient's capacity status specifically, were raised by defense counsel. Reportedly due to the lateness of the hour (9 P.M.—the deposition had started at 2 P.M.), the deposition was adjourned, to be rescheduled and continued at a later date. However, the deposition was never re-noticed and thus I was never asked to testify regarding my capacity opinions. In retrospect, the defense counsel's decision to avoid specific capacity issues and opinions at the deposition appeared to be a tactic designed to avoid the ultimate issue and enhance his client's bargaining position in subsequent mediation negotiations.

OUTCOMES OF THE CASE

As noted above, Ms. Patient passed away prior to the conclusion of the civil legal proceedings and prior to my involvement as a consultant and expert.

The family's legal action against SRNH and its parent company was settled out of court approximately a month after my deposition.

With respect to Mr. Lucky, the State of Iowa brought criminal charges against him for kidnapping, sexual assault, and rape. Mr. Lucky now conceded that he and Ms. Patient had left the unit and had sex, but he asserted that their relations were completely consensual. Mr. Lucky was subsequently tried and convicted on these criminal charges. He is currently serving a 10-year sentence in the Iowa state prison system.

CLOSING THOUGHTS

This was a memorable case in almost all respects. The dramatic events on November 22, 2000, involving abduction and illicit sexual activity, with resulting civil and criminal legal actions and outcomes, made this a competency case of first instance. The family's proactive step in immediately videotaping Ms. Patient, followed the very same day by the nursing home's neuropsychological consultation on consent capacity, provided a contemporaneous, rich, and also highly conflictual evidentiary context for analysis of the decisional capacity issues. This conflictual context was further amplified by the subsequent test results and conclusions of Dr.

Veteran, which formed an interesting and opposing counterpoint to those of Dr. Psychologist.

However, putting the drama and conflict to one side, the case demonstrated the importance of the forensic expert bringing a sound conceptual model of decisional capacity to the case at hand. Although I had not previously encountered a matter of sexual consent capacity in dementia, my familiarity with the general model for decisional capacity allowed me to apply it successfully to the unique circumstances of this case. The model allowed me, with some confidence, to formulate and analyze relevant issues of sexual consent capacity in the context of advanced AD, and in turn, to understand how the cognitive deficits in advanced AD would and did impact Ms. Patient's different consent abilities in November 2000.

ACKNOWLEDGMENTS

Preparation of this chapter was supported in part by an Alzheimer's Disease Research Center (1P50 AG16582-01; Lindy E. Harrell, Principal Investigator), and the Alzheimer's Disease Cooperative Study (U01 AGO10483; Leon J. Thal, Principal Investigator).

REFERENCES

Appelbaum, P., & Grisso, T. (1988). Assessing patients' capacities to consent to treatment. *New England Journal of Medicine, 319*, 1635–1638.

Dymek, M., Atchison, P., Harrell, L., & Marson, D. (2001). Competency to consent to treatment in cognitively impaired patients with Parkinson's disease. *Neurology, 56*, 17–24.

Folstein, M., Folstein, S., & McHugh, P. (1975). Mini-Mental State: A practical guide for grading the cognitive state of the patient for the physician. *Journal of Psychiatry Research, 12*, 189–198.

Grisso, T., & Appelbaum, P. (1995). The MacArthur Treatment Competence Study: III. Abilities of patients to consent to psychiatric and medical treatments. *Law and Human Behavior, 19*, 149–169.

Marson, D. C., & Briggs, S. (2001). Assessing competency in Alzheimer's disease: Treatment consent capacity and financial capacity. In S. Gauthier & J. L. Cummings (Eds.), *Alzheimer's disease and related disorders annual 2001* (pp. 165–192). London: Dunitz.

Marson, D. C., Chatterjee, A., Ingram, K. K., & Harrell, L. E. (1996). Toward a neurologic model of competency: Cognitive predictors of capacity to consent in Alzheimer's disease using three different legal standards. *Neurology*, *46*, 666–672.

Marson, D. C., Huthwaite, J., & Hebert, K. (2004). Testamentary capacity and undue influence in the elderly: A jurisprudent therapy perspective. *Law and Psychology Review*, *28*, 71–96.

Marson, D. C., Ingram, K. K., Cody, H. A., & Harrell, L. E. (1995). Assessing the competency of patients with Alzheimer's disease under different legal standards. *Archives of Neurology*, *52*, 949–954.

Marson, D. C., Sawrie, S., Snyder, S., McInturff, B., Stalvey, T., Boothe, A., Aldridge, T., Chatterjee, A., & Harrell, L. (2000). Assessing financial capacity in patients with Alzheimer's disease: A conceptual model and prototype instrument. *Archives of Neurology*, *57*, 877–884.

Morris, J. (1993). The Clinical Dementia Rating (CDR): Current version and scoring rules. *Neurology*, *43*, 2412–2414.

Roth, L., Meisel, A., & Lidz, C. (1977). Tests of competency to consent to treatment. *American Journal of Psychiatry*, *134*, 279–284.

Wechsler, D. (1997a). *Wechsler Adult Intelligence Scale–Third Edition*. San Antonio, TX: Psychological Corporation.

Wechsler, D. (1997b). *Wechsler Memory Scale–Third Edition*. San Antonio, TX: Psychological Corporation.

II

CIVIL CASES
Pediatric

10

On the Far Edge of the Last Frontier

The Alaska Experience

PAUL L. CRAIG

A lark! That's what it was—a lark!—a 9-month lark in Alaska that somehow evolved into 24 years of practice on the Last Frontier with many more years to come. In 1980, I was completing an internship in health psychology at the University of Minnesota Health Sciences Center. Dr. Manfred Meier, fondly known as "Mannie," was my primary supervisor in clinical neuropsychology. Although I was intellectually enamored of the burgeoning field of human neuropsychology, I was equally attracted to the field of rural community mental health. I had come of age in rural Nebraska and had attended the doctoral program in clinical–community psychology at the University of Wyoming—a program that emphasized rural community mental health. Somewhat ironically, it was during this rural mental health training in Wyoming that a graduate school classmate, Dean Delis, first introduced me to clinical neuropsychology following a summer practicum he had completed with some of the giants in the field at the Boston Veterans Administration Hospital. Neuropsychology fit perfectly with my undergraduate roots in biopsychology. Following the internship in Minnesota, working in a practice setting sounded interesting, but I wanted to remain closely affiliated with academia and

167

research. An advertisement in the *APA Monitor* caught my eye. The opportunity described therein integrated everything I was ambivalent about into one postdoctoral training opportunity.

In 1980 the University of Washington Department of Psychiatry and Behavioral Sciences was funded to send one postdoctoral fellow to the Gateway Community Mental Health Center in Ketchikan, Alaska, for 9 months. The remaining 3 months of the fellowship were to be spent in Seattle at the medical school campus. The fellowship was characterized as involving exposure and training at a rural community mental health center working with Alaska Natives, fishermen, loggers, and the occasional cruise line passenger needing some crisis intervention while the ship was at the dock in Ketchikan. The icing on the cake was the fact that the fellowship would also involve research and training in clinical neuropsychology! It was as if the fellowship were structured with all of my various interests in mind.

I applied and was accepted for the fellowship. Upon completing the program, I decided to accept a job offer to serve as the psychologist and program director of the South Peninsula Community Mental Health Center in Homer, Alaska—a small community on the Alaska Kenai Peninsula surrounded by unsurpassed natural beauty. After 3 years of serving a broad spectrum of rural mental health clients located in the Homer area, I decided to return to academia in order to complete a more traditional postdoctoral fellowship in clinical neuropsychology at the University of Oklahoma Health Sciences Center, under the supervision of such notables as Oscar Parsons, Bruce Crosson, Russell Adams, and others. During this postdoctoral fellowship, I was introduced to forensic consultation. While collaborating with Dr. Adams on some forensic cases, I learned the importance of intellectual integrity, scientific objectivity, and ethical comportment when navigating in the forensic environment—an environment rife with adversarial relationships and a press toward advocacy. Upon conclusion of the fellowship, I felt a strong urge to return to the Last Frontier. Alaska had found its way into my heart and was not about to let go. I returned to Alaska, set up an independent neuropsychology practice in Anchorage, including hospital and outpatient services, and have considered Alaska my home ever since that fateful "lark" that took me to Ketchikan—for 9 months!

Soon after my return to Alaska from the fellowship at the University of Oklahoma Health Sciences Center, I began receiving requests for forensic evaluations of patients with known or suspected brain disorders. These activities included evaluating individuals for whom a petition for guardianship had been filed with the court as well as evaluating accused criminals awaiting trial. I frequently found myself serving as a fact witness relative to traumatic brain injury patients whom I had evaluated at one of the inpatient rehabilitation programs in Anchorage. Likewise, legal counsel, representing either plaintiff or defense, occasionally retained me to evaluate individuals alleging brain injury following an accident. Parenthetically, in Alaska the causes of a traumatic brain injury can be somewhat unique (e.g., "The patient received a blow to the occiput when a 600-pound pot was swinging from the winch above the deck, while fishing for king crab during a storm with 14-foot waves in the Gulf of Alaska during January"). Other than the fact that I was frequently asked to evaluate culturally and linguistically unique individuals (e.g., Alaska Natives of various heritages, including Inupiat, Yup'ik, Siberian Yup'ik, Athabascan, Aleut, Tlingit, Haida, and others), most of these forensic evaluations were conducted in my office under similar circumstances and constraints as would be expected for any other clinical neuropsychologist providing forensic services in the Lower 48 states. However, some requests for my services could be classified as unique.

CASE BACKGROUND

On a dark and stormy afternoon during October 1999, an attorney from Aniak, Alaska, called my office. Gazing out my office window around 3:00 P.M., all I could see was snow whipping around a street light in the blustering wind. The stormy weather apparently was creating a lot of static, which was interfering with our satellite-mediated telephone connection (satellites are used for transmission of telephone calls to and from the Alaska bush). In Alaska any sparsely populated community or village that is accessible only by boat or plane—read, about 99% of the state—is referred to locally as the *bush*. Aniak is a bush village located on the Kuskokwim River. Theoretically, a person could travel to Aniak in a boat during the summer. But for practical purposes, a flight on a bush plane is the only way to travel to or from Aniak as well as most other bush villages. This attorney had previously retained me as an expert in a few other cases. He is an example of a very bright and well-trained professional who has deliberately chosen the path less traveled by others among the baby boom generation—life in the Alaska bush. Mushing dog teams had captured his spirit many years earlier. A few years ago, I visited this attorney at his log home in Aniak. About 20 malamutes were howling beside or on top of their respective doghouses strewn around his yard—although suburbanites in the Lower 48 would hardly call it a "yard."

Anyone unfamiliar with the Alaska bush may find it difficult to understand the lure of having 20 dogs howling in the yard while living amid some of the harshest circumstances known to humans. In the recently published book *The Cruelest Miles,* Salisbury and Salisbury (2003) tell the gripping story of the heroic mushers who relayed a lifesaving serum to Nome in 1925. The lead dog, Balto, guided the final sled team into Nome to deliver the medicine in time to save the children of the community from the "strangler," better known as diphtheria. Balto became a national hero, and his statue can be found in New York City's Central Park. *The Cruelest Miles* captures the historical role of sled dogs in the bush. Dogs are to the bush what camels are to the desert—well-adapted animals that were essential for human survival in an inhospitable environment prior to the introduction of modern technology. Reading this book will give even the most calloused urbanite a glimpse into the allure of the Alaska bush.

The attorney served as counsel for six teenagers from two tiny villages, Sleetmute and Nightmute, located on the coastline of the Bering Sea close to Kotzebue. These youth were of Inupiat heritage, although all were fluent in English. The six students had been selected to participate in a 2-day training program in "peer conflict mediation" in Kotzebue. During March 1998 these teenagers and a chaperone were returning from a school function in Kotzebue. At about 4:30 on a Friday afternoon an air taxi service was scheduled to fly these six students from Kotzebue back to Sleetmute in a single-engine Cessna 207 airplane. The two students living in Nightmute were planning to travel the last 5 miles on snowmachines (i.e., snowmobiles) to reach their village. The weather was fierce—a strong southerly wind was whipping up the snow on the ground creating poor visibility. Worse yet, any pilot familiar with the region would know that those southerly winds suggested that the landing strip at Sleetmute would be cursed with a crosswind, making a landing difficult, at best.

No flights had landed at Sleetmute that day. The weather forecast suggested more of the same for several days, with a high probability of deteriorating conditions. The pilot on duty for the air taxi service that day was relatively young and fairly new to Alaska. As is common among novice commercial pilots, he had accepted a job in the bush in order to log as many flight hours as possible in the hope of expanding his career options. Although Alaskans frequently joke with one another that an "*old* bush pilot" is an oxymoron, we feel safest flying with a bush pilot who has many years of experience. These pilots have proven their ability to stay alive. One trait of older bush pilots is that they know not only how to land a plane, they also know when *not* to fly.

Dr. John Middaugh (1986) of the Alaska Office of Epidemiology, Division of Public Health, published *The Epidemiology of Involuntary Injuries Associated with General Aviation in Alaska, 1963–1981*. In 1983 there were 10,250 pilots in Alaska. In other words, one person among every 45 Alaskans was a pilot—by far, the highest percentage anywhere in the United States. In *Coming into the Country*, John McPhee (1977) deftly captured the role that small aircraft and bush pilots play in the daily life of Alaskans. Unfortunately, aircraft accidents have played an even bigger role in the lives of all too many Alaskans.

Between 1963 and 1981 an average of 72 pilots died each year as a result of aviation accidents in Alaska; the fatality rate was 799 per 100,000 pilots per year. During the same period, there were an average of 117 traffic fatalities per year among drivers in Alaska; the fatality rate was 39 per 100,000 licensed drivers per year. Thus, the rate of fatalities among general aviation pilots was 21 times greater than the fatality rate for drivers on the roads of Alaska (Middaugh, 1986, p. 3). Based upon analyses of all aviation accidents in Alaska between 1963 and 1981, Middaugh described the profile of a high-risk flight as follows:

> A male pilot, age 25–39 years, who has fewer than 100 hours of flight time in type, flying a PA-18 float-equipped aircraft, on a hunting trip in September or October who overloads the aircraft and crashes on takeoff or during initial climb after failing to attain adequate flying speed. (p. 16)

I am a fisherman, not a hunter. Nevertheless, when I think about how many float plane flights I have taken during my 24 years in Alaska that generally fit this profile, I shudder and count my blessings. Although aviation accidents reportedly peaked in the late 1970s, a follow-up study conducted by Middaugh and colleagues (1991, p. 17) indicated that no fewer than 584 individuals died as a result of aviation accidents in Alaska between 1980 and 1989. These data help others understand why Alaskans frequently quip, "A good landing is one you can walk away from!"

Thankfully, the teenagers from Sleetmute and Nightmute did not become more entries in the database of aviation fatalities in Alaska. However, the flight from Kotzebue to Sleetmute was ill-fated. Despite the conditions, the novice bush pilot decided he could land at Sleetmute. One of the female students from Sleetmute had a longstanding fear of flying and was reluctant to board the Cessna 207 in Kotzebue. The chaperone was in a somewhat untenable situation. The air taxi pilot was willing to fly and all of the other students and the chaperone were eager to go home. The prospect of the weather becoming worse overnight and remaining inclement for the next several days raised the possibility that the entire group could be marooned in Kotzebue for several days before another flight could be attempted. Leaving a female high school student to fend for herself in Kotzebue was not an option. Hence, the chaperone ignored this student's preferences and required her to board the plane, despite her anxiety about doing so.

Takeoff was uneventful. The flight was bumpy due to turbulence, but the plane was able to reach the airspace over Sleetmute without incident. However, the instant the wheels touched the runway at Sleetmute, a strong gust of crosswind caught the wing of the Cessna 207 and instantly flipped it. The plane skidded upside down until it came to a halt on the snow-packed runway. Although it was almost a "good landing," one of the students did not walk away. She reported leg numbness immediately after the accident and needed to be carried to a van that was waiting to pick up the students. She was able to ambulate fairly soon thereafter.

Shortly before I was called, the attorney from Aniak had negotiated a financial settlement, on behalf of all six students, with the insurance company that had issued the liability policy to the air taxi business based in Kotzebue. This attorney has represented many plaintiffs from the bush. He is known throughout the bush for being sensitive to the Alaska Native culture and is respected by defense counsel insofar as he typically makes reasonable claims on behalf of plaintiffs.

In this case, the attorney wanted to retain me as an expert in neuropsychology and clinical psychology to screen all six students. He wanted to ensure that the settlement he had negotiated was sufficient in relation to any damages they had sustained. He did not tell me the amount of the negotiated settlement, nor did I ask. He told me that through his contact with all six students and their families, he had concluded that each student had been shaken up physically and psychologically but that none of them was seriously scarred in either the physical or psychological domain. He was not concerned about any as yet unnoticed orthopedic or soft-tissue injuries among the six students, because each student had been carefully evaluated from a medical perspective. The attorney simply wanted my expert opinion regarding whether any of the students had suffered from a mild traumatic brain injury and/or persisting psychological sequelae that had been overlooked. In his typically ethical style, he indicated that he was not asking me to find problems to promote his litigation agenda. Rather, he simply wanted to know whether any legitimate psychological or neuropsychological problems had occurred. If so, were the problems persistent and functionally significant in the lives of one or more of these youth? In the event that I identified persistent and significant problems, he requested that treatment recommendations and prognoses be forwarded as part of my expert opinion.

The attorney requested that I travel to Sleetmute to complete screening evaluations with each of the six teenagers from the two villages. I agreed to be retained as a psychological and neuropsychological expert for this purpose. My office manager faxed a copy of my retainer agreement to him disclosing my fees and policies. The attorney remitted payment for the retainer and arrangements were made for me to travel to the far north of Alaska. Early one morning during late November 1999, I flew from Anchorage to Kotzebue on an Alaska Airlines jet that was configured to carry containerized cargo in the front of the fuselage and a few passengers in the rear. While the front of the aircraft was being loaded with cargo, I descended some stairs from the airport departure lounge to the ice-covered tarmac and then ascended a mobile staircase leading to the rear door of the jet.

At 66°53′ north latitude, Kotzebue is precisely 20 miles north of the Arctic Circle. For several days around winter solstice, the sun doesn't even peek over the horizon. Locals call this interval of time "The Tunnel." Otherwise, during the long winter months, late in the morning—long after the spellbinding curtains of dancing colored light known as the *aurora borealis* have enjoyed their grand finale overhead in the wee hours of the morning—a dusky tinge of light begins to bathe the environment. The stars eventually fade from sight as pastel pink and azure hues emerge in the sky. On most winter days, the air is too frigid to contain any moisture and the sky is sparkling clear. Eventually, the sun briefly rises along the southern horizon and dips down again shortly after noon. Rather than being called "Land of the Midnight Sun," Alaska might just as aptly be named "Land of the Noon Moon!"

I boarded the Boeing 737 jet in Anchorage at 6:00 A.M. and landed in Kotzebue almost 3 hours later in the total darkness of the arctic morning. The next flight to Sleetmute was scheduled to depart at noon. I had 3 hours to burn. An Alaska Native woman behind the Alaska Airlines counter summoned a taxi for me on a CB radio. I headed for the Arctic Beach Café to savor some coffee and local culture. Anybody who wants to enjoy a well-written description of life in bush Alaska should read *Going to Extremes* (McGinnis, 1980), a travelogue that captures life as it was a quarter century ago in the harsh but enticing land called Alaska. McGinnis writes about his experiences and the characters he encounters in Nome, Homer, and many points between. On this particular morning at the Arctic Beach Café, I found a perch at a table near a window overlooking the moonlit frozen Bering Sea. Against the far wall of the café was an enormous salt-water aquarium containing live coral and several tropical fish. To this day, I wonder how that tank and those fish ever found their way to Kotzebue. Purely by coincidence, the book I was reading at that time was *The Wisdom of Insecurity* (Watts, 1951)—a fitting title for the adventure ahead. After placing my order for scrambled eggs and reindeer sausage, I pulled out Watts's book and began reading. The large round table between the aquarium and me began filling up with five or six locals who obviously met there most mornings before sunrise (read, before noon). Clearly, I was at risk of being classified as an interloper at the Arctic Beach Café. Therefore, I attempted to remain inconspicuous behind my book while surreptitiously savoring the conversation that unfolded within the coffee klatch—"Engine wouldn't start . . . " "Did you hear about Imogene and Matt?"

Again, a CB was used to summon the taxi and I returned to the airport terminal—a small metal building next to the airstrip—to await my flight. I sat down in a well-used overstuffed chair that appeared to be a remnant of the 1950s. A young Eskimo man, neatly dressed in his Army National Guard uniform, was standing next to his green duffle bag. Elvis's voice singing "Blue Moon" was wafting from a CD player behind the counter. The small metal building was full of stale, smoky air. Through a hole in the frost on a window, I could see the twin-engine plane in which I would be flying as it was being loaded with cargo destined for Sleetmute. While boarding, I casually asked the female pilot about the content of the boxes. She replied, "Soda pop." The left half of the plane was stacked with boxes filled with cans of carbonated sugar water and the right side was lined with about six passengers, most of whom were Inupiats returning to Sleetmute.

As is typical in Alaska Native culture, few words were exchanged onboard. Paradoxically, it was apparent to me that everybody was being very friendly and cordial, albeit quietly. In Nebraska where I was reared, people jabber with each other until they are comfortable, then they can be silent together. In Alaska Native culture, people are quiet until they are comfortable, then they can talk. In Alaska nomenclature, a new arrival to Alaska is called a *cheechako*. When a *cheechako* meets an Alaska Native from the bush, it is not uncommon for each to leave the interaction believing that the other was unfriendly, rude, and socially inappropriate. The *cheechako* tries to be polite by using a firm handshake and an incessant flow of words while trying to fill those uncomfortable gaps of silence. The Alaska Native politely remains quiet, diverts his or her gaze, and is silently aghast at the apparent rudeness of the *cheechako*. If you are aware of these cultural differences, rapport can be enjoyed. Although I usually experience some feelings of insecurity due to my cultural heritage, I find that if I remain fairly quiet when encountering an Alaska Native, usually he or she will initiate a conversation—sometimes in a very witty way. As an example, I was once flying to Seattle and was seated next to an Inupiat gentleman from Barrow. After reading the morning newspaper, I placed it on the empty seat between us. He eventually turned to me and asked if I would mind if he read the sports section. In an attempt to establish rapport, I inquired, "Sure. I take it you like sports?" Without missing a beat, he replied in a deadpan manner, "No." I asked, "Why do you want to read the sports section then?" Again, without cracking a smile, he replied, "It's the only part of the paper that tells the truth." I laughed and his eyes twinkled, expressing appreciation that I understood his subtle humor. When *cheechakos* do not chuckle in response to such wit, I suspect that Alaska Natives silently feel sorry for our humorless souls.

As might be expected, I was particularly interested in the Sleetmute runway. The pale midday light dimly illuminated the treeless snow-covered tundra. As you move from the equator toward the poles, the altitude of the timberline descends accordingly. By the time you reach Sleetmute, the timberline has descended below sea level! The visual environment was so unfamiliar that it felt as if the plane were landing on a different planet. The snow-packed runway was as white as the surrounding hills but was otherwise unremarkable. The landing was smooth. There were virtually no signs of civilization in the vicinity other than our plane and a passenger van awaiting our arrival. I briefly tried to assist the pilot and driver with transferring the boxes of soda from the plane to the back of the van. A few inches of skin were exposed on my face, and I felt the burning sensation of frostbite penetrating my flesh. My urge to be helpful was quickly supplanted by a desire to get out of the elements. I jumped into a passenger seat inside the van and the Inupiats, already in the van, knowingly smiled at me, raising their eyebrows in a manner that nonverbally communicates understanding within their culture. My eyebrows were also raised—but for a different reason!

As we drove a couple of miles along the snow-packed road into Sleetmute, a few English words were exchanged, and it quickly became apparent to me that everybody in the van knew who I was and why I was there. Confidentiality is not a familiar concept in a remote bush village. When trying to explain the need for a signed release of information to an Alaska Native living in the bush, the villager usually appears perplexed and probably wonders why the professional is concerned about such matters, given that everybody in the village already seems to know everything about him or her.

I was driven to one of two general stores servicing this village of 200 residents. The proprietor was a Caucasian man who had moved to the bush and married an Inupiat woman. Their son was one of the teenagers involved in the crash. The attorney from Aniak had made arrangements for the proprietor to coordinate my schedule and arrangements in Sleetmute. I was planning to spend at least one night in the village, so he drove me in his pickup to the only business with rooms for rent. I was given my choice of any one of 10 identical small rooms located along a long narrow hall in a former work camp building. There was one bathroom in this building. Thankfully, it had running water and a flush toilet rather than a "honey bucket" (an "in-house," as it were, comprised of a five-gallon bucket containing some liquid toilet chemicals; the bucket is usually covered by a toilet seat that is supported by a makeshift chair or wooden frame). The only furniture in each room was a single bed made of metal struts and a flat web of interconnected springs supporting a thin cotton mattress. When traveling to the bush during the winter, it is wise to pack a sleeping bag. Thankfully, I had done so. I was the only resident in the building for the night. The gentleman who drove me in his pickup to the bunkhouse stated that he would not go inside with me when I registered for my room. Apparently, he and the owner of this bunkhouse had gotten into a fistfight several years ago and had assiduously avoided seeing each other ever since. I had a difficult time fathoming how two grown men could *not* see each other in a remote bush village of 200 people. But apparently they had been successful in doing so.

There are no restaurants in Sleetmute. I purchased a few food items from the proprietor's store to make sure I would have something to eat back at the bunkhouse. Then I was taken to the village health clinic where an office had been vacated for my use. While driving toward the clinic, the gentleman who was coordinating my schedule advised me that one of the Inupiat teens from Nightmute had given birth 3 days earlier and that I would need to travel to her village to see her. While I was there, I would also be able to meet with the other student from Nightmute. He pointed to the end of the street toward the frozen Bering Sea while commenting that I could use one of his snowmachines to get there. All I could see beyond the end of the street was a vague trail in the snow leading onto the frozen sea. The afternoon sky was quickly growing dark. Swirls of snow whipped into the air by the arctic winds obscured the vista. The wind chill factor was so low that any exposed skin would begin freezing immediately. I looked at the driver and said, "I have only driven a snowmachine once several years ago. I cannot travel to Nightmute alone." He looked slightly surprised at my reluctance, as if he had just been told that I was afraid to cross a city street by myself, but politely replied, "We'll figure something out."

At the clinic I spent an hour interviewing each of the teenagers from Sleetmute. At my request, the village health aide at the clinic contacted the proprietor at the store on the CB radio. When he arrived to pick me up, I was relieved to learn that an Inupiat man from Nightmute would be making the journey with me. The village was now so dark that it appeared as if an octopus had squirted ink in the sky. As we approached the store, two snowmachines were warming up on the pitch-black street. I followed the proprietor inside his store and began donning arctic gear, including an insulated helmet, bunny boots (massive white rubber boots that use a layer of air trapped within the boots to provide remarkably effective insulation), and multiple layers of protective clothing. While suiting up for the ride across the frozen ocean, I was introduced to the Inupiat man from Nightmute with whom I would be traveling. He had a pleasant glint in his eye and appeared to be about 40 years old. He appeared healthy and still had all ten digits on his hands. In short, he appeared to know how to survive in the Arctic, and I felt very comfortable traveling with him. However, he made a couple of brief comments that led me to believe that he felt deferential to me as "Doctor Craig." I quickly reframed his assumptions by letting him know that he was the captain of this mission and that I was relying entirely upon him and his knowledge of the Arctic to make sure I survived as we crossed the frozen Bering Sea. He raised his eyebrows and smiled. It appeared that he appreciated my humility and felt confident about being my guide. When I was finished dressing, my head was completely covered with the helmet, face shield, goggles, and various layers of wool and down insulation. I was able to breathe, but was unable to talk audibly through all the layers covering my face and head. My hearing was completely muffled as well. Not one square millimeter of skin was exposed to the ambient air. The huge mittens I was wearing allowed for gross hand gestures but no finger signals. Due to the multiple layers of insulated clothing around my torso, my arms protruded at a 45-degree angle away from my torso. Other than the fact that my suit was not pressurized, I felt prepared for a stroll on the moon.

The proprietor waved me toward the door and the three of us emerged into the frigid darkness where the snowmachines were purring away. He gestured for me to throw a leg across the seat to prepare to drive the snowmachine to Nightmute. As soon as I nervously straddled the seat, the engine died. I could see that the owner was surprised and perplexed. He began tugging at the starter rope, to no avail. I glanced toward the dark heavens above and silently thought, "There is a God!" Without missing a beat, the proprietor and the Inupiat gentleman knowingly signaled one another and walked between the store and the adjacent building to retrieve a wooden sled that would normally be used for dog mushing. They found a rope and tied the front of the sled to the back of the Inupiat gentleman's snowmachine. Next, I saw them retrieving a large orange plastic tarp. With deft movements that reminded me of two housekeepers placing a sheet on a hotel bed, they worked together to line the sled with the tarp. The proprietor grabbed the shoulder bag in which I was carrying a few neuropsychological screening instruments and placed it in the front of the sled. Then the two men signaled me to lie down on the tarp. While contemplating the wisdom of my insecurity, I succumbed to the social cues and trusted that these two men knew what they were doing. Soon I found myself supine in the dog sled and wrapped from head to toe inside the tarp. I heard the snowmachine engine rev, felt the sled bouncing toward the frozen sea ahead, and smelled the odor of two-cycle engine exhaust fumes wafting through the air. The headlight of the snowmachine created a diffuse orange glow through the tarp. About halfway through the journey across the frozen Bering Sea, my anxiety waned and I found myself giggling while thinking a variety of thoughts such as: "I wonder if this is what it is like to be abducted by aliens like those people from the cover of *The National Enquirer*?" and "I feel like a human burrito all rolled up in this tarp!" and "Bering Sea . . . Polar bears . . . maybe I'm not at the top of the food chain, after all!" and, finally, "I wonder how many other neuropsychologists are going to work today in a dog sled pulled behind a snowmachine across a frozen arctic sea?"

Upon arrival in Nightmute, the Inupiat gentleman unwrapped me from the tarp that had become a large orange tortilla in my now vivid imagination. He led me into the largest of the handful of tiny buildings in this village, population 50. Once I was inside what appeared to be the main building for the community, I noticed a group of about five teenage lads socializing on the far side of the room. I began doffing the several layers of clothing and protective gear so that they could see my countenance. The snowmachine driver walked over and spoke with them briefly. As he departed the building, he made eye contact with me but uttered nothing. I quietly sat in a chair on my side of the room. I did not want to be yet another obnoxious *cheechako* forcing myself upon the lads in the room. After a couple of minutes, one of them strolled over toward me. Before beginning his retreat toward his friends, he quietly and monotonically stated, "My aunt is coming." I replied in a friendly tone, "Thank you." We were all getting comfortable.

After a few more minutes, the matriarch of Nightmute arrived and was very accommodating. She gave me an office to use and told me that the young woman who had recently given birth would be seen first. Next I would see a 14-year-old lad who was the youngest person involved in the accident.

Obviously, when evaluating personal injury plaintiffs, a neuropsychologist must remain vigilant for purposes of detecting objective and subjective data indicative of symptom magnification and motivational deficits, as well as frank malingering. The naiveté of the 14-year-old Inupiat lad was refreshing in this context. When I asked him about his feelings regarding being involved in the accident, a spark of excitement spread across his face, he leaned forward in his chair, and he said with complete sincerity, "That was fun! I want to do it again!" as if he were describing a roller coaster ride! I stifled the laughter that I felt surging from my belly and continued asking him questions about blows to his head, retrograde or anterograde amnesia, symptoms of anxiety or depression following the accident, changes in his school performance, etc. He was very forthcoming, and it was readily apparent that he was neuropsychologically and psychologically intact. Although he was physically shaken during the "good landing," he was doing fine. Certainly, all Alaska plaintiffs are not always so transparent with their feelings, but it was very refreshing to have the opportunity to interview somebody who was so completely honest. Obviously, the attorney in Aniak had not coached him. Also, he was not motivated by, or perhaps even aware of, the possibility of enhancing the size of the green poultice that he would be receiving consequent to his involvement in the aviation accident.

After I completed the interviews in Nightmute, the matriarch of the village used the radio to contact the proprietor in Sleetmute. He drove a snowmachine to pick me up and arrived in Nightmute sooner than I thought possible. What I had not yet learned about him was that his avocation was snowmachine racing. He waited outside to avoid becoming overheated in his garb while I finished suiting up for the ride. Once again, we could not exchange words. He signaled for me to sit behind him on the snowmachine and then tugged on my arms indicating that I should hug his back as tightly as possible. I soon found out why. We screamed back across the frozen Bering Sea traveling well over 70 mph. Each time we hit a mogul on the trail we flew into the air. At such moments, butterfly wings seemed to flutter against the lining of my stomach until the snowmachine finished its arc through the air and once again settled firmly on the frozen sea. I glanced over the driver's shoulder as we raced forward through the arctic darkness and gazed longingly at the twinkling lights of Sleetmute a few miles ahead. Upon arrival at his store, I thought, "Cheated death again."

The next day I flew back to Kotzebue with the air taxi service. The pilot asked me to sit in the co-pilot's seat. In order to get there I wiggled my way past three middle-aged Inupiat women who were already seated and then belly-crawled over some cargo and finally wrenched myself into the seat. I asked the pilot whether he needed me to sit in the front of the plane for purposes of balancing the weight, fore and aft. He replied, "Nope. I just wanted to be able to chat. You must be a psychologist or a social worker or something." I complimented him on his ability to read people and quietly chuckled about his reason for asking me to be a contortionist through the fuselage in order to reach the front seat! An Inupiat woman seated behind the pilot explained to him why I had been in Sleetmute—even though I had never seen her before. Once again, the cloak of confidentiality had been instantly stripped away by others. The pilot used the opportunity to launch into his story about that fateful day in March 1998. He told me that he had 25 years of arctic flying experience and had advised the novice pilot not to attempt to fly to Sleetmute on the day of the accident. As suggested previously, one reason he was alive after 25 years of being a bush pilot was that he knew when *not* to fly. Unfortunately, the errant pilot had not yet learned that important lesson.

CROSS-CULTURAL EVALUATIONS
WITH ALASKA NATIVES

When evaluating Alaska Natives in a neuropsychological context, several unique issues arise. First, the norms for this population are sparse. Beginning in 1960, the Alaska Area Native Health Service, in collaboration with the Epidemiology Program of the Arctic Health Research Center, launched a prospective population study (Bender, Williams, & Hall, 1984) involving all 696 pregnancies occurring within the study period (October 1, 1960, through January 2, 1961) among the Alaska Native women residing in the Yukon–Kuskokwim Delta region of Alaska. In addition to biomedical data, intellectual functioning was sequentially assessed using the Stanford–Binet Intelligence Scales, Form L–M followed by the Wechsler Intelligence Scale for Children later in childhood. In 1976 the Wechsler Adult Intelligence Scale, Draw-A-Person Test, and the Bender–Gestalt Test were administered to the surviving youth from this cohort. Some summary statistics regarding these psychometric data were presented at a circumpolar health meeting in 1984 (Doak & Nachmann, 1984). Otherwise, these normative data remain sequestered, apparently out of respect for the confidentiality of the participants who reportedly have grown weary of being research subjects over their lifespan. Other than these data and the clinical data collected from patients referred for neuropsychological evaluations due to known or suspected brain disorders, norms for this population simply do not exist. Knowing that the recent versions of the Wechsler scales have included a representative sample of the U.S. population does not translate into meaningful norms when evaluating an Alaska Native from the bush who speaks English as a second language. A neuropsychological evaluation report regarding an Alaska Native must contain a caveat disclosing this issue with regard to interpreting the diagnostic validity and functional significance of the findings.

During a clinical interview with an Alaska Native, I always begin by apologizing for being rude. I explain that I am aware that it is impolite for me to barge ahead asking so many personal questions so quickly after meeting him or her. I then explain that doing my job properly and professionally requires me to ask these questions, and I request his or her forbearance in this context. By acknowledging the mores and norms of the Alaska Native culture, rapport is improved and I am almost always allowed to proceed with my standard set of questions regarding health and psychosocial history.

FINDINGS AND OPINION

None of the teenagers involved in the aviation accident reported significant blows to the head or amnesia during or around the time of the accident. All of them recalled the accident very well. Nobody endorsed
postconcussive symptoms following the accident. The girl who was
already fearful about flying before the accident was still somewhat psychologically distressed. However, she had already begun flying again—an
activity that is as necessary in the Alaska bush as riding in a car is for a
suburbanite—and was tolerating the flights with less anxiety each time she
flew. Each of the students noted that his or her comfort level in airplanes
was altered consequent to the accident, but none of the students was so
anxious that he or she was unable to board a small aircraft. None of them
had sought psychotherapy or treatment with psychotropic medications
for any purpose following the accident. All of the students were moving
forward constructively with their respective lives and academic pursuits.
The fact that these students had been chosen for "peer conflict mediation" training at their respective schools suggested that they were viewed
by others as being among the most psychologically healthy teenagers in
Sleetmute and Nightmute. Perhaps, they were also the most psychologically resilient among their peers.

Insofar as there was no reason to suspect brain injury after a screening interview with each of these students, no neuropsychological tests
were administered. Symptoms of depression were denied, although vary-
ing levels of anxiety were extant among most of the students. However,
none of them met diagnostic criteria for posttraumatic stress disorder.

I indicated in my written consultation report that it would be sensi-
ble to provide each of these students with reasonable access on a prospective basis to psychological services including, but not limited to, training
in progressive relaxation, biofeedback, and cognitive-behavioral techniques to help them learn how to recognize and manage anxiety. Some
education regarding flight safety was thought to be appropriate, so that
they would have a better sense of awareness and control if another naive
pilot appeared to be making bad decisions about when, how, and where
to fly and land. Training in assertiveness skills was also recommended so
that if any of these students ever encountered a similar situation in the
future, he or she would have the necessary communication skills and
knowledge to firmly and consistently say, "No."

After submitting the written consultation report and conferring tele-
phonically with the attorney in Aniak, no further services were requested

of me regarding this accident. Prior to writing this account, I contacted the attorney to request his permission to write about the students involved in this aviation accident. I explained that the dates, village names, and associated identifying information regarding the accident would be altered to protect the privacy of the involved parties. I also inquired about the status of the case. He informed me that my consultation report had been helpful in relation to settling the case. The six students and their respective families were satisfied with the outcome. The attorney had discussed my recommendations with the plaintiffs and their families at the time of settlement. These students enjoy unencumbered access to a broad spectrum of high-quality health and mental health services provided to Alaska Natives through the Public Health Service at no expense to the individual. Hence, the attorney was certain that professional services would be available to address any current or emerging mental health issues experienced by any of these six students. The insurance carrier apparently perceived the settlement to be fair and agreed to settle shortly after my consultation report was produced rather than proceeding with discovery followed by trial.

CONCLUSION

Most forensic neuropsychological evaluations are completed in my office in Anchorage. These evaluations typically fall within the same rubric as would be the case in an office in other parts of the United States. However, the forensic consultation I've described demonstrates some of the unique circumstances in which I find myself as a neuropsychologist practicing in Alaska. As I reminisce about the adventure described above, I find myself leaning forward in my chair, smiling, and thinking, "That was fun! I want to do it again!" Therein lies the reason why a 9-month lark evolved into a career on the Last Frontier.

AUTHOR NOTE

All of the village names have been altered to maintain confidentiality. The village names used are actual village names from Alaska but are geographically remote from the villages in which the attorney and the clients resided. The dates and facts regarding the accident and consultation have also been altered for purposes of protecting the privacy and confidentiality of all parties involved.

REFERENCES

Bender T. R., Williams, C. J., & Hall, D. B. (1984). Study of a cohort of Yukon–Kuskokwim Delta Eskimo children: An overview of accomplishments and plans for the future. *Circumpolar Health,* 115–119.

Doak, B., & Nachmann, B. (1984). *The psychometric component of the infant mortality and morbidity cohort study.* Paper presented at the Sixth International Symposium on Circumpolar Health, Anchorage, AK.

McGinniss, J. (1980). *Going to extremes.* New York: Knopf.

McPhee, J. (1977). *Coming into the country.* New York: Farrar, Straus & Giroux.

Middaugh, J. P. (1986). *The epidemiology of involuntary injuries associated with general aviation in Alaska, 1963–1981.* Anchorage: Epidemiology Office, Division of Public Health, State of Alaska.

Middaugh, J. P., Miller, J., Dunaway, C. E., Jenkerson, S. A., Kelly, T., Ingle, D., et al. (1991). *Causes of death in Alaska 1950, 1980–1989: An analysis of the causes of death, years of potential life lost, and life expectancy.* Anchorage: Section of Epidemiology, Division of Public Health, State of Alaska.

Salisbury, G., & Salisbury, L. (2003). *The cruelest miles: The heroic story of dogs and men in a race against an epidemic.* New York: Norton.

Watts, A. W. (1951). *The wisdom of insecurity.* New York: Pantheon Books.

11

The Evolution of a Forensic Case
A Transition from Treating Clinician to Expert Witness

LYNN BENNETT BLACKBURN

I never set out to practice forensic neuropsychology. Forensic neuropsychology found me. I eased into the forensic arena while working as part of a pediatric neurology department. The neurologists were usually the ones to be retained to offer expert testimony. My role in each case was not significantly different from my role in clinical cases. I was asked to characterize the child's pattern of strengths and weaknesses. The neurologist would then incorporate the information into his testimony. After a few years of providing this service, my role changed. Attorneys began to contact me directly to serve as an expert witness. For the first few cases, I was able to provide this service without ever being called to do a deposition. The work provided different challenges than my clinical cases. My clinical cases focused on answering the questions of "What is it?" and "What do we do about it?" Forensic work added very different questions. I was asked to sort through all the clues in the history and assessment data to answer the questions of "How did the child get this way?" and "What will the future hold?

When I was called to give my first deposition, no one prepared me for what it would be like. No one explained that you swear to "tell the truth, the whole truth," but the reality is that you get to tell as much of the truth as the lawyer allows. No one suggested that the *Miranda* warning should be given before being deposed, to remind me that comments, when taken out of context by a lawyer, can (and would) be used against me by significantly altering my testimony. No one told me what to do when an attorney enthusiastically stated "I object!" but then told me to answer the question if I was able to do so. No one explained that you should ask the attorney requesting the deposition to bring a check along so that you are paid immediately.

As I learned the process, I found legal work to be fascinating. Not only did I get to use all of my neuropsychological knowledge, but I also got to practice my psychotherapy skills. Each lawyer conducting a deposition became a client in my mind. My job was to understand their construction of reality, while helping them to accept a more accurate construction—mine. There was the constant mental challenge of attempting to figure out what the attorney was trying to get me to say, so that I could make a conscious decision about whether or not I wanted to say it. Much like teaching graduate students, I found that legal work forced me to stay current in my field, reading research in a critical fashion so that I knew which findings I could trust and defend, if necessary, in deposition or court. After about 10 years of involvement as a consultant and occasionally being deposed, I became involved with the patient that would serve to give me my first courtroom experience.

BACKGROUND INFORMATION

The call came from "Joe," a colleague practicing in a rural area. He was the only neuropsychologist for miles. Although the majority of Joe's training focused on adults, he found himself drawing on his pediatric training rotations to meet the needs of his community. "I'm faced with a puzzling case," he said. "I've got this little boy who was referred to me for possible ADHD [attention-deficit/hyperactivity disorder]. I know that he has all the symptoms, but there has to be something else going on. He has had strange reactions to stimulant medication. Even when medication is working, he is just not like the typical child." Joe concluded: "If he was older, I would think he had frontal dysfunction. Can that be seen in a 6-year-old?" I agreed to help, starting by reviewing Joe's reports and reports of assessments conducted by the child's school. He obtained all the appropriate releases from the parents. Thus my involvement with Richie had begun, with no warning of the forensic component to come.

According to the reports I received, Richie presented with a history of normal development up to about 2 years of age. A skull film was obtained at 20 months of age due to concerns regarding his slow growth in head size. The films at that time were read as normal. By 4 years of age, Richie's small head size, increasing behavioral problems, and head-aches caused his parents to return to the pediatrician. They were greeted with reassurance and offered the option of obtaining skull films if they wished.

Skull films revealed craniosynostosis, a syndrome involving prema-ture closure of the skull's sutures, areas that allow the skull to expand in response to brain growth. For some children, the premature closure involves only a single set of sutures. As the brain grows, the skull expands where it can, resulting in a misshapen head. For some children the synostosis involves all sutures, preventing significant skull growth. As the brain continues to grow within the small skull, increased intracranial pressure may result. When this occurs, surgical intervention is necessary to prevent brain damage and allow for normal brain development. For other children, normal brain development continues within the confines of the small skull.

In addition to the closed sutures, Richie's skull films revealed evi-dence of "convolution markings" in the inner surface of the skull, result-ing in a scalloped appearance. This finding suggested that the brain was exerting sufficient pressure on the skull to alter the development of its inner surface. In spite of this finding, the treating physician made a deci-sion to monitor Richie's brain and skull growth. This decision became a key issue in the eventual malpractice case. As I was reading this history in my colleague's report, I did not know that I had taken the first step on the road to becoming an expert witness in this case.

The parents had reported to Joe that Richie had begun to display impulsive and hyperactive behavior between 2 and 4 years of age, reflect-ing a significant change when compared to his adjustment during the first 2 years of life. Richie began to complain of headaches around age 2, with a gradual increase in frequency between the ages of 2 and 4. He underwent a series of ophthalmological exams looking for evidence of papilledema as a sign of increased intracranial pressure. His parents con-tinued to receive reassurance that everything was all right. At almost 5 years of age, Richie was admitted to a hospital for intracranial pressure monitoring. The monitoring revealed spikes in pressure during sleep to a level four times normal values. Surgical release of sutures and skull remodeling were conducted shortly after this monitoring. Although the frequency of headaches improved following the release procedure, behavior remained a significant problem.

For most clinical cases, I do not request all of the child's medical records. Because Richie was a clinical case, I accepted the history outlined in past reports, feeling that I could fill in additional details when I met with the family. After all, the question was what the parents and school could do to help him, not why he had developed the problems he was experiencing. Records provided by the school indicated that Richie had been placed in a prekindergarten program at 4 years of age. The school staff described him as showing an extremely short attention span and impulsive, hyperactive, and aggressive behavior. A trial of Ritalin had been initiated prior to his first neuropsychological assessment. Although Ritalin was of some benefit, his behavior remained significantly atypical for his age. For example, the teacher described him as stepping on other children, not to be mean, but because he was focused on getting an object and did not appear to be aware that they were in his path.

Richie's first neuropsychological assessment was conducted at 5 years of age. According to his parents, he did not play with toys at home but would become focused on a single toy and carry it around the house the entire day (*carry it* but not play with it). The parents informed Joe that Richie no longer was interested in cuddling or affection. He spent most of his day on the move, impulsively pursuing whatever caught his attention. Taking 7.5 mg of Ritalin twice a day made Richie "initially subdued," but this effect was gone within 3 hours, when he would then experience a rebound effect, becoming more disruptive and difficult to control. The Child Behavior Checklist revealed concerns in the areas of aggressive behavior, social immaturity, and depression.

During testing, Richie's behavior had a driven quality, with minimal evidence of inhibition. He demonstrated a limited range of affect. Although he would occasionally emit high-pitched laughter, this did not appear to be a reflection of pleasure. Richie's intellectual ability, language skills, and visual–motor control fell in the average range (see Table 11.1). He was able to repeat sentences accurately. Although he could remember details from a story, he could not sequence them. Richie offered isolated words and phrases, as they occurred to him. All the facts were there by the time he finished, but the story was lost.

An attempt was made to quantify attention and inhibition through administration of the Gordon Diagnostic System. Overall, performance

TABLE 11.1. Scores from Evaluation at Ages 5 and 6

Scaled score		Standard score	
WISC-III (WPPSI-R)			
Information	7 (10)	Verbal IQ	81 (95)
Similarities	7 (11)	Performance IQ	104 (104)
Arithmetic	5 (9)		
Vocabulary	5 (8)	PPVT-R	110 (97)
Comprehension	9 (9)	EOWPVT	104 (91)
		VMI	88 (85)
WRAML			
Story Memory	10 (10)		

Note. Scores from evaluation at age 5 are in parentheses. WISC-III, Wechsler Intelligence Scale for Children–III; WPPSI-R, Wechsler Preschool and Primary Scale of Intelligence–Revised; PPVT-R, Peabody Picture Vocabulary Test–Revised; EOWPVT, Expressive One-Word Picture Vocabulary Test; VMI, Developmental Test of Visual Motor Integration; WRAML, Wide Range Assessment of Memory and Learning.

fell in the borderline range only because Richie was provided with frequent reminders of the "rules." Richie talked constantly, although his comments were unrelated to the task. Joe made sure that Richie stayed in the room but could not keep him in a chair. At times, Richie became so frustrated with the task that he struck the equipment with his fist.

Joe concluded that Richie's cognitive skills were a strength for him. His severe impairment of self-regulatory behavior was noted to be a limiting factor in his ability to demonstrate his learning, as well as affecting his ability to acquire play skills, both for solitary play and for peer interaction. Joe recommended placement in a highly structured educational setting, with clear behavioral routines to help Richie stay organized throughout the day. Speech therapy and occupational therapy were recommended to help him learn to organize and sequence output (e.g., coherent expressive language, motor planning for academic tasks and activities of daily living). His parents were encouraged to work with a behavioral therapist to address the behavioral concerns in the home setting.

Richie was already involved in a prekindergarten program. The school district evaluated him for therapy services, but he failed to qualify for occupational therapy; however, a significant delay in the development of his articulation skills qualified Richie for speech therapy. The therapist tried to address Richie's larger problems with language by using pragmatic language tasks as a means of working on articulation. The school also administered the Vineland Adaptive Behavior Scale. Functioning fell below the level expected based on documented intellectual ability (Communication Domain standard score = 81; Daily Living Skills Domain standard score = 77; Socialization Domain standard score = 73). His delays in adaptive behavior reflected his need for one-to-one supervision to complete any task, including play activities.

Richie's second evaluation was conducted a year later (age 6). He was still in a prekindergarten setting due to concerns that his behavior could not be effectively managed in a mainstream kindergarten setting. At the time of assessment, he was being treated with a 10 mg. Ritalin dose, administered three times per day. This treatment had resulted in a significant behavioral change—but not a change for the better. Richie's parents described him as spending his day "in a world of his own." His behavior had become rigid and inflexible; he could not tolerate changes in his routine or transitions from one activity to another. Responses to the Child Behavior Checklist identified concerns in the areas of withdrawal, obsessive–compulsive behavior, and hyperactivity.

Joe found Richie to be subdued to the point of having difficulty initiating action. He demonstrated a flat affect and very limited eye contact. Richie did not initiate conversation but would respond to direct questions, typically in the form of phrases, with only intermittent use of full sentences. His prosody had a robotic quality. At times, Richie would mimic Joe; at other times, his responses reflected clear echolalia. Richie found the testing setting to be anxiety provoking, and he responded to the anxiety by engaging in rocking behavior and becoming increasingly restless. Richie relied on the structure Joe provided to help him focus and sustain attention. He demonstrated perseverative behavior, becoming focused on a question and repeatedly asking it, even though it had been answered.

Test results from the second assessment are summarized in Table 11.1. Richie demonstrated a decline in Verbal IQ, possibly related to the change from the Preschool to Children's form of the Wechsler and/or the deterioration in expressive language skills. For the most part, Richie's scores continued to fall in the average range. However, the way that he achieved the scores was anything but average. Achievement on memory tasks continued to be affected by problems with organization and sequencing of verbal output. Joe worked hard to provide sufficient structure to help Richie compensate for his impairment of attention and self-regulatory behavior. His performance would abruptly deteriorate and anxiety increase whenever Richie was expected to develop a strategy. On the other hand, he seemed relieved when Joe's directions defined a strategy for him. Joe concluded that Richie's problems went beyond ADHD.

Behavior in the second assessment session had qualities consistent with frontal dysfunction as well as with pervasive developmental disorder. Based on the results of the evaluation, Joe encouraged the parents to get a second opinion from a neuropsychologist who specialized in pediatrics. Joe called me, and Richie was soon on his way to my office.

Changes in Richie's medication had occurred before Richie reached my door. Ritalin was discontinued due to concerns that the high dose was contributing to the emergence of autistic-like behavior. Richie was started on dexadrine but stopped after 4 days due to a worsening of problems with initiation of sleep. All medication was discontinued for 2 weeks. The autistic-like behavior resolved, but his impulsivity and hyper-activity worsened. At the time of my evaluation, he was being treated with a 5 mg dose of Ritalin, given twice a day.

THE NEUROPSYCHOLOGICAL EVALUATION

Behavioral Observations

If you saw Richie sitting in my waiting room, you might not have noticed his somewhat cupped ears and narrow head. He was by no means a funny-looking child. However, if you watched him in the playroom or lis-tened to him, you would have immediately known that something was very different about him. Richie handed me a small rock as we met in the waiting room. He explained this gift in one long disjointed sentence that went something like this: "I needed a rock and you needed a rock and I saw a store and the mall was big and the toys in the store, lots of toys, but I needed a rock and you needed a rock and I saw a rock . . . and . . . and Mom said we should go, and you needed a rock and I needed a rock and so I got a rock, my rock, and you got a rock. Here!" The story from his mother was just a little different. They had been walking around a local mall and gone into a science/learning store. Richie was happily touching everything within reach, moving within seconds from one item to the next. He then came upon a small bin of polished stones. Richie became fixated on the stones. He would not stop talking about them and manipu-lating them. Attempts to get him to leave the store prompted crying and physical resistance. The only way to get him to leave the store was to allow him to pick out a rock. Knowing that he was seeing a new doctor the next day, he insisted that he get me a rock as well. The rock remains on my bookshelf as a reminder of the power of overfocused, inflexible, perseverative behavior.

I had plenty of test scores from the previous evaluations. It was a clinical case, and I was pretty sure that I already had the answer to "What it is?" I needed to interact with Richie, to get a behavior sample, and to try some interventions in order to answer the question "What do I do about it?" I chose a test battery that would allow me to see how he handled demands for mental flexibility and strategy generation. I wanted to see how he reacted to a variety of interventions to support his ability to meet task demands. I got the data I needed for the clinical question. Unfortunately, his problems with mental flexibility and the anxiety elicited by such tasks prevented me from completing the entire battery I had planned (see Table 11.2).

Richie and I gave our rocks to his mother for safe keeping. Consistent with previous testing, Richie was restless. His body was constantly moving, but he was able to maintain his attention on the tasks. His spontaneous speech was effective in communicating his desired intent, in marked contrast to his difficulty in organizing verbal output in response

TABLE 11.2. Neuropsychological Test Battery

Kaufman Assessment Battery for Children			
Sequential tests	Scaled score	Simultaneous tests	Scaled score
Hand Movements	4	Gestalt Closure	9
Number Recall	7	Triangles[a]	9
Word Order	9	Matrices[b]	
		Spatial Memory	7
		Photo Series[c]	

Test of Language Competence

Ambiguous Sentences[c]

California Verbal Learning Test–Children's Version

	Z-score
Trial 1	4.0
Trial 5	0.0
List B	0.5
Short Delay Free Recall	−1.5
Short Delay Cued Recall	−0.5
Long Delay Free Recall	1.5
Long Delay Cued Recall	−0.5
Recognition	−4.0

[a]Administered in a nonstandardized manner.
[b]Unable to complete the task due to increasing anxiety.
[c]Administered in a nonstandardized manner; discontinued due to increasing anxiety.

to a question. Richie's anxiety was a limiting factor in testing. He would immediately respond "I don't know" to each question presented. We had a little discussion about what it meant to guess, and that I expected a response to each question, so he needed to guess. He said he understood. He continued to say "I don't know" to each question. I would remind him to guess and then watch him squirm in his chair or walk around the room. Eventually, he would guess.

Test Results

The novelty of tasks on the Kaufman Assessment Battery for Children proved very effective in eliciting Richie's problems with strategy generation, mental flexibility, and inhibition. For Hand Movements, Richie was able to copy the movement sequences, but he started with the last movement I made and then repeatedly cycled through the sequence until I told him to stop. He could do the motor planning, but not inhibition. He could maintain sequence and inhibit when presented with verbal sequential memory tasks. Richie had no difficulty with visual integration (Gestalt Closure) or with visual memory.

Richie's difficulties with Triangles, Matrices, and Photo Series summed up his problems. On Triangles, he learned to build the two triangle designs through repeated demonstration and guided practice on the practice item. When the task shifted to building with three triangles, Richie was totally at a loss. At that point, I had a choice. I could have continued testing in a standardized manner, and Richie would have immediately failed. Instead, I chose to test limits. Repetitive teaching on the first three-triangle item helped him to generate a strategy that he was able to apply to other items using three triangles. We went through the same process when a fourth triangle was added, and when the middle and top triangles were rotated 90 degrees. Richie was capable of doing the visual analysis and reproducing what he saw, but he was immobilized by his lack of a strategy. The Matrices subtest was given in a standardized fashion; Richie was unable to shift strategy from one item to the next,

On Photo Series, Richie was required to sequence a set of photographs to reflect an evolving event. I demonstrated the sample item, then asked Richie to do the item. Instead of sequencing the pictures, Richie randomly selected a picture, held it up and identified what he saw, then put it down and picked up another. However, if I reminded him that all the pictures were part of one story and asked "What comes next?" after each picture selection, he was able to effectively perform the task.

Richie made it through the California Verbal Learning Test—Children's Version with continuous reassurance that it was OK if he did not remember all the words. He did fantastic on the first trial, recalling 9 of 15 items. However, his achievement declined over subsequent trials, appearing to reflect the effects of interference (order of words on the list did not match his ordering of words on recall). He appeared to have some difficulty shifting between immediate and longer-term memory stores. He had no difficulty in the single trial of list B, but he had problems shifting back to list A for the short delay trial. He recalled few words. Semantic cues helped him to locate the information. The opposite pattern was evident on long delay tasks and on recognition testing. His excellent recall (10 of 15 words) appeared to "set" the list in his mind, but he could not regroup the list to match the semantic cues. On the Recognition subtest, Richie also had difficulty, confusing list items with the distracter items. As a result, he accurately identified only 4 of 15 items. The recognition list produced interference, whereas the cued recall trials reflected his limited mental flexibility.

To give him a break from tasks with right or wrong answers, a few cards from the Roberts Apperception Test were presented to Richie. My goal was to elicit a story so that I could observe his organization and sequencing. He responded with a series of short descriptive phrases but failed to integrate the components he identified into a cohesive story. He was totally unable to add information that would go beyond the picture, that is, to use imagination. When this information was presented to his mother, she reported that Richie failed to demonstrate imagination in his free play. His lack of imagination had been one roadblock to developing interactive play skills.

Richie and I made it through one more task before his anxiety became overwhelming. I had planned to administer the entire Test of Language Competence. We made it through the first subtest—Ambiguous Words. Richie could recognize the ambiguous word in the sentence and provide one meaning for it, but he was unable to provide a second meaning. At his age level, four pictures are presented after the child's descriptive response, and the child is asked to select the two out of four pictures that reflect the meaning of the sentence. Once again, Richie could choose one but not two.

After testing was completed, I met with Richie's parents to review the results. We discussed what they could do and what the school could do to help Richie function to the best of his ability. I called Joe and reassured him that frontal dysfunction can occur in 6-year-olds. Joe resumed

Richie's care, agreeing to help the parents locate a behavioral therapist to show them behavior-shaping paradigms and to provide periodic reassessments to track their son's development. Richie was also referred to a pediatric neurologist to titrate medication to support attention and inhibition.

THE CLINICAL CASE BECOMES A FORENSIC CASE

Months after the assessment was completed, I received a letter requesting my report from the attorney representing the family in their medical malpractice case. Shortly after I sent the report, I changed jobs. I still had the rock to serve as a reminder of Richie, but I thought that my involvement with him had ended. I was wrong. Much to my surprise, I received a call from the law firm representing Richie and his family. An efficient voice greeted me: "We have a report that you have written. We would like to schedule your deposition. Would 2 weeks from Friday work for you?" I assumed that I was being deposed as a fact witness. I assumed I would be asked questions about my evaluation and my recommended interventions. I was about to learn an important lesson about forensic work: *never assume*.

I explained to the efficient voice that I had changed jobs and no longer had access to Richie's file. I explained that the parents would have to sign a release so that my previous employer could send me a copy of Richie's file. The file arrived containing a copy of my handwritten notes and my report, but no test forms. My previous employer followed the established policy of not releasing raw data. I wasn't concerned. Richie was a memorable child. Since I thought I was a fact witness, I felt that I had all the information I needed. It turned out that I had been listed as an "expert witness" by Richie's attorney and was about to be treated as such by the defendant's lawyer. In fact, I became aware of my expert witness status about 60 minutes into the deposition.

In preceding depositions, I had had the chance to meet with the retaining attorney in advance to review the case. I had never been deposed as a fact witness, but I assumed that the plaintiff's attorney would do the same. Once again, my assumption was wrong. For this deposition, I walked into a room full of strangers. The friendliest looking person in the room was the court reporter. I learned another valuable lesson: Always at least meet the retaining attorney (or plaintiff's attorney when called as a fact witness) at some point prior to the deposition. If I

had done so, I would have come better prepared. Although I came prepared to answer questions about diagnosis and interventions for this
child, these questions took only minutes out of a deposition that went on
for 2 hours.

As I was adjusting to the sudden change in my perceptions of my
role in the case, the differences between a forensic assessment and clinical assessment became increasingly clear to me. I had relied on records
of previous evaluations and a parent interview for my clinical assessment.
Those were fine for answering the "What is it?" and "What do we do with
it?" questions of clinical work. I never considered the possibility that
Richie's parents might be distorting the history to meet their needs, but
the deposing lawyer certainly had. I wrote the report for the parents and
for the school staff. My practice was, and still is, to include definitions of
terms in parentheses to make sure that the reader understands them.
The definitions are informal; they are my way of communicating. My
forensic reports no longer contain informal definitions. The deposing
lawyer in Richie's case asked me to site sources for the informal definitions, questioning my qualifications to write any explanation on my own.

Had I known that this was a forensic case, I would have asked for all
past medical records in advance. Had I known that this was a forensic
case, I would have gotten additional school records. Had I known this
was a forensic case, I would completed a typed summary of the content
of the parent interview. Had I known that I was going to have to defend
my conclusions in court, I would have had Richie come back for as many
sessions as it took to complete my initial test list, giving all tasks first in a
standardized fashion to get standardized scores and then testing the limits. But I didn't know it was a legal case. When it became one, I had to
live with the information that I had from the evaluation.

THE DEPOSITION

In a deposition, you are at the mercy of the lawyer deposing you. We
spent the first 30 minutes going through my CV in excruciating detail.
This included a considerable amount of time discussing the 1 month
break in my employment history that occurred with my job change. I suspect that the questions were an attempt to aggravate me. It almost
worked, until I shifted my thinking. Instead of viewing the attorney's
questions as intrusive, I decided that if he wanted to pay me to talk about
my summer vacation, it was an easy way to make money. We covered the
journals I read, the meetings I typically attended, and who I knew in the

neuropsychology community. I was asked if I knew and received referrals from a very well-known neuropsychologist whom I shall call "Dr. Brain." Since Dr. Brain lived about 900 miles away from where I was practicing at the time, I replied: "We don't really cover the same catchment area."

We talked about ADHD, including a stroll through the DSM-IV definition. As the discussion shifted to ADHD research, the lawyer stated: "Don't you agree that Dr. Brain is the definitive authority in the field of ADHD?" I said, "No." Although I have a world of respect for Dr. Brain's work in other areas, I pointed out that there were other neuropsychologists whom I viewed as authorities in ADHD. I found out later that the defense had tried to retain Dr. Brain for this case. I never found out why the defense expert at trial was a less well-known neuropsychologist.

As the first hour of the deposition drew to an end, I was still thinking I was a fact witness. I figured that the deposing lawyer was either incredibly thorough or was being paid more per hour than I was. As hour 2 approached, we finally got into what I had come to discuss. The content shifted to the child, the evaluation, the treatment recommendations, and the prognosis. My moment of insight, "Oh no, I'm an expert witness," occurred as we began to go through my report sentence by sentence. All the pieces fell in place. The questioning of my definitions, my reading preferences in journals, the lengthy stroll through DSM-IV, and now the questioning of every word I wrote suggested to me that I was no longer being asked the "What is it?" and "What to do about it?" questions, we were heading toward "Why?"

In forensic cases, I include a list of records reviewed and identify sources for what I view to be key facts in the report. In clinical cases, I do not engage in that level of detail. The attorney began to ask for the source of every piece of information in the history. When I replied, "The mother," he would counter with "Just how did you phrase that question?" I repeatedly responded, "I don't recall." Each "I don't recall" would prompt the question, "Well, how do you typically get that information?" We covered my "failure" (his term, not mine) to review the medical records. In a tone of voice that suggested I was a gullible fool, he said, "So you simply took her word for it?" Sometimes brevity is best. With the most confident tone of voice I could muster, I responded "Yes." Finally we moved out of the background section.

We moved on to the testing and results. I was finally beyond Mother's report and into my own experience. My feelings of relief ended with his first question: "Now, just what score or scores in your testing provide evidence of frontal lobe dysfunction?" "The scores were not important. What was more important was watching Richie's approach to tasks," I replied. I provided him with a top-notch description of Richie's problems with strategy generation, perseveration, and cognitive rigidity. "So what does all that mean?" he asked. I knew at that point that we had a long road to travel before we were done. Time was spent defining executive functions and frontal lobe syndrome. Next, we dealt with the issue of whether any child of 6 had these functions. With confidence, the lawyer stated that the frontal lobes don't begin to work until adolescence, so how could I possibly diagnose frontal dysfunction in frontal lobes that aren't supposed to be working at Richie's age. Suddenly, I was in the position of knowing something to be true and having to prove it. I needed research references.

Now, when I elect to become involved in forensic work, I come prepared with selected references to support my position. I learned never to come with a "comprehensive review." When you do, you can count on the lawyer deposing you to refer to some obscure journal containing an article that you didn't include and that contradicts your opinion. Smugly the lawyer then concludes: "If you are an expert offering a comprehensive review, why haven't you seen this article?" I had a different problem in this deposition. I hadn't brought a list of selected references. Even worse, at the time of the deposition, there was a lot of monkey literature, but the amount of published work with preschool children was limited. I did the best that I could, while confessing my inability to remember names of authors. Luckily, I can remember book titles and journal names.

When the deposition ended, I was exhausted. I worked hard to explain that executive dysfunction was not evident in a test score, it was evident in how the child achieved the score. I did my best to communicate the limitations that result from executive dysfunction. I felt that I had failed this child and his family because no matter how hard I tried, the deposing attorney just didn't seem to understand. Much to my surprise, my new acquaintance, the attorney from the firm representing Richie, shook my hand, said it was nice to meet me, and told me I had done a good job. She said she would be in touch.

PREPARING FOR TRIAL

It was over 2 years later that I received a phone call from the paralegal for Richie's attorney. Attempts at settlement had failed and the case was going to trial. She gave me a choice of 2 days and told me that the plane tickets would be in the mail. It was the first time any of my cases had got-ten this far. It was clear that I was going to testify in court. Even though 2 years had passed, I had held on to all the material I had gathered for the deposition. Since I had never received a copy of my deposition, I asked for it. This time I knew I was an expert witness, not a fact witness. I asked for all the medical records as well.

In a deposition, the lawyer is discovering your "likely testimony" and developing a strategy for managing it. You can use the deposition in the same way. What had I learned? As I read through the deposition, themes emerged. The lawyer was concerned about my knowledge of the medical records. He seemed concerned about my ability to interpret intracranial pressure readings. Although there was no arguing the fact that Richie had craniosynostosis, he was seeing how far he could go to argue that the increased pressure that Richie experienced was "not that bad." I could see his argument. If there were no significant and prolonged increased pressure, then there would be no brain damage. The neurologist that continued treating Richie was going to testify the day after my testimony. If questions about intracranial pressure were raised, I planned to defer to the neurologist.

The lawyer had focused on my experience with ADHD, and we had agreed that Richie met diagnostic criteria for ADHD. He focused on other etiologies, including genetics. He focused on the fact that all of the family history and syndrome-onset history I had came from Richie's fam-ily. He implied that they had strong motivation to be less than honest with me. He was building the argument that Richie is suffering simply from ADHD, something that happens to lots of children, something that might run in the family, and therefore is unrelated to his cranio-synostosis. I couldn't do anything with the issues of my sources for family history. It was clear that I had to paint of picture illustrating how differ-ent Richie was from the typical child, even the typical child with ADHD.

If those two arguments failed, the defense lawyer was developing an argument to undermine my finding of frontal lobe dysfunction. He wanted to argue that Richie was too young to allow anyone to make such a diagnosis. In trial, the "burden of proof" clearly rested on me. I needed to find a credible source to back up my assertion that the frontal lobes were functioning in most children of Richie's age, and that the quality of that functioning could be evaluated. I turned first to the medical records, then to a literature search, then to the library to get the articles I needed to support what I already knew clinically. There was not a lot of litera-ture, but I tracked down every reference I could find.

THE TRIAL

The trial was being held in a small city (hereafter called Smallville) that became somewhat isolated in the winter due to frequent snowstorms. The trial was scheduled for January. The last 300 miles of my plane trip was on a small, 30-passenger plane, flying at night through one of their typical storms. When we took off, the pilot indicated that he couldn't guarantee that we would land in Smallville, but he was sure he could get us within 100 miles of it. I felt lucky to land in Smallville, even though we were a few hours late.

Court testimony is really a team effort. The lawyer that has retained me has the responsibility to help me understand the issues of the case and the legal burden of proof. The lawyer has the responsibility of helping me know what part my testimony plays in his overall game plan. My first job is to translate what I know into language that made sense to the attorney. Part of my role is to be the attorney's teacher or guide through my area of expertise. My second job is to help the lawyer know what questions to ask me so that I have an opportunity to explain my findings to the jury.

Our pretrial testimony conference was scheduled for 7:00 P.M. the evening prior to my court testimony. In reality, with my plane being late, our conference began around 10:00 P.M. and wrapped up close to midnight. What I remember most from this conference was a discussion of the example I frequently use in describing the limitations that frontal dysfunction places on adult employment opportunities. I typically talk about the importance of routine and structure in eventual employment. As an example of a rule-bound job, I often use employment by the Postal Service. In Smallville, where most people were involved in blue-collar jobs with few fringe benefits, working at the post office is considered a job to which children are encouraged to strive. You need to know the community and the culture to be effective. I developed another example.

In addition to covering my testimony, the lawyer offered me a strategy for testifying. He suggested that I turn slight toward the jury and make eye contact with them as I testified. It validates the jury's role and keeps them interested. However, when being cross-examined, he suggested that I look at the defense attorney. It suggests that the cross-examination is just a time when the defense attorney and I are having a chat, a conversation that doesn't really involve the jury. This strategy has continued to work well for me over the years.

At the end of our meeting, the lawyer pointed out that my testimony and that of the neurologist would be the keys to his success in the case. He pointed out that the neurologist often used dry humor, something that would not be well received by the jury. He concluded: "We are counting on you." Those words gave me something to think about as I tried to sleep. Up until now, Richie had been a fascinating case. The forensic aspects had been an intellectual challenge. Suddenly we were talking about a child's future.

Richie's lawyer did a good job restoring my focus by the end of breakfast the next morning. Joe had already testified as a fact witness, and now it was my job to give his insights validation from the perspective of a pediatric neuropsychologist. I felt prepared; I felt confident. I approached the cute little-old courthouse prepared to do my job. I was greeted by Richie's parents. They expressed gratitude for the help I had given them, and for my willingness to travel. It was reassuring to know that they only expected me to try. They were not holding me accountable for the outcome. The jury filed in, the judge arrived and we were ready to go. I had chosen a flannel dress rather than my fancy suit, thinking that they might relate better to my testimony if it was not coming from an obvious outsider. I had grown up on a farm outside a town much like Smallville and remembered how we viewed big-city folks. Given that the snow storm was still raging and the temperature was barely above zero, the only ones in the courtroom not dressed in flannel were the two lawyers. I couldn't tell what the judge was wearing, but would not have been surprised if flannel lined pants were warming his legs under his robe.

I was not to be the first to testify. Two teachers currently working with Richie were to testify before me. At the request of the defendant's attorney, one teacher and I were asked to step out of the courtroom so that we would not be biased by the testimony of the other teacher. One teacher and I left the courtroom, being guided to a small room nearby. I do mean small. The room held four chairs, and a little end table with one old magazine. There was no room for anything else.

The judge provided no directions regarding what we could or could not discuss. Well, we covered the weather (it was still snowing), how we had chosen our careers, and where we had gone to school. We spent a few minutes comparing public and parochial education (Richie was in parochial school). After 10 minutes, we were down to the only subject we had in common. We talked about Richie and his family. We did not share expected testimony. I answered her questions relating to teaching strategies for Richie. She got a free neuropsychological consult and I got a sense of Richie's current functioning. In the time left, we reverted back to the weather ("Just where do you put all the snow?"). The teacher was called to testify and I was left alone in a small room with only my thoughts and an old magazine to keep me company.

Then it was my turn. I had frequently gone to Juvenile Court during my early years working in a community mental health setting. Juvenile court is nothing like civil court. Everything is relaxed, informal, and you are never asked to swear to anything. Smallville was a great place to be for a "first court" experience. The judge looked kind. The jury looked just like my old neighbors when I was growing up on a farm. I felt like I had come home.

As the testimony began, I realized that I was being asked to do the same thing I do at the end of every evaluation. I was doing a feedback session, converting my test findings into words that a parent can understand. When I communicate with anyone, I tend to gesture. I talk with my hands, using them to demonstrate concepts and for emphasis. All of this occurs automatically, as it did during my testimony. It was brought to my attention by the defense lawyer suddenly jumping up and offering a firm "I object!" For a few seconds, no one in the courtroom knew just what had set him off. All I was doing was describing the result of closed sutures when the brain is attempting to grow. I had interlaced my fingers and may have also moved them to suggesting "squished." The defense lawyer pleaded: "She is using her hands. Her hands aren't reflected in the record. She cannot use gestures." "Objection overruled!" responded the judge, "Her gestures match her words. If they don't match, I will tell her to stop." The judge leaned toward me and in a soft, encouraging tone told me to just keep going.

The team worked well. The lawyer posed the questions that allowed me to describe all of the behavior that made Richie different from other children. I stayed focused on his behavior, referring to test scores only in terms of how different Richie's behavior was from what would be expected based on his test scores. His scores said he had the same skills as other children his age, but his behavior said he couldn't use them. The term "executive dysfunction" was introduced to the jury at the end. By that point, I was giving them a shorthand term to use for all the behavior that I had just described.

The lawyer allowed me to create a picture of Richie, a picture that the jurors could apply when they eventually got to meet Richie. They knew what to look for, and they saw it. The defense attorney and I had a nice discussion about the development of the frontal lobes. We explored the research showing that executive function is evident in young children. The jury had the mental picture. It was stronger than the academic discussion of research.

The cross-examination focused on the issues that I had anticipated. When my use of the mother's history was questioned, I responded: "She wanted help for her child, and the only way to get help was to be honest with me. I trusted her." I also pointed out that a subsequent review of the medical records supported her report. "Aren't we really just talking about ADHD?" he asked. I kept it brief and stated, "No." He had no choice at that point but to ask me "why?," giving me another change to talk about executive deficits. Then he asked the question for which I was waiting. "Isn't it true that the frontal lobes don't function until you are an adolescent and that you can't measure executive functions in a child of Richie's age? I again chose the simple answer, "No." When he asked me to prove it, I was ready. An issue of *Developmental Neuropsychology* devoted to research on executive functions in children had come out about four months prior to the trial. I had the reference in front of me, including a list of the contents. Obviously, he didn't know about that issue, but it's very existence seemed to be enough for the jury.

I suspected I had done my job well as the cross-examination drew to a close. The defense lawyer asked, "Just how many times have you testified in court?" I suspect he was getting reading to suggest that I was a "hired gun," a professional plaintiff's witness. "You, sir, have the privilege of being part of my first experience." I replied. He turned to walk back to his table mumbling, "Then why are you so good?"

When you do clinical work, your involvement in the case is measured in hours and days. When you do forensic work, the case can become a part of your life for years. Suddenly the testimony is done. You are dismissed. You are expected to walk out the door, forget the case, and dive into the next one.

Along with the check reimbursing me for my court appearance, I received a short note from the attorney. He indicated that the jury had arrived at a "favorable settlement." I don't know exactly what a "favorable settlement" means in the eyes of the attorney, but I suspect that it would be sufficient for a family living simply in Smallville. I don't know exactly what happened to Richie. I only know that I helped to make sure that his needs would be met for the foreseeable future.

LESSONS LEARNED

The experience of having a clinical consultation become a forensic case has had a lasting effect on my clinical practice. My intake coordinator routinely asks parents if they are involved in litigation whenever referral concerns involve the effects of traumatic injury.

I now treat every case as if it could become a forensic case. In preparing for the patient, I request copies of original records for any medical or educational history that is relevant to the case. I do not rely on summaries by others, even my trusted colleagues, for this information. During interviews, I clearly document the informant (child, parent, parents' summary of a teacher's comments, teacher, etc.). I review my handwritten notes for completeness immediately after seeing the patient. If I could not reconstruct the interview from my notes or feel that my notes could be easily misunderstood by others, I transcribe the notes.

During my assessment of Richie, my compassion for his struggle caused me to stop test administration when I felt I had enough behavioral information to address the question raised by my colleague. I now judge the adequacy of my behavioral data and supporting test scores in the larger context of its ability to demonstrate the reasons for my conclusions to others beyond the referral source. While remaining compassionate to the child's struggle, incentives are offered to support continued effort instead of prematurely ending a testing battery. I remain amazed at the power of juice and animal crackers or a sticker chart to reengage the overwhelmed, tired, or noncompliant child.

12

Childhood Malingering
Faking Neuropsychological Impairment in an 8-Year-Old

GEORGE K. HENRY

Your children are not your children.
They are the sons and daughters of Life's longing for itself.
They come through you, but not from you,
And though they are with you yet, they belong not to you.

You may give them your love, but not your thoughts,
For they have their own thoughts.

You may house their bodies, but not their souls,
For their souls dwell in the house of tomorrow,
Which you cannot visit, even in your dreams.

You may strive to be like them, But seek not to make them like you.
For life goes not backward nor tarries with yesterday.
                              —KAHLIL GIBRAN, *The Prophet*

For those of us who have children, or work with children, the quote from Kahlil Gibran's *The Prophet* conveys both truth and wisdom. Being both a parent and a pediatric neuropsychologist, I like to think that I have acquired a certain level of sophistication and understanding regarding children's behavior. But just when I think "I have seen everything," something happens that catches me by surprise and causes me to reorder my thinking and remember that life is a lifelong process of learning. It is in this context that I present the following case study. I hope that this case will not only help pediatric neuropsychologists to think more deeply about behavior in children, but also facilitate discussion pertaining to test-taking effort in children.

BACKGROUND INFORMATION

This case began with a phone call from an attorney, stating he had obtained my name from a colleague of mine, and that I came highly recommended. When I hear this comment during the initial contact I usually translate it into "What can you do for me?" I am also somewhat angered and annoyed, because I see this as a veiled attempt to gain some modicum of favor with the retained expert from the very beginning. However, my anger and annoyance quickly gave way to feelings of gratitude and good fortune as the referral source asked if I would be willing to conduct an independent medical examination (IME) on an 8-year-old child. To those of us who perform evaluations in the forensic area, an IME means that we are not only going to be paid for our time, but that our fees will be paid in full irrespective of the outcome of the case. Normally, we are not asked to reduce our fees for our time—although occasionally a plaintiff's attorneys have asked me to reduce my fees when a verdict was not reached in their favor or when a settlement amount was less than they had anticipated. I am sure we can all look back and share amusing anecdotes regarding the trials and tribulations of embarking on a forensic practice. But being paid for our time and structuring financial agreements in a way that is reasonable and fair (for both parties) is critical to maintaining an active forensic practice.

Approximately 15 years ago when I began my involvement in the forensic arena, every referral from a plaintiff's attorney was secured on a lien basis. I guess I am a slow learner, or perhaps simply trusted others at their word, but I actually believed that I would be eventually compensated for my time when the case ended. I found out the hard way. By working on a lien basis, not only was I not being paid for the time spent in record review, consultation, testing, scoring, report preparation, and preparation for deposition or trial, but I was often asked "to cut my fees" when a case settled, or worse yet, to "go after the plaintiff" when their attorney did not prevail at trial. It also occurred to me that working on a lien basis produced a potential "conflict of interest," because I could be perceived as an advocate or having a personal interest in the outcome of the matter before the court. If I was asked under cross-examination, "Then, Doctor, isn't it true that if the plaintiff does not win this lawsuit, you don't get paid?" So for at least the past 10 years, and continuing currently, I no longer work on a lien basis for referrals from plaintiff attorneys. Rather my services are secured under a written Professional Service Agreement (PSA) between attorney and doctor. The PSA sets forth the fees and conditions of the attorney–doctor relationship and eliminates "the patient" as the responsible party for payment of fees. The PSA also guarantees payment for my time irrespective of the outcome of the case. This arrangement has resulted in a much higher rate of return for my time. In the three cases where the PSA was not honored, I prevailed in small claims court. This, of course, is all academic when retained by the defense, because I told the defense attorney I would be interested in working on this case.

He began to provide the usual preliminary details and associated requests. He stated that the child had not been previously evaluated by a neuropsychologist, and that the father was suing "Quick Transit," a bus company, for "damages" the child, "Johnny," had sustained when struck by an automobile as he was attempting to cross the street and board the bus. The attorney wanted me to fax to him a copy of my current CV and fee schedule as well as provide some dates for conducting the evaluation. At this point, as I do with all defense referrals, I advised him of the conditions under which the IME would go forward; no audio or video recording of test-administration procedures and no third parties present during the testing process. I did not object to either having the plaintiff's attorney present during the interview or recording of the same. He reminded me of the requirements "under the Code" and to "etch it in my brain." It was plain what his position was; however, rather than get into a debate on the conflict between ethics and law, I agreed to proceed with the examination with the understanding that the conditions I had requested may eventually require a written declaration for the court or at least a stipulation from the plaintiff's attorney following consultation with his expert. In the interim, he was going to send me "all records in his possession," but when I asked if he also had educational records, he informed me that they had not been subpoenaed. I told him that the educational records would be important. I offered possible dates for the evaluation, and a date for the examination was set.

The records arrived several weeks before the scheduled examination and included the paramedic's report, hospital records, and deposition transcripts of Johnny and his father, but no school records. A review of available records revealed that Johnny was an 8-year-3-month-old right-handed Caucasian boy who 2 years earlier, while crossing the street, was struck by an automobile traveling approximately 25 mph. He had sustained a left femur fracture, a closed head injury with skull fracture, and loss of consciousness for less than a minute. Paramedics reported a Glasgow Coma Scale (GCS) score of 14. At the hospital, he was amnesic for the event, with a GCS of 15. A CT (computed tomography) scan of the head revealed a left frontal nondepressed linear skull fracture, but no evidence of intracranial abnormality. A CT scan of the abdomen revealed a splenic laceration, and a CT scan of the leg confirmed a left femur fracture. He was hospitalized for approximately 3 weeks and discharged home. An EEG (electroencephalogram) at 14 months postinjury was normal. Review of Johnny's deposition transcript indicated that he did not recall the accident, and no family member ever told him what had happened. In his deposition Johnny's father said that "no doctor has ever told me that Johnny had brain damage," but a number of behavioral changes were reported postinjury, including enuresis, nightmares, insistence on sleeping in his father's bed, refusal to ride in an automobile or a bus without his father present, increased aggression with his brothers, stealing, lying, temper tantrums, and sullenness at times.

NEUROPSYCHOLOGICAL EVALUATION

Interview

Johnny arrived at 10 A.M., 1 hour late for his 9:00 A.M. scheduled IME. He was accompanied by his father. There was no attorney present, and no request was made to record any portion of the examination. Johnny and his father had driven to the Fresno area the day before and spent the night at a nearby hotel. Johnny reported that he had gone to bed at 10 P.M. and slept alone in one of two double beds. He said that he slept through the night and felt rested upon awakening at 6:00 A.M.. After he washed and dressed, he went out to a local restaurant with his father for breakfast. He then went to a place called "Pyramid," which is like an indoor jungle gym for children. He played there awhile and then went with his father to Starbucks before finally leaving for the examination.

The interview was conducted conjointly. Johnny stated that his father drives him to school, and that he was in the second grade at "Maxine Elementary School." His teacher, "Mrs. Chambers," was "nice." He added that he was not receiving any special education services, but attended a class before school to get help with his homework. He denied school-related problems, but said that he did not like school. His father reported that Johnny receives "speech therapy" twice a week at school for a total of 3 hours. He also said that the teacher was having "lots of trouble with him"—that is, Johnny does not sit still in class; he leaves his seat and goes to the window to look out. Johnny also has difficulty with attention and listening, as well as problems comprehending questions. A home tutor was recommended by the family physician postinjury, but Johnny never received any tutorial assistance. Johnny's father stated that his son "struggled in school" before the accident, in that he was behind in his reading, but his academic performance had gotten worse following the accident. When I heard this description, I wondered if perhaps there were some premorbid "weakness," as opposed to a frank learning disability, which may have been exacerbated by the injury. Once again, the importance of reviewing educational records was evident. In my experience, these kinds of records can provide additional insight into a child's academic performance, although they also tend to be somewhat limited because teachers are often reticent to record negative comments or criticism that then become part of the child's permanent cumulative school record. I find that reviewing deposition transcripts of the teachers, when they exist, to be more informative, with the most helpful information derived via direct interview of the teachers. Unfortunately, the examiner usually does not have the benefit of conducting teacher interviews in the process of conducting a defense IME because the examination is usually "limited to the plaintiff" by plaintiff's attorney. Furthermore, in my experience most plaintiff's attorneys will not allow any parental, let alone teacher interviews.

Psychosocial history revealed that Johnny was the middle child in a family of three brothers. He had an older 10-year-old brother, "Kevin," and a younger 3-year-old brother, "Otto." The parents were married in 1990 and separated in the late 1990s following an alleged episode of infidelity. Johnny's mother moved out but maintained visitation rights, and the children stayed in the family home with their father. On several occasions between 1999 and 2000, Johnny's mother refused to return the children, following visitation, to their father's home, prompting police intervention. Then in February 2001, she attempted to "kidnap" the children and take them across state lines where her parents resided. She was apprehended by the state police, and the children were reunited with their father, who was granted a restraining order. Johnny's mother was allowed only monthly supervised visits. She moved to another state during the summer of 2001 but continued to call them on the phone once or twice weekly. Johnny's parents divorced in October 2001, approximately 18 months postinjury. When Johnny was asked about his mother, he reported that he speaks with her once a week when she calls, but he does not want to visit her. He added that he had not seen her since his accident, and hoped that his father would "find another mommy." Johnny appeared to be excited that his father was moving to a new home and that he would get his own bedroom. He stated that when he was not attending school, he liked to skateboard and go Rollerblading; he wore a helmet when he engaged in these activities. He also played organized baseball and enjoyed watching the Dodgers and professional wrestling on television. Johnny reported that he enjoys wrestling "WWF style" with his older brother, Kevin, and occasionally "fights" with him, which he described as pushing and yelling, but no punching. In contrast, Johnny's father said that Johnny does punch his older brother, as he did before his injury, but it has become more frequent.

On interview, the only accident-related residual symptom Johnny identified was transient left-leg pain that occurs spontaneously at a rate of once a week, lasts for 5–10 minutes, and is not related to physical exertion such as walking or running. He denied problems with cognition, learning, or behavior, in stark contrast to his father, who reported myriad persistent accident-related sequelae. Specifically, the father reported that Johnny displays enuresis at a rate of five times weekly, which occurs at home and school. He added that the family physician had determined that the enuresis had no organic etiology. He complained that Johnny does not use silverware in restaurants but eats with his fingers, despite multiple prompts and requests. Johnny also "wanders off" when he is with his father at malls, parks, or stores; he requires constant parental surveillance, refuses to ride the school bus, and crawls into bed with his father at around 2 A.M. each night. His father described Johnny as displaying a lot more emotion since the accident, in that he cries more easily and is more aggressive with his older brother. In contrast to Johnny's report, Johnny's father described Johnny's residual leg pain as constant, adding that sometimes other children ridicule Johnny because he walks with a slight limp. Lastly, the father reported that Johnny was not taking any prescription medications.

Behavioral Observations

Following the conjoint interview, which lasted approximately 90 minutes, Johnny's father was asked to return to the waiting room and fill out some behavioral questionnaires. Johnny separated easily from his father, and testing commenced. Although I usually like to begin the test administration portion of the evaluation with a task that is nonverbal and fun (i.e., the Beery–Buktenica Developmental Test of Visual–Motor Integration [VMI]), on this occasion I began with the Test of Variables of Attention (TOVA) because the norms were derived on children during the morning hours, and it was approximately 11:30 A.M. when testing started. After test instructions were provided, Johnny was given the standard 3-minute practice trial to ensure comprehension and compliance. During the practice trial, he incorrectly pressed the hand-held control to the nontarget, not the target, which was exactly opposite to the test instructions provided by the examiner. After completion of the practice trial, Johnny was asked to reiterate the test instructions. With a sheepish grin he incorrectly stated that the "target" was when the small black square was at the bottom of the large white square (which is really the nontarget stimulus!) I then spent several minutes reexplaining the instructions to him before he correctly identified the target. Once it was clear that he understood the task demands of the TOVA, the test was administered. Just as he had done during the practice trial, Johnny incorrectly pressed the button nearly every time the nontarget stimulus appeared on the screen. At that point it dawned on me that I may be observing a child who was deliberately performing poorly, so I decided to administer several measures of symptom validity.

Tests Administered

Johnny was administered two measures of symptom validity (i.e., Test of Memory Malingering [TOMM]; Tombaugh, 1996) and Computerized Assessment of Response Bias [CARB]; Condor, Allen, & Cox, 1992) to evaluate effort, as well as a flexible battery of neuropsychological tests to assess intelligence, academic achievement, attention, receptive and expressive language, and visual–motor integration. Measures included the Wechsler Intelligence Scale for Children—Third Edition (WISC-III; Wechsler, 1991), Wide Range Achievement Test—Third Edition (WRAT-3; Wilkinson, 1993), Test of Variables of Attention (TOVA; Greenberg, Kindschi, Dupuy, & Corman, 1996), Receptive One-Word Picture Vocabulary Test (ROWPVT; Brownell, 2000a), Expressive One-Word Picture Vocabulary Test (EOWPVT; Brownell, 2000b), and the VMI (Beery, 1997). Testing was terminated earlier than planned due to Johnny's performance on the symptom validity measures, as well as the nature of his responses on standardized tests, indicating very poor effort. Given the medical–legal nature of the case, the child and father were not confronted. Whereas other neuropsychologists may have handled this aspect of the case differently, it is my custom and practice to not share my opinions of the examinee's effort with the examinee, because I perceive my role as an expert is to assist the trier of fact in matters of causation and alleged damages, and not as a patient–litigant advocate.

TEST RESULTS

On both measures of symptom validity, Johnny scored in a range consistent with definite malingering (i.e., below chance). For example, on trial 1 of the TOMM, he obtained 14 out of 50 correct (28%), and only 5 out of 50 correct (10%) on trial 2. On the CARB he obtained scores of 29.7% correct on block 1, 2.7% correct on block 2, and 10.8% correct on block 3. The number correct across all trials was 16 out of 111, which is 14.4% and significantly below the average of 97.5% correct ($SD = 3.8$) in nonlitigating patients with moderate to severe traumatic brain injuries (Green & Iverson, 2001). On a measure of reading ability, the WRAT-3, he pronounced *cat* as *dog*, *book* as *pack*, *tree* as *try*, *now* as *here*, and *even* as *odd*. When asked to spell to dictation, he spelled the word *and* as *nqd*, *in* as *nq*, *him* as *ham*, *make* as *meak*, *cook* as *kek*, and *must* as *mqsk*. On written arithmetic problems, he computed the following: $1 + 1 = $ "3," $5 - 1 = $ "10," $2 + 7 = $ "11," $8-4 = $ "100," and $9 + 3 = $ "20." On the WISC-III, he obtained a Verbal IQ of 74, Performance IQ of 80, and Full Scale IQ of 75. The lowest WISC-III age-corrected subtest scores of 1 were displayed on Digit Span, Arithmetic, and Digit Symbol. On Digit Span, he recalled only two digits forward and none backward. During completion of the sample portion of the Digit Symbol subtest, he committed four transpositional errors, which were pointed out to him by the examine; Johnny continued to transpose numbers during the actual test portion. Scores on a measure of sustained attention, the TOVA, were well below the 1st percentile; Johnny committed 155 errors of omission and 267 commission errors. On the VMI, which required him to copy designs, Johnny drew a vertical line when shown a horizontal line, a circle when shown a square, a triangle when shown an *X,* and an *X* when shown a triangle. On a test of receptive language, the ROWPVT, he pointed to a picture of a sock when the word *shoe* was shown, to a train when the word *car* was given, and to a sailboat to the word *spoon.* Expressive language, the EOWPVT, was likewise replete with bizarre and implausible responses. For example, when he was shown the picture of a dog, he answered *cat,* a toe was called a *leg,* a house was a *tree,* eyes were *feet,* and eating was *drinking.* See Table 12.1 for a listing of tests administered, raw scores, and standard scores.

TABLE 12.1. Neuropsychological Test Results in Raw and Standard Scores

Test	Raw score	Standard score
TOMM Trial 1	14	< 45
TOMM Trial 2	5	< 45
CARB Block 1	11	< 45
CARB Block 2	1	< 45
CARB Block 3	4	< 45
CARB Total	16	< 45
WISC-III VIQ	NA	74
WISC-III PIQ	NA	80
WISC-III FIQ	NA	75
WISC-III VCI	NA	81
WISC-III POI	NA	90
WISC-III FDI	NA	50
WISC-III PSI	NA	61
WRAT-3 Reading	16	63
WRAT-3 Spelling	11	58
WRAT-3 Arithmetic	0	< 45
VMI	2	< 45
ROWPVT	0	< 45
EOWPVT	0	< 45
TOVA Omissions	155	< 45
TOVA Commissions	267	< 45

Note. TOMM, Test of Memory Malingering; CARB, Computerized Assessment of Response Bias; WISC-III, Wechsler Intelligence Scale for Children–Third Edition; VIQ, Verbal IQ; PIQ, Performance IQ; FIQ, Full Scale IQ; VCI, Verbal Comprehension Index; POI, Perceptual Organization Index; FDI, Freedom from Distractibility Index; PSI, Processing Speed Index; WRAT-3, Wide Range Achievement Test–Third Edition; VMI, Beery–Buktenica Developmental Test of Visual–Motor Integration; ROWPVT, Receptive One-Word Picture Vocabulary Test; EOWPVT, Expressive One-Word Picture Vocabulary Test; TOVA, Test of Variables of Attention; NA, not applicable.

DISCUSSION

This case represents an example of extreme exaggeration of cognitive impairment by an 8-year-old undergoing forensic neuropsychological assessment. Below-chance performance was displayed on two measures of symptom validity, and rather bizarre and implausible answers were given to questions on standardized neurocognitive measures. Following the completion of testing, I contacted the defense attorney and informed him that the testing was invalid.

Johnny's level of performance was clearly very poor and rendered the entire data set unreliable and invalid. What remains less clear are the factors responsible for such behavior. Some understanding might be gleaned from looking at such behavior from the perspective of contingencies of reinforcement. Children, like adults, may engage in disingenuous or deceptive behavior due to some perceived positive reinforcer (i.e., some secondary gain such as money, attention, or approval) or to avoid some perceived negative consequence or punishment (i.e., the testing situation). An example under a positive reinforcement paradigm might include malingering by proxy; that is, receiving attention and approval for poor performance due to parental or attorney coaching. However, under coaching conditions, the feigned performance is usually more subtle and not so obvious, and therefore probably does not explain the obvious behavior exhibited by Johnny in this case. An example of dissimulation under a negative reinforcement condition might include oppositional behavior, wherein the child avoids or terminates a situation perceived to be aversive by deliberately refusing to comply with requests or rules set forth by the authority figure in the testing room (i.e., examiner). Although this hypothesis is certainly plausible, I believe it is less tenable, because such children do not usually display such behavior during interactions with strangers, and Johnny was fairly cooperative during the interview portion of the examination. Another possibility is that Johnny was malingering; that is, he engaged in conscious manipulation of the testing session due to some secondary gain. Although Johnny's performance was obviously disingenuous to this "seasoned" examiner, it is not known if Johnny actually thought he was faking "believable" deficits. The only way to know for sure would be if Johnny were to "confess," and this did not happen.

A final and somewhat intriguing theory by which to try to understand Johnny's behavior might involve the role of emotion and how the brain makes moral decisions. Research efforts such as those of Antonio

Damasio at the University of Iowa (Damasio & Van Hoesen, 1983) have shown how emotions can control choices or decisions even when they may be morally wrong. Thus, in Johnny's case, although he may have behaved in an immoral manner (i.e., misrepresenting his true abilities), his decision to do so may have been driven by strong underlying emotions that had more to do with psychosocial dynamics related to family and parenting factors than seeking financial gain (as is often the case in adult personal injury cases). A report was never prepared because the defense attorney told me to "hold off" on any report at this time. The attorney contacted me approximately 2 months after my evaluation and informed me that the case had settled.

The literature on malingering and deception in children is rather sparse. There are a few clinical case studies of faking or exaggeration of psychiatric symptoms or illness (Greenfield, 1987; Cassas, Hales, Longhurst, & Weiss, 1996; Roberts, 1997; Heubrock, 2001). One study (Faust, Hart, & Guilmette, 1988) showed that children and adolescents are capable of feigning cognitive deficits, and a recent case report (Lu & Boone, 2002) indicated that a child as young as 9 is capable of feigning cognitive impairment. Although this was my first professional experience with an individual this young giving such grossly distorted responses during testing, there is some evidence that children between the ages of 2 and 3 years old are capable of engaging in deceptive behavior. This case clearly represents gross faking; however, it is not known if more sophisticated patterns of faking exist in young children. There is evidence that sophisticated symptom fabrication can occur in some adolescents, and neuropsychologists are rather poor at identifying such individuals (Faust, Hart, Guilmette, & Arkes, 1988).

Some may question the reliability and validity of utilizing adult symptom validity measures in cases of child neuropsychological assessment. Preliminary efforts in this area have been equivocal. One study of the CARB and WMT has shown that children below the age of 10 perform more poorly compared to children older than 10, whereas children 11 years and older perform similar to adults (Courtney, Dinkins, Allen, & Kuroski, 2003). However, this study did not control for reading level. A more recent study of the WMT (Green & Flaro, 2003) that controlled for reading level demonstrated that children as young as 7 years old did not score any lower than older children. Intelligence level was not related to effort scores, whereas reading below a third-grade level was associated with a drop in WMT Immediate Recall (IR) and Delayed Recall (DR) scores.

LESSONS LEARNED

Although unexpected, very young children can score below chance levels on tests of symptom validity that have traditionally been associated with definite malingering in the adult forensic arena. Given the emerging clinical research data in children, symptom validity measures that have been standardized with adults may have applicability in cases of child forensic assessment. Over the past year, I have routinely administered symptom validity tests to children as part of my neuropsychological evaluation. To my surprise, there have been two additional children, ages 12 and 16, who have scored below recommended cutoffs for these tests but not below chance. Thus, clinically I am seeing kids in forensic neuropsychology situations who are not putting forth adequate effort, as measured by symptom validity tests. Obviously, this behavior renders the associated data base unreliable and invalid. It remains to be determined what the base rate might be for such behavior, and more importantly, why children as young as 8 years old engage in such disingenuous behavior.

Given these clinical experiences, I believe it is necessary for neuropsychologists who evaluate children within a forensic context to routinely include measures of symptom validity, and that examiners include such tests in their test battery in order to provide an objective basis for evaluating effort and establishing confidence in the reliability and validity of the data set. This routine practice might be particularly helpful in cases where more subtle forms of dissimulation occur, as opposed to the gross and extreme exaggeration that characterized this case. In the absence of such effort measures, examiners will be forced to rely upon subjective factors such as clinical judgment, which historically has been shown to be quite poor, when rendering opinions regarding a child's level of effort and validity of test scores. The current case study clearly demonstrates that an 8-year-old child can fake neuropsychological impairment, but the reason he did so is less clear. The utility of effort measures in children warrants further study, especially in young children who have the capacity to fake cognitive impairment.

REFERENCES

Beery, K. E. (1997). *Beery–Buktenica Developmental Test of Visual–Motor Integration.* Parsippany, NJ: Modern Curriculum Press.
Brownell, R. (2000a). *Receptive One-Word Picture Vocabulary Test.* Novato, CA: Academic Therapy Publications.

Brownell, R. (2000b). *Expressive One-Word Picture Vocabulary Test*. Novato, CA: Academic Therapy Publications.

Cassas, J. R., Hales, E. S., Longhurst, J. G., & Weiss, G. S. (1996). Can disability benefits make children sicker? *Journal of the American Academy of Child and Adolescent Psychiatry, 36,* 700–701.

Condor, R., Allen, L., & Cox, D. (1992). *Computerized Assessment of Response Bias*. Durham, NC: Cognisyst.

Courtney, J. C., Dinkins, J. P., Allen, L. M., & Kuroski, K. (2003). Age effects in children taking the Computerized Assessment of Response Bias and Word Memory Test. *Child Neuropsychology, 9*(2), 109–116.

Damasio, A. R., & Van Hoesen, G. W. (1983). Emotional disturbances associated with focal lesions of the limbic frontal lobe. In K. Heilman & P. Satz (Eds.), *Neuropsychology of human emotion*. New York: Guilford Press.

Faust, D., Hart, K., & Guilmette, T. J. (1988). Pediatric malingering: The capacity of children to fake believable deficits on neuropsychological testing. *Journal of Consulting and Clinical Psychology, 56,* 578–582.

Faust, D., Hart, K., Guilmette, T. J., & Arkes, H. R. (1988). Neuropsychologists' capacity to detect adolescent malingerers. *Professional Psychology: Research and Practice, 19,* 508–515.

Green, P., & Flaro, L. (2003). Word Memory Test performance in children. *Child Neuropsychology,* 9(3), 189–197.

Green, P., & Iverson, G. L. (2001). Validation of the Computerized Assessment of Response Bias in litigating patients with head injuries. *The Clinical Neuropsychologist, 15*(4), 492–497.

Greenberg, L., Kindschi, C., Dupuy, T., & Corman, C. (1996). *Test of Variables of Attention*. Los Alamitos, CA: Universal Attention Disorders.

Greenfield, D. (1987). Feigned psychosis in a 14-year-old girl. *Hospital and Community Psychiatry, 38,* 73–75.

Heubrock, D. (2001). Münchhausen by proxy syndrome in clinical child neuropsychology: A case presenting with neuropsychological symptoms. *Child Neuropsychology, 7*(4), 273–285.

Lu, P. H., & Boone, K. B. (2002). Suspect cognitive symptoms in a 9-year-old child: Malingering by proxy? *Child Neuropsychology, 16,* 90–96.

Roberts, M. D. (1997). Munchhausen by proxy. *Journal of the American Academy of Child and Adolescent Psychiatry, 36,* 578–580.

Tombaugh, T. (1996). *Test of Memory Malingering*. North Tonawanda, NY: Multi-Health Systems.

Wechsler, D. (1991). *Wechsler Intelligence Scale for Children–Third Edition*. San Antonio, TX: Psychological Corporation.

Wilkinson, G. S. (1993). *Wide Range Achievement Test–Third Edition*. Wilmington, DE: Wide Range.

13

—

Lead Astray

The Controversies of Childhood Lead Poisoning

LISA D. STANFORD

As in every other forensic neuropsychology case, childhood lead poisoning cases do not offer immunity from the battle of the contradiction: advocacy, boundaries of competency, expert versus treating witness, clarification of the client among multiple contacts, maintenance of data integrity, comorbid factors of influence, and, most importantly, knowing when to say you do not know something. I often have the fantasy that childhood lead poisoning cases would be so much more relevant for a pediatric neuropsychologist if they were only about determining if a ubiquitous agent has negatively impacted a particular child's developing brain. However, the issue is embedded in a huge social context of industry versus ecology; law firm versus law firm; expert witness versus expert witness; and who can accumulate the most number of articles and cite the strongest case for the inverse relationship between IQ scores and blood lead levels, regardless of the clinical utility of those changes in scores. Somewhere it seems that the emphasis on the data is lost in a whirl of competition for some sort of external reward.

I am very clear on the point that my role in the case often has little bearing on the outcome, regardless of how strong the data are and how complete my testimony. Still, the challenge of each case has helped me grow as a neuropsychologist, recognize the boundaries of testimony that allow me to sleep soundly at night, and continue to strive to present the data in the most direct and unbiased manner possible. However, it is still easy to be seduced by the phrases "more likely than not" or "with a reasonable degree of psychological certainty" that elevated blood lead levels (BLLs) may have contributed to a child's identifiable deficits when accepting a childhood lead poisoning case for forensic evaluation.

The first lesson that I learned very quickly about serving as a forensic consultant was that, with every impending childhood lead poisoning case, the role of the child advocate has little place in the legal arena. It is all about the data—even when the data can be confusing and the signature pattern of childhood lead poisoning elusive. I consistently find myself engulfed in massive amounts of literature (presented to me by both plaintiff and defense attorneys) about the lowered IQ scores, "threshold of safety," generalizability of individual data in the context of group data, trajectories of development, and contribution of maternal IQ to a child's current level of functioning. Then come the continual practical issues associated with many pediatric cases, such as comorbid attention-deficit/hyperactivity disorder (ADHD), historical developmental delay, variable cooperation, and retrospective information obtained during clinical interview with the parent. The case I have chosen to present is not unique or unusual. It simply illustrates the common controversies that come with childhood lead poisoning cases and further demonstrates the need for continued examination of this area in pediatric neuropsychology.

BACKGROUND INFORMATION

This lead poisoning case started out like other forensic neuropsychology cases that I had seen—which, in itself, was a unique occurrence. As part of my position at my previous place of employment (large tertiary medical center), I had it in my mind that I needed to do an incredible amount of work, and that I should be reimbursed 100% for that work. Thus, in a moment of significant capitalistic weakness, which was of no personal financial benefit to me, I agreed to see a case of childhood lead poisoning referred from one particular law firm. What I did not realize at the time was that this referral source would soon generate 45 more cases, each individual cases rather than class action, related to lead poisoning in the Cleveland Public Housing System. By the time this case came around, I already had a few of them under my belt, but I was blissfully unaware that at least 40 more cases would follow. However, none of them would hold quite the challenge for me that this first one did.

When dealing with an extremely large and wealthy law firm, you very frequently receive initial contact from support staff, and often never meet the attorney until the day before your deposition. Thus, I had received all referral source and initial information regarding this 7-year-old male child via overnight mail with the directive to call some unknown attorney whom I had never met with additional questions, as needed. I always work under a retainer fee that is sent prior to my reviewing any records or seeing the child for evaluation in order to avoid bias associated with a lien or with collecting a fee for service following completion of the evaluation. My fees for hourly rates for the process (e.g., review of records, evaluation, testimony) are sent ahead of time, and I prepare an invoice as each service is provided. One of the "perks" of my previous place of employment was that I could not personally receive renumeration for any forensic services delivered. This condition proved advantageous in depositions and trial testimony, because I was never perceived as the "hired gun" and never had to justify the amount billed per hour. Also, I found it appropriate and useful to charge the same amount for the testing (technician fee) and clinical interview time across forensic and regular clinical cases (although my rates for attorney consultation and record review were somewhat higher).

As with the previous lead poisoning cases I had seen, "Frank" proved very similar in that he came from a low-income family from a minority group, with very few options for moving out of the Cleveland Public Housing System. Additionally, according to the attorney's letter, he was being serviced through the special education program in the Cleveland Public School System, with current classification under Specific Learning Disability (SLD), despite the fact that his previous level of intellectual functioning had been within the "mentally impaired" range, he had no identifiable discrepancy between IQ and achievement (the accepted special education eligibility criteria of SLD at the time), he was only in the first grade, and he had a history of significant behavioral difficulties. Additionally, Frank had been diagnosed with ADHD by a pediatrician whom he had seen a few years prior to this evaluation. No one else in his family had been exposed to the lead or had elevated blood lead levels, no one else had symptomatology of ADHD, no family members reportedly had developmental delay or below average intellectual functioning, and the family had only lived in one place during the time of his reported lead exposure and elevated blood lead levels. Thus, the case seemed somewhat straightforward, and I agreed to take the case.

The records arrived in their usual form, on a CD-ROM that was easily readable and printable from my desktop computer. The law firm most graciously created this format so that the records could easily and inexpensively be sent to me from their office out of state. There was something reassuring about having this compact disc with huge amounts of data at my fingertips, which allowed ease of cataloguing and marking of more pertinent documents and efficiency for quickly scanning through less relevant ones. Plus, the size and portability of the CD rendered storing records in my office or reviewing the records away from the office a much less cumbersome task. As with every other lead case that I had received from this law firm, I was assured that the biggest issue was to determine if it was more likely than not, or with a reasonable degree of psychological certainty, that Frank's behavioral and cognitive deficits as well as his language delay could be, *in part,* due to his elevated blood lead levels. It always sounds so easy when the attorney presents it in this way, and the neuropsychologist must be vigilant to guard against the effects of bias toward the attorney's agenda even at the onset of the case.

The neuropsychological test battery for the evaluation was chosen in advance and was fairly fixed (although not a published fixed battery) to cover all neurobehavioral domains, in contrast to a flexible battery constructed to further examine deficits after having met the child. I prefer the broad approach of evaluating strengths and weaknesses in a standardized manner, and I conduct a forensic evaluation in the exact same way as with any clinical case that is not forensic. I use a well-trained neuropsychology technician to conduct the testing (to minimize my own bias and to allow me time to interview, without interruption of the evaluation or adding to the time a family must stay at the office). The evaluation is completed in 1 day so that I can examine the role that fatigue and fluctuating attention have on the child's functioning. I use the most current version of well-accepted tests that are age appropriate and appropriately normed. (As an aside, the use of technicians frequently comes up in depositions, so I come prepared with the position statements from the American Academy of Clinical Neuropsychology [1999] and the National Academy of Neuropsychology [2000] regarding the acceptable use of technicians in neuropsychological evaluations. This saves a lot of time and unnecessary discussion during the deposition about issues of individual or site-specific practices.) Finally, I do not allow third-party observers (which I specify before I agree to take a case) unless the presence of a parent in the evaluation is necessary to gain compliance or best effort from the child. I fully explain to the family (and to all parties involved) the purpose of the evaluation; to whom the report will be sent; that, regardless of who hired me, I am concerned with the data and not with furthering any attorney agenda; my role and that of my technician; and that I would not be offering additional treatment or assistance with securing any clinical/educational services for the child based on the results of the testing, so as not to conflate expert versus treating witness roles. At my former place of employment, we found it very useful to put all of these issues in writing as part of informed consent long before the Health Insurance Portability and Accountability Act (HIPAA) guidelines existed. Clearly stating your position and procedures up front, without apology, also goes a long way in preventing further explanation or challenges later in the forensic process.

NEUROPSYCHOLOGICAL EVALUATION

Clinical Interview

Frank was accompanied to the neuropsychological evaluation in early February of 2002 by his mother, several siblings, and a few cousins. As is often the case with pediatric cases, I had to demonstrate extremely flexible interviewing skills to talk over the roar of several small children under 5 years of age, who were playing at high decibel levels in my office, while conducting a clinical interview with Frank's mother. Over the years, I have become quite adept at dodging flying objects, racing after a child who has headed straight for my computer keyboard, and nodding supportively as the parent attempts to answer my thoughtful questions in the midst of multiple distracters. Based on interview with Frank's mother and review of his available medical records, he had elevated BLLs ranging from 67 in March 1997, 40 in July 1997, 30 in September 1997, and 18 in July 1998. His mother indicated that the family had lived only in one place during that time period (although I have never made it my position to discuss the issue of *where* a child was exposed as part of the litigation—that is for someone else to prove), and that his elevated BLLs were discovered during a routine physical when he was 2 years old. Frank's mother recalled that there had been some discussion about hospitalizing her son for treatment due to his high BLL, but instead he was put on iron supplements and did not receive any other oral medication or chelation treatment. Frank's mother also expressed concerns that he did not talk or say an intelligible sentence until well after 2 years of age. She also recalled that he had begun to display frequent tantrums, was very hyperactive, and had demonstrated significant behavioral problems at home and school during the time period of the exposure. She noted that it was still very difficult to get him to follow instructions, that he frequently talked back to her, and that he misbehaved in public places.

Fortunately, Frank's birth records revealed no prenatal complications, a full-term pregnancy, and Apgar scores at 9 and 9 for 1 and 5 minutes, respectively. There were reportedly no postnatal complications, Frank's mother had not used any medications or substances (i.e., drugs, alcohol) during her pregnancy, and both mother and child had been discharged 2 days following his birth in good health. This information allowed me to rule out most congenital or perinatal influences on the data. Frank's mother also indicated that he had been relatively healthy throughout his childhood, with the exception of lead poisoning. Gross and fine motor developmental milestones were reportedly reached within normal limits, but he was delayed in his acquisition of speech. The only other issue was the diagnosis of ADHD and treatment with Ritalin, which was initiated approximately 7 months prior to the current neuropsychological evaluation.

My impression from the interview was that Frank's mother was extremely sincere, certainly had the welfare of her children at heart, and was motivated and capable of providing a fairly accurate and distortion-free history. I had only briefly scanned the CD-ROM of records so as not to bias or lead me during the clinical interview. Instead, as with every other pediatric neuropsychological evaluation that I conduct, I encouraged her to relate her presenting concerns, historical information in response to my questions, and to put the recollection of facts in her own words. I have consistently taught my trainees and students that a clinical interview is not solely for the purpose of gathering information. Instead, it is also a venue for (1) applying clinical judgment in determining the psychosocial and dynamic issues of the family system, (2) conveying to the person that he or she has been heard, and (3) allowing the opportunity for subtle information to surface that has not been presented on the forms or in medical records. Additionally, I asked Frank's mother to complete a history form as well as several behavioral checklists to provide additional objective information with regard to her concerns about her son's presentation. She relayed the information to the best of her ability, in the context of the multiple siblings and cousins who were roaming about my office, and I believe that I had obtained an accurate recollection of the events leading up to this child's referral for an evaluation.

Behavioral Observations

At the morning break in testing and after the clinical interview, I was able to discuss with my technician the behavioral observations made of Frank during the first part of testing. The technician indicated that Frank was social, cooperative, talkative, but physically active. As the morning had progressed, he became increasingly more active, and his attention to task was very short. He needed ongoing redirection back to task, but he maintained a cooperative effort throughout the day. He was also noted to have difficulty in comprehending and abstracting complex instructions, and instructions often needed to be simplified. He was observed to give up easily and quickly as tasks became more difficult. The test results were believed to be an accurate representation of his functioning, because Frank's behaviors were consistent with those described as occurring across other settings, such as school and home environments.

By the lunch break, I took inventory over the morning events. I had to juggle the three or four other patients whom I was seeing during that day (which opposing counsel always want to know so that they can question my ability to pay adequate attention to the case being brought to trial) with the use of additional technicians. Nevertheless, I believed that I had obtained an accurate clinical history and a valid and representative performance from Frank during testing, and had chosen the appropriate battery of tests with which to evaluate his overall pattern of cognitive strengths and weaknesses. The same battery chosen for most children his age that come to our service for evaluation was used with Frank, because he did not have any specific limitation that would prohibit him from participating. It is always a good day when a pediatric neuropsychological evaluation occurs without major incident, such as test refusal, losing a child, racing down the hall, or having to tell a parent that his or her child has inadvertently swallowed a piece of test material.

My complacency was short-lived. By the early afternoon, Frank was unable to sit in his chair to complete tasks, his attention span became more variable, and I was receiving complaints from the support staff at the front desk about the state of the waiting room in the wake of the multitude of children accompanying the parents whom I was seeing for the day. Fortunately, the "major tests" (i.e., intelligence, memory, academic) had been accomplished without significant incident during the morning session, and I had an adequate behavioral sample with which to discuss the deterioration of Frank's behavior and his variable attention span throughout the day, in essence, simulating his school environment. We also discovered that Frank had not been given his Ritalin on the morning of testing. Thus, the rest of the evaluation had to continue without implementation of this medication so as not to artificially influence the test results. I always have my technician write the exact time of day each test was given and when it ended. This information has proven to be very helpful to me when opposing counsel brings up the issue of undue fatigue on memory or some other cognitive ability that might have been assessed later in the day. I try to have the most effort-demanding tasks administered in the morning, after sufficient rapport has been established, and I try to avoid having a memory test given right before lunch when a child seems to be most distracted by his or her hunger. Whereas the position of a certain test during the day is an important consideration, I have found it additionally helpful to know exactly what time a test was begun and concluded so that I can more accurately talk about the evaluation in a deposition.

We sent the family on their way at the conclusion of testing, and I began the arduous task of reviewing the case records. I had become accustomed to the ways of this particular law firm, given that I had already seen five or six of their clients claiming lead poisoning, and I was able to quickly scan my computer screen to find those documents that were relevant to my portion of the case. I reviewed the child's birth records, prenatal care records, pediatrician progress notes, school records, and the Cuyahoga County Health Department reports listing BLLs, procedures, and dates of testing for lead. I soon discovered that Frank had an Individualized Education Program (IEP) under the label of Severely Behaviorally Handicapped (SBH) and that he was currently attending a day treatment center for children with behavioral problems. He had been initially referred for testing by his school back in kindergarten, when he could not follow single-step instructions, was running around the room and making noises, and needed to be excluded from the larger group. It was also noted that he had to be physically removed from the class and restrained by a staff assistant in order to keep him under control and safe. His school progress notes indicated that the kindergarten teachers said that he had the most extreme behavioral problems that she had ever seen, and that his behavior made him unable to function in the kindergarten setting. His attention was described as only

"momentary" during the standardized testing session, and previous testing could not be completed due to his inability to follow directions, sit in
the seat, or stay on task. He was described as exhibiting limited expressive vocabulary, difficulty with receptive vocabulary, and a short attention
span. Although no formal data could be collected, Frank was described as
needing therapeutic language instruction because his speech and language skills were adversely affecting his educational development. On his
IEP, additional testing at a later date reportedly revealed a level of intellectual functioning in the "mildly impaired range," but no test data were
available for review. None of these facts was mentioned during the clinical interview with Frank's mother, nor had the attorney specified the
severity of these issues in the initial retainment letter.

I had just evaluated a child with severe behavioral problems, who was
not taking his medication on the day of the evaluation, and whose
mother may not have been as reliable as I had hoped with her description
of her child during the clinical interview. Thus, it was a fairly representative evaluation in pediatric neuropsychology and fairly typical of childhood lead poisoning cases. My task was to determine if Frank's behavioral difficulties, cognitive delay, language difficulties, and short attention
span were more likely than not, or with a reasonable degree of psychological certainty, related in part to his previously elevated BLLs.

Test Results

Frank was administered the Wechsler Intelligence Scale for Children–
Third Edition (WISC-III; Wechsler, 1991) in order to assess his current
level of intellectual functioning. Results indicated overall abilities in the
intellectually deficient range (Full Scale IQ = 59, < 1st percentile), with
slightly better developed verbal intellectual ability in comparison to nonverbal intellectual ability. Factor indices of the WISC-III revealed mildly
impaired verbal comprehension and expression ability (Verbal Comprehension Index = 68, 2nd percentile) and mildly impaired nonverbal and
visuoperceptual reasoning ability (Perceptual Organization Index = 62,
1st percentile). On subtests particularly susceptible to fluctuations in
attention and requiring working memory skills, Frank also performed in
the mildly impaired range (Freedom from Distractibility Index = 61, < 1st
percentile). He also demonstrated mildly impaired performance on tasks
requiring speeded mental and motor processing (Processing Speed Index
= 67, 1st percentile). Examination of the verbal subtest scatter revealed
relative weaknesses for word definition skills and verbal comprehension.

He demonstrated relative weaknesses for attention to visual detail and for speeded clerical ability on nonverbal subtests. He had significant deficits in receptive and expressive language on measures of confrontation naming, oral fluency, repetition, and auditory comprehension. His performance on memory testing was also extremely poor but consistent with his measured level of intellectual ability. Academic achievement skills were strengths for Frank, although he performed at almost greater than 1 year below his chronological age and grade across all tasks. He was mildly suppressed for bilateral fine motor coordination and dexterity, although fine motor speed was within normal limits bilaterally. He was also noted to be less efficient on tasks requiring working memory and mental flexibility, and he became frustrated as the tasks increased in complexity.

Frank's behavioral presentation during the evaluation, at home, and at school (according to the records) was significant for distractibility, hyperactivity, and impulsivity. He had significant difficulty working in a one-on-one distraction-free setting during the evaluation, and he was reportedly more hyperactive and impulsive at home and at school. In my opinion, his IQ was more significantly suppressed secondary to language disruption as well as unmedicated (on the day of the evaluation) ADHD. I was left to consider the comorbidity issue of ADHD, the disproportionate suppression of his language abilities relative to other cognitive skills, the impact of his behavior on the validity of test results, the duration of his exposure to lead, his BLLs, the critical period of development during which he was exposed to lead, the relationship of his functioning and behavior to other family members, and all of these factors in the context of an increasingly controversial literature regarding threshold of safety and contributing factors in childhood lead poisoning cases (e.g., maternal IQ, socioeconomic status, and individual vulnerability). Then, of course, there was the ever-present reevaluation by another neuropsychologist hired by the defense attorney.

I kept telling myself that I only had to determine if Frank's deficits were more likely than not, or at least in part, due to Frank's previous elevated BLLs, so I proceeded to interpret the data in the context of the fact that none of Frank's siblings displayed symptomatology of ADHD or had been diagnosed as such, that no family member had learning or behavioral difficulties in school, there was no history of language delay in any family members, and Frank was the only sibling who had been exposed to high levels of lead and then documented to have high BLLs. Additionally, his BLLs were significantly higher than the previously established threshold of safety of 10 µg/dl (Centers for Disease Control and

Prevention, 2000), and the duration of his exposure appeared substantial enough to make a statement with regard to a likely causal relationship. Additionally, he was exposed to lead and had high BLLs, based on medical records, during critical periods of language development. Thus, I noted in my report that the pattern of his test results, his behavior during the evaluation and in other settings, his emotional lability, and his language difficulties were consistent with what has been observed in children who have a history of significantly elevated BLLs during critical periods of development. Based on numerous articles in the childhood lead poisoning literature, I noted that attentional difficulties and an inverse relationship between IQ and BLLs have been seen in children with lead levels as low as 10 µg/dl and that Frank's BLL was substantially higher for an extended period of time. Thus, I believed that I was able to say with reasonable certainty that my neuropsychological opinion was that Frank's neurocognitive and behavioral deficits were, in part (although attorneys always want to know what percentage, which is a slippery slope that I never climb), a result of his elevated BLLs and previous lead exposure rather than a product of genetic or other environmental factors given that his biological parents did not reportedly experience attentional or behavioral problems, there was no family history of ADHD in non-lead-exposed family members, and that Frank had had no perinatal complications to suggest other neurological contributions to his difficulties.

DEFENSE EVALUATION

The next step was to wait for the defense neuropsychologist to evaluate Frank. This evaluation occurred approximately 1 year later from my evaluation and 4½ years after Frank had first been identified as having elevated BLLs. Review of the other neuropsychologist's history indicated that Frank had spoken single words at 24 months of age, combined words at 30 months, and was noted to be hyperactive by the time he was about 2 years of age. So far so good. The neuropsychologist also noted that Frank's mother indicated that she had left high school during the 11th grade and had not pursued a GED. However, no parental academic records were available for review. Interestingly, during my clinical interview with her she had indicated some difficulty in mathematics but relative strengths in reading and related skills. She reported to the other neuropsychologist that she was a below-average student with particular difficulties in mathematics, and that she had received special education services in math and English during middle school and high school (contrary to what she indicated to me during clinical interview).

This discrepancy raises the issue that an interview, conducted either by plaintiff- or defense-retained neuropsychologist, is vulnerable to the effects of the bias and undue influence that may accrue when the interviewer suspects difficulties or seeks to uncover facts that support his or her position. The neuropsychologist must always be cognizant of how questions are worded, which questions are pursued, and leaving no stone unturned. I always cringe and hold my breath when another neuropsychologist describes a previous evaluation conducted by me—not because I question my competence or the procedures used, but because there seems to be an inherent bias, despite best intentions, to critiquing work that might be in contradiction to one's own opinion or even a possible threat to another's source of income.

I should note that I had received, prior to Frank being seen for the defense's neuropsychological evaluation, an extensive list of all possible tests that might be administered during that evaluation, because the plaintiff's counsel had requested a list of all anticipated procedures to be administered by the defense expert. Surprisingly, this letter had been sent directly to me at my new place of employment. After a brief scan of its contents, I resealed the FedEx package and immediately called the plaintiff's counsel, who had retained my services. He indicated that the letter should not have been sent directly to me and would I kindly forward it to the attorneys. I subsequently received a phone call from the defense's neuropsychologist, apologizing for sending the contents of the FedEx package directly to me rather than to the plaintiff's counsel. I had a sneaking suspicion that this telephone call was also something that would not be readily appreciated by the plaintiff's counsel, and it seemed somewhat inappropriate given the circumstances of the evaluation. The neuropsychologist ended the call by saying that he/she had noticed that I had recently seen the child and he/she just wanted to make sure he/she was not repeating any tests that I had given. In the future, I will heed my own advice to end these calls as courteously as possible without discussing the case.

The defense neuropsychologist's report indicated that Frank had been taking Ritalin at the time of my evaluation (which was contrary to what actually had occurred), and that his behavior had undermined his test performance and suppressed his test scores on most of my procedures. During the defense neuropsychologist's evaluation, Frank was inattentive and increasingly fidgety from the start and more difficult to redirect as testing continued. He was readministered the WISC-III and obtained a Full Scale IQ of 79, composed of a Verbal IQ of 85 and a Performance IQ of 77, placing him in the low-average to borderline impaired range of intellectual functioning, relative to others his age. The neuropsychologist noted that the scores were noticeably better than those obtained during my evaluation approximately 1 year prior and likely reflected Frank's improved attentiveness and cooperation when treated with Adderall. No mention was made of practice effect. Frank reportedly demonstrated no observed deficits in manual motor speed, strength, coordination, and persistence, and there were no observed difficulties with fine touch, positional sense, astereognosia, or finger localization. He also performed in the average range of the sensorimotor domain using the NEPSY (Korkman, Kirk, & Kemp, 1998). He demonstrated a low-average performance on tasks of receptive and expressive language but noticeable deficits on tests of two- and three-dimensional constructions, visual synthesis, special orientation, and attention to visual detail. The report further indicated that "what few inefficiencies there were in memory skills" were attributed to Frank's language and attentional deficits, and that the previous neuropsychological evaluation (conducted by me) had been compromised by Frank's hyperactivity, inattention, and oppositionality. He was found to be under better behavioral control then he was the year before, likely due to more effective medication management.

The report contended that, although Frank's lead level was significantly elevated, it had remained so for only a short while and only when he was "already" 4 years of age. His history of overactivity appeared to have predated his first lead exposure (which is questionable, given that the first detected BLL does not specify duration and when initial elevation occurred). The neuropsychologist continued to cite a number of other risk factors for the development of intellectual, academic, and behavioral disorders (which were certainly true) and indicated that there is an active debate in the professional literature suggesting that family socioeconomic status, qualitative nurturing environment, maternal IQ, and other developmental medical factors are more important than low-level lead burden in predicting eventual functioning. There was no compelling evidence, the report contended, that "these behaviors of attentional deficits and developmental spatial problems" were linked to his relatively brief and relatively late onset lead exposure, and, in fact, there was little peer-reviewed replicated research suggesting a link between ADHD or specific behavioral disorders and early childhood lead exposure.

I was left to consider my thoughts regarding what I perceived to be a somewhat long duration of lead exposure (over 4 years) and exposure during critical periods of language development (prior to 2 years of age, up until at least 5 years of age); the incidence of behavioral difficulties occurring at age 2, during the time Frank was exposed to lead; in the context that none of Frank's siblings had severe deficits, and all had been exposed to the same nurturing environment, the same maternal IQ, and the same socioeconomic status. Certainly, Frank's test performance during my neuropsychological evaluation had been negatively impacted by his behavior, but negative behavior, in and of itself, is a relevant clinical observation that could be caused by some intervening event—which, for Frank, was only elevated BLL. Although very aware of the current controversies discussed in the childhood lead poisoning literature, I still believed that I could say, with confidence, that Frank's difficulties were *at least in part* due to lead poisoning and elevated BLLs experienced in early childhood. I could attribute the improvement in his scores during the second evaluation to some test practice effect and improved behavioral control secondary to a change in medication, as well as developmental maturity, given that the testing occurred approximately 1 year later. However, I was surprised by the low-average to average scores on many of the tests that Frank was administered, given his significant difficulties on these tasks prior to any behavioral interference in our neuropsychological evaluation. I believed my interpretation and conclusions were justified given that there is an extensive literature on the psychological effect of lead poisoning that clearly indicates that most lead poisoned children suffer a loss of IQ, although the literature does not clearly indicate that there is a consistent and reliable degree of loss corresponding to the degree of elevation of BLLs.

Since I had left my previous place of employment for my current position during the time this case was coming to deposition and trial, the attorneys who hired me had the additional burden of requesting all copies of previous records (i.e., protocols, previous test results, and evaluation report) related to Frank's neuropsychological evaluation, because I did not bring any data or patient information with me to my new position. I was subsequently served with an affidavit from the attorney with whom I was working, so that he could verify that I was who I said I was, that I was a board certified clinical neuropsychologist, that I had a PhD, and that I was licensed as a clinical psychologist in both Illinois and Ohio. I also had to verify my current place of employment and my previous place of employment, under which the previous evaluation had occurred. The affidavit further indicated that a copy of the patient file had been requested, with the plaintiff's permission, from my previous place of employment because the file had remained the property of that clinic after I had moved to Chicago. I also had to confirm that I had received the patient file in Chicago on such and such date from my previous place of employment, and that I had been requested to forward my raw test data to the defense's neuropsychologist (rather than to defense attorneys, so as to protect the security and integrity of the tests and interpretation of the data). So, I signed my life away after carefully changing many of the words in the affidavit to reflect my most accurate position.

DEPOSITION AND TRIAL TESTIMONY

The deposition was draining but exhilarating. The first hour focused on my background, training, publications, etc. (I am always amused that defense attorneys like to ask if I am married and have children—I rarely see those questions asked of a male expert neuropsychologist—and I have yet to convincingly explain that such information really bears no relevance on my ability to testify.) Typical questions included the relevance of board certification in clinical neuropsychology, how many cases I have done for defendant versus plaintiff counsel, what percentage of my income results from forensic work (which was zero, given that I was not allowed to keep any of the money retained at my previous place of employment), did I have any particular articles or books that I routinely rely upon to form my opinions, what were the duties of each employment position I have held since graduate school, and what population of patients do I typically see in my day-to-day practice. Then there were the questions related to the diagnosis and etiology of ADHD, and the difference between a behavioral diagnosis and a documented neurological cause of a disorder. It was well into the second hour of the deposition that defense counsel asked me to verify that the report submitted into evidence was my evaluation report and that it summarized my opinions. Then I was asked to repeat what records I had reviewed, had I seen the child since, and had I been given any additional information that would change my opinion. As an aside, it is advisable to put a statement at the end of your report stating that you reserve the right to amend or append your opinion, should you receive additional information. I was then asked to read my findings, discuss each test given, why it was chosen, and what I hoped to assess with each particular test.

The deposition turned to issues relevant to the literature and controversies regarding the threshold of safety, the magnitude of the inverse relationship between BLLs and IQ, and whether all "brain injury" of lead poisoning occurs at initial exposure or is cumulative. It was fortunate that a pediatric neurologist had also been retained by the plaintiff's law firm. I did not have to get into issues regarding my boundaries of competency. Indeed, it is critical to know your limits with regard to medical issues, including the mechanism of pathology, medication effects on behavior, and percentage of causation from lead poisoning, so that you may defer to other experts who practice in areas beyond your competence to provide testimony. I tried to limit my testimony to the data, a balanced review of relevant literature, and acknowledgment of other factors that can impact data interpretation. And I tried to avoid speculation and "crystal ball interpretation" on whether a child will be able to get married, complete college, and make an adequate living. Yet making some statements about predictive validity is not out of bounds. I also illustrated how, when a child is developmentally delayed, he or she will continue to make progress but will do so at a slower rate, widening the gap or lag compared to other children his or her age.

Then there was the whole discussion about the differences in my evaluation and the other neuropsychologist's evaluation. I stuck to the data, explained the reasons why our neuropsychological evaluations might be different, restated my opinions about "more likely than not" and "with a reasonable degree of psychological certainty," and refrained from making any pejorative comments about my colleague. I knew that the bigger argument of whether the elevated BLLs had caused Frank's problems was not going to be decided on that day, and that my testimony was just a small piece of mounting evidence that would be presented by both sides, should this go to trial.

Trial was scheduled to commence 3 weeks later. I prepared for trial by reviewing the key cases in the literature, studying the mechanisms of pathology, and rehearsing in my mind all the details of both neuropsychology reports. I felt ready and looked forward to the challenges of courtroom testimony and presenting a very academic and scientific topic in a meaningful and understandable way to the jury. I was flown to Cleveland from Chicago, I met with the plaintiff's counsel for several hours to review the case issues, and I headed back to my hotel room with a new binder of material to consider. Then the case settled on the night before the trial.

LESSONS LEARNED

As stated previously, I did not choose this case because of its uniqueness. Rather, I chose it because it illustrates the dilemmas frequently encountered in childhood lead poisoning cases. It is not my intent to advance a position agenda, describe my personal opinions regarding childhood lead poisoning, or offer myself as an expert in the area. Instead, my hope is that this case brings to mind many of the issues facing pediatric neuropsychologists who have decided, for one reason or another, to participate in forensic evaluations and to highlight areas of discussion specific to childhood lead poisoning. Despite the literature on childhood lead poisoning and the apparent impact it has on the developing brain, a signature neuropsychological profile eludes us at this time. We do not fully understand the clinical utility of the inverse relationship of elevated BLLs to cognitive and behavioral functioning, a threshold of safety with regard to BLLs has not been established, and it remains very difficult to definitely state causation of brain damage in children with elevated BLLs at the current time. We must attempt to make sense of the neuropsychological data on a case by case basis, while trying to understand the impact on functioning across large groups of patients or cohort studies. In doing forensic work, it is important that we practice in our areas of competence, suppress our role as child advocates, and render opinions based on what we have learned and been trained to do about a child's level of functioning, in the context of standardized data that we believe have been obtained in a reliable and valid manner. It is more likely than not, and with a reasonable degree of psychological certainty, that we will be faced with the recurring issues of data integrity, boundaries of competence, how much is attributable to a known cause, and what measurable impact childhood lead poisoning actually has on the developing brain. The jury is still out on this one.

REFERENCES

American Academy of Clinical Neuropsychology. (1999). American Academy of Clinical Neuropsychology policy on the use of non-doctoral-level personnel in conducting clinical neuropsychological evaluations. *The Clinical Neuropsychologist, 13*(4), 385.

Centers for Disease Control and Prevention. (2000). Blood lead levels in young children—United States and selected states, 1996–1999. *Morbidity and Mortality Weekly Report, 49*(50).

Korkman, M., Kirk, V., & Kemp, S. (1998). *Manual for NEPSY: A developmental neuropsychological assessment.* San Antonio, TX: Psychological Corporation.

National Academy of Neuropsychology. (2000). The use of neuropsychology test technicians in clinical practice: Official statement of the National Academy of Neuropsychology. *Archives of Clinical Neuropsychology, 15*(5), 381–382.

Wechsler, D. (1991). *Manual for the Wechsler Intelligence Scale for Children–Third Edition.* San Antonio, TX: Psychological Corporation.

III

CRIMINAL CASES

14

Boyfriend Busted in Fatal Stabbing

WILLIAM B. BARR

Through daily reading of *The New York Times*, I follow the progress of local crime stories. I would not label myself as a true "crime buff," but I do admit to becoming rather intrigued by the range of behaviors reported in news accounts of murders and other crimes committed daily in New York City. I find myself rather lucky to have worked with the Manhattan District Attorney's Office on a number of murder cases, including some that have received coverage in the local newspapers. I do not regard myself as a forensic psychologist but rather as a clinical neuropsychologist with an expertise in evaluating the validity of "extreme behaviors." I developed these skills through research on patients with a variety of neurological and psychiatric conditions and by performing clinical evaluations on a range of patients, from those with severe brain disorders to neurologically intact individuals attempting to malinger effects of cerebral dysfunction.

BACKGROUND OF THE CASE

On October 29, 2001, slightly before 2:00 P.M., an unidentified man called the City of New York's 911 number and in a calm voice reported, "I killed somebody." He stated that the deceased was his common-law wife and that he had stabbed her with a knife. His thought processes were intact. He was able to recite his correct location and phone number. There were no sounds of any emotional outburst or crying. The voice remained calm and relaxed.

Officers responded to the scene at "West 47th Street" within minutes. Their notes indicate that they apprehended a Caucasian man in his mid-40s, later identified as "Oscar Maldonado," attempting to leave the vicinity with blood on his clothes. They found the victim, "Kim Martin," inside apartment #6B lying face up on a bed. The EMTs (emergency medical technicians) pronounced her dead at the scene. A white metal knife with a brown handle was retrieved from under the bed. Shortly after his arrest, Maldonado passed out at the 17th Precinct Station from an apparent drug overdose. He was taken to Roosevelt Hospital in an unresponsive state. Upon waking, he admitted to having stabbed Ms. Martin and attempting to kill himself with a drug overdose. The New York *Daily News* reported the story with the headline, "911 caller admits deadly gal-pal stabbing."

Learning the Facts of the Case

When I received a telephone call from Assistant District Attorney (ADA) Vincent McKinney in July 2002, I had no knowledge of the murder of Kim Martin. Mr. McKinney was inquiring about my availability to serve as an expert witness for the prosecution of murder charges against defendant Oscar Maldonado. Mr. McKinney, a young attorney working for the Manhattan DA's Office, was given my name by his bureau chief. He informed me that he had no prior experience with psychological experts. He stated that the defendant had completed a psychological evaluation by an expert retained by his counsel. The test results had apparently shown that the defendant was unable to appreciate the nature of his actions at the time of the murder as a result of psychosis. I advised Mr. McKinney to forward me a brief outline of the facts of the case and a copy of the psychological report. I told him that I would contact him with my impressions after reading this material.

A few days later a package arrived at my office containing copies of the indictment, police records pertaining to the arrest, and a rap sheet on the defendant. It turns out that Maldonado and Martin had been in a relationship for 17 years. The couple met while working together at one of the Manhattan branches of Crate and Barrel, the retail furniture and home goods store. Martin was in sales, Maldonado worked in accounting. They had lived together in the same one-bedroom apartment for 12 years, in the same location where Martin's life eventually came to an end. Over the course of her relationship with Maldonado, Martin's career had advanced to a level of sales executive for another large firm in the furniture industry. She was making a "six-figure" income at the time of her death. Over the same period of time, Maldonado had been continuously unemployed. He belonged to health clubs and spent his time buying and selling a collection of comic books on the Internet.

I learned that Maldonado had an arrest record dating back to 1972 that consisted of seven arrests and five convictions. Prior charges for assault and grand larceny had been dropped for undisclosed reasons. He had been convicted for petit larceny, possession of stolen property, and disorderly conduct. Most importantly, there were records, in 1985 through 1987, that he had issued a plea of guilty to several misdemeanors related to harassment of Ms. Martin. These included assault, destruction of property, contempt of court, and tampering with a witness. The court had issued an order of protection that had been violated on a number of occasions. As a result, he had served a sentence of 6 months in prison. In a note accompanying the records, the ADA informed me that he was in possession of much more material on the relationship between Maldonado and Martin. He recommended that I come to his office to review Martin's diaries and letters, which documented the level of harassment that she had experienced during this period.

The records indicated that Maldonado also had a significant history of drug abuse, mostly involving the use of cocaine and heroin. He was arrested in 1994 for drug possession. He had completed rehabilitation through a series of well-known drug treatment programs and had apparently been drug free for 3 years prior to the arrest for murder. During the period of sobriety, he participated in an outpatient methadone maintenance program through Bellevue Hospital. There was no mention of any past psychiatric history. However, in August 2001, the summer before the murder, the defendant had presented to St. Vincent's Hospital indicating that he was hearing voices. He also described a delusion in which he had previously killed somebody in a subway station. He was admitted for an inpatient evaluation and treatment on a psychiatric unit and was discharged 2 weeks later with a range of diagnoses, including schizophrenia, panic disorder, opioid dependence, and head injury.

Acquiring the Background Data

"Dr. Derek Sandelson," a psychologist whose work I had encountered on other criminal cases, conducted the defense's psychological evaluation.

Dr. Sandelson is well known to the New York legal community for his work with criminal defendants. He had examined Maldonado on two occasions. The first was in January 2002, over 2 months following the arrest. The second evaluation was in May 2002. A 19-page report was issued shortly afterward, outlining the defendant's social, educational, and medical history and summarizing some of the details of the complicated 17-year relationship between the defendant and victim. I had many questions regarding how the defense would argue for insanity in this case. I sat down to read this report very carefully.

Dr. Sandelson reported that, in the initial interview, the defendant stated for the first time that he had been hearing voices for at least 1 or 2 years prior to October 2001. On the day of the murder, he had heard voices telling him to do "stupid things." In more detail, he stated that the voices had commanded him specifically to "choke Kim Martin." He also claimed that he was under the influence of medications prescribed to him by the doctors at St. Vincent's a few weeks earlier. The report mentions that the defendant had told police that he had seen Ms. Martin exiting the car of another man on the night before the murder. At one point, he had informed the police that he had murdered her out of "jealousy." However, in the second interview with Dr. Sandelson, conducted 4 months later, the defendant totally denied having any involvement in the murder. The same behavior was exhibited in meetings with his attorney, occurring at approximately the same time. It persisted even when he was confronted with details from the police records.

The report went on to review the results of psychological testing that had been completed over the course of the two meetings with the defense expert. The results had indicated that the defendant's intellectual functioning was at the level of mental deficiency (Full Scale IQ = 66, < 1st percentile), representing the effects of severe cognitive decline. Profound deficits were found in attention/concentration, suggesting compromise by functional psychopathology. Confused and defective performances on other tests were felt to represent the effects of neuropsychological impairment. Scores on procedures utilized to assess attitude and motivation were all considered normal, indicating to the examining psychologist that the poor test scores were not an artifact of uncooperativeness or a concerted effort to malinger symptoms of cognitive deficiency.

The results of personality testing were considered to represent the presence of "pseudo-neurotic schizophrenia." The defendant was considered to have a severe schizotypal personality organization compounded by anxiety, depression, and neuropsychological deficits. It was argued that the presence of the latter was supported by neuroimaging results (computed tomography [CT] scan) indicating frontal atrophy. The proposed mechanism of neuropsychological impairment was considered to be the result of a combination of factors, including drug abuse, head injury, chronic schizophrenia, and possibly HIV.

The expert's final conclusion was that the defendant had acted as a result of both insanity and extreme emotional disturbance. The report portrayed Maldonado as someone who had been experiencing symptoms of a severe psychotic illness with paranoid features for a number of weeks prior to the murder. He argued that the nature and extent of the psychosis were documented in great detail in records of the psychiatric admission at St. Vincent's Hospital. The expert concluded that the defendant had attacked Ms. Martin out a combination of both rage and paranoia. At the time of this attack, he was confused and psychotic and lacked the capacity to react to, or control, his impulses. He was unable to appreciate the nature of his actions as a result of being "overwhelmed" by psychosis.

In reading the report, I had noted that a number of important details had been omitted or had not been emphasized. There was little mention of the drug history or Maldonado's history of harassing Ms. Martin in the past. A number of other items included in the report, particularly the arguments for the presence of neuropsychological impairment, seemed implausible to me. I was eager to go further with this case and get my hands on the raw data from the psychological evaluation to determine what evidence Dr. Sandelson possessed with which to document the presence of psychosis and this vague description of neuropsychological impairment. I was also eager to review the psychiatric records from St. Vincent's Hospital to see what actually had occurred when Maldonado presented for admission in August 2001.

I gave Mr. McKinney a call to communicate my initial skepticism about the defense's case and told him that I would be willing to serve as the prosecution's psychological expert. I informed him of my need to obtain copies of Dr. Sandelson's complete interview notes and raw data. I also requested copies of all of the available medical records. He stated that he would get me these as quickly as possible. We made an appointment to meet in his office 2 weeks later to review what I had found. He also repeated that I would be very interested to get a look at the material that had been obtained from the victim's apartment following the murder.

A box of medical records arrived in my office by express mail the next day. A few days later, I received a call from Dr. Sandelson's office indicating that the psychological test data were available. His office is close to mine on the east side of Manhattan. Since it was a nice day and lunchtime was approaching, I decided to pick up the records personally rather than waiting to receive them by mail. After returning to my office, I opened the package and looked over the data. I found it odd that I had been provided with the original copies of the data, rather than photocopies. I wondered whether there had been a mixup. I called the office and they told me not to worry about it. I documented this call and went on to engage in my usual activity when receiving test data for forensic cases: have all of the data rescored by one of my postdoctoral fellows or psychometricians. I noticed that the package included response forms for two objective measures of personality functioning. I had both of these faxed to a computer scoring service to obtain formal copies of their forensic and correctional reports.

Once all of the data had been rescored, I sat down to review them. A summary of the cognitive test data is provided in Table 14.1. The first point I noticed was that the range of scores on the Wechsler Adult Intelligence Scale–III (WAIS-III) was much lower than I had expected for a man who had completed high school, worked in an accounting department, and had a relationship with a rather accomplished woman such as Kim Martin. After reviewing some of the other data, I began to wonder whether these test results provided an accurate or valid measure of Maldonado's intellectual functioning.

Turning to data from other tests, I noticed that the total score from the Raven Progressive Matrices was also very low. I found that the profile of obtained scores did not meet the pattern of consistency reported in the test manual, rendering the test administration invalid. It took the defendant an exceedingly long time to complete the Trail Making Test's Parts A and B. His copy of the Rey Complex Figure Test appeared much worse than I have seen in patients with severe disorders of visual–spatial functioning following strokes involving the right cerebral hemisphere.

I had recalled that Dr. Sandelson's report included a statement ruling out the presence of malingering. I found among the raw test data forms for tests that I had never encountered. One appeared to be a facsimile of the Rey Dot Counting Test, using only two presentations each of grouped and ungrouped dots. The other forms involved some type of forced-choice procedure for responses from the WAIS-III. In a quick computer search, I was unable to find references of any published studies using these procedures. I soon realized that the defense expert had apparently ruled out the presence of malingering based on the use of some homespun techniques, rather than employing test measures that

TABLE 14.1. Cognitive Test Results for Defendant O. M. Obtained from Defense Expert

Wechsler Adult Intelligence Scale–III	Scaled scores
Vocabulary	8
Similarities	3
Arithmetic	4
Digit Span	6
Information	7
Comprehension	4
Letter–Number Sequencing	7
Picture Completion	4
Digit Symbol Coding	3
Block Design	5
Matrix Reasoning	5
Picture Arrangement	4
Symbol Search	4
Verbal Comprehension Index	78
Perceptual Organization Index	69
Working Memory Index	73
Processing Speed Index	68
Full Scale IQ	66
Raven Progressive Matrices	Raw score = 6
Trail Making Test	
Part A	114 seconds, 0 errors
Part B	232 seconds, 0 errors
Rey Complex Figure Test (copy)	Raw score = 13

had been validated empirically. According to my analysis, he had also failed to look for possible signs of malingering on the "standard" tests included in his test battery.

In the psychological examination, the defendant had completed both the Minnesota Multiphasic Personality Inventory–2 (MMPI-2) and the Millon Clinical Multiaxial Inventory–III (MCMI-III) (see Table 14.2). There was no indication that he had the responses read to him, nor was there any sign that the questions were provided to him on an auditory tape. There was apparently no concern about whether this man with a Full Scale IQ in the "defective" range could read and understand the test questions. It turns out that the response profiles on both tests were valid, according to conventional analysis. The MMPI-2 profile was indicative of chronic psychological maladjustment with features of anxiety, tension, and depression. The MCMI-III profile showed no signs of a discrete DSM-IV Axis I disorder, although anxiety disorder and major depressive

**TABLE 14.2. Personality Test Results for
Defendant O. M. Obtained from Defense Expert**

Millon Clinical Multiaxial Inventory–III
  Modifying Indices

X	120	BR = 73
Y	8	BR = 39
Z	18	BR = 74

  Clinical Personality Patterns

1	17	BR = 96
2A	20	BR = 101
2B	10	BR = 71
3	14	BR = 84
4	1	BR = 4
5	5	BR = 23
6A	10	BR = 72
6B	11	BR = 80
7	18	BR = 55
8A	7	BR = 52
8B	9	BR = 72

  Severe Personality Pathology

S	7	BR = 63
C	8	BR = 58
P	7	BR = 63

  Clinical Syndromes

A	13	BR = 98
H	8	BR = 69
N	2	BR = 24
D	16	BR = 91
B	4	BR = 60
T	15	BR = 82
R	13	BR = 75

  Severe Clinical Syndromes

SS	7	BR = 64
CC	15	BR = 78
PP	3	BR = 63

Minnesota Multiphasic Personality Inventory–2

VRIN	5	$T = 54$
TRIN	7	$T = 64F$
F	7	$T = 58$
F(B)	9	$T = 79$
Fp	3	$T = 63$
L	6	$T = 61$
K	18	$T = 56$
S	23	$T = 48$
FBS		
Scale 1 (Hs)	9	$T = 57$
Scale 2 (D)	28	$T = 70$
Scale 3 (Hy)	20	$T = 47$
Scale 4 (Pd)	23	$T = 67$

(continued)

TABLE 14.2. *(continued)*

Minnesota Multiphasic Personality Inventory–2 *(cont.)*

Scale 5 (Mf)	16	$T = 30$
Scale 6 (Pa)	14	$T = 64$
Scale 7 (Pt)	18	$T = 70$
Scale 8 (Sc)	23	$T = 75$
Scale 9 (Ma)	11	$T = 39$
Scale 0 (Si)	41	$T = 68$

Rorschach Inkblot Test
  Number of responses = 5
  Number of rejections = 5

disorder were offered as possible diagnoses. There were indications of some Axis II features consistent with an avoidant or schizoid personality. Diagnostically, there appeared to be no signs of any severe psychosis, but the objective test findings did raise some question about tendencies for confusion and disorganization.

Unlike many neuropsychologists, I believe that there is a role for using the Rorschach, especially when it is scored and interpreted within the confines of empirically based methods. I have found this procedure to be especially helpful in forensic cases involving the insanity defense. In this case, the defendant provided single responses to only five of the ten cards; he rejected five others. There was no inquiry. By all standards, this was not a valid protocol due to the lack of responding. The defense expert interpreted this lack of response as representing Maldonado's extreme confusion. In looking at the protocol, I believed that he simply did not want to do the test.

Turning the to medical records, I was eager to see what actually happened in the summer of 2001. Did Maldonado really have a psychotic episode warranting a hospital admission? The records from St. Vincent's were 2 inches thick. I was hoping that the majority consisted of laboratory results, but I would not be so lucky. There were many pages of progress notes that had to be reviewed carefully. The documents indicated that Maldonado had presented to the emergency room on August 19, 2001, stating that he was hearing voices. He also stated a belief that he had killed a man by pushing him in front of an oncoming subway car. There had been no report of such an occurrence at that time. He experienced some seizure-like event in the emergency room that was later diagnosed as a nonepileptic seizure. Electroencephalogram (EEG) results showed slowing from apparent medication effects and no epileptiform abnormality. A CT scan of the brain was notable for some mild frontal atrophy. The emergence of psychosis was noted to have coincided with a tapering of the defendant's methadone dose. He was transferred to the psychiatric unit for inpatient treatment.

The inpatient progress notes provide descriptions of reported auditory hallucinations and delusions that apparently persisted throughout the 2-week hospital stay. Maldonado was noted by the hospital staff to be withdrawn and guarded. His grooming was described as "very good." He had received regular visits from his "wife" during the admission. It was discovered that she had been bringing him unauthorized Xanax. When confronted about this, he filed a 72-hour letter for release and consulted with a lawyer. He later agreed to remain in the hospital to complete the full course of treatment. He was placed on lower doses of methadone and was also prescribed Risperdal, Zyprexa, nortriptyline, alprazolam, and sodium valproate. He exhibited little change in his reporting of "psychotic" symptoms in response to treatment. He continued to report hearing voices and stated that he felt "radioactive." In contrast, there were no signs of any other unusual behavior. He showed little interaction with patients or staff members. He preferred to spend time sitting alone and reading, minding his own business.

Maldonado left St. Vincent's on September 2, 2001. Discharge records listed a primary diagnosis of schizophrenia, paranoid type. There were no indications of any previous psychotic behavior in Maldonado's past. There was no family history of schizophrenia. This psychiatric admission appeared to me to have come "out of the blue." At the age of 45 years, Maldonado was rather old to be presenting with a first episode of schizophrenia. Furthermore, the behavior described in the hospital records was not typical of that seen in other psychotic individuals I had encountered in the past. Maldonado reported the presence of "positive symptoms" of schizophrenia, such as hallucinations and delusions. However, there were no observations of any emotional blunting or other "negative symptoms" that are also known to characterize the disorder. There was also a notable lack of response to standard treatment. After looking at all of these elements together, I started to become skeptical about this hospital admission.

A few days later, I hailed a cab to One Hogan Place, the renowned location of the Manhattan District Attorney's Office. After passing through a security check with metal detectors, I met with ADA Vincent McKinney on the sixth floor. Mr. McKinney is a polite young man who offered me a seat in his cluttered office. The wall was plastered with *Godfather* posters and newspaper clippings of Yankees World Series victories—decorations I have found common to many of these offices. After initial pleasantries, I informed Mr. McKinney of my doubts on the validity of Maldonado's insanity defense. We discussed the options of how I should proceed in my role as a psychological expert in this case. I explained the pros and cons of simply having me prepare a report based on available records. He was rather insistent that I meet with the defendant directly and examine him through methods of my choice. We made an appointment for me to return in 3 weeks to perform an interview and neuropsychological testing.

The other goal of my visit was to review additional records. Mr. McKinney told me that he had a lot of information on this case. He asked me, "What do you want to see?" My response was, "Everything." This is a topic where the opinions of psychologists working in a forensic setting tend to differ. Many believe in the sanctity of the direct examination of the defendant. They feel confident that the information that they obtain in the interview and testing will provide them with all of the elements they need to fully understand the intentions and state of mind of the defendant at the time of the incident offense. Others extend the scope of their investigations to include a complete review of the forensic evidence, which enables them to provide a larger context for interpreting the results of the psychological examination. The goal is to see if all of the pieces fit. This second group of practitioners is often accused by the other group as trying to be "gumshoes"—amateur versions of the forensic investigators seen in popular television shows.

My approach to both clinical and forensic work is more consistent with that of the latter group. I have found it valuable in previous cases to visit crime scenes, view relevant photos, and read autopsy reports. In this case, I was taken to an empty office. Mr. McKinney wheeled in a cart of boxes filled with records and other evidence. He smiled and said, "Dig in, Doc." I started with the tape of Maldonado's initial call to 911. In listening to it, I had the chilling experience of hearing his calm voice explain everything to the operator in an organized and sequential manner. At one point, there was a long delay on the operator's end, and he correctly reminded her of where they had left off. This was clearly not the voice and behavior of a man who was in the midst of psychosis.

I pulled out an envelope labeled "Crime Scene Photos." The first consisted of a partially clad blonde in her late 40s lying face up on a convertible bed. This was my first introduction to Kim Martin. In seeing her face, my view of her was transformed from the vague concept of a victim in this case to that of a person with a life that was ended abruptly at that moment in time. Other photos depicted a medium-sized studio apartment in disarray. I was struck by the fact that the apartment was filled with piles of comic books. Some were in plastic wrappings displayed throughout the room, on shelves. The image of a dead woman lying amidst these comic books was a bizarre sight that will haunt me forever. The autopsy report indicated that the cause of death was strangulation and multiple stab wounds to the torso. There were a total of 16 stab wounds, including defensive wounds to the left hand and right leg.

I proceeded to review a folder of financial records. According to the credit card statements, Maldonado had been supplied for many years with a steady flow of men's clothing from Bloomingdale's and Saks Fifth Avenue. There were also numerous purchases from comic book stores and online vendors. The couple had apparently gone on a 2-week Caribbean cruise in February 2001. Pharmacy records from the local drug store indicated that Maldonado was receiving regular prescriptions for Xanax from a "Dr. Brown" on the Lower East Side. I learned that Xanax is a popular drug of abuse among methadone users. I was informed by my colleagues in the psychiatry department that Dr. Brown is a notorious "psychiatry whore" who essentially sells prescriptions to those willing to pay. The pharmacy records indicated that Maldonado had been receiving a steady stream of prescriptions from Dr. Brown for at least 2 years. The large number of prescriptions for Xanax, filled at a variety of drug stores, provided a quantity of medication that would exceed what Maldonado could consume himself. It made me think that he was probably selling some of these drugs on the street. Regardless, I wondered whether Dr. Brown could shed some light on Maldonado's psychiatric history and the likelihood of the "psychotic break" in August. Mr. McKinney told me that he had left numerous messages with Dr. Brown's answering service and had not yet received a return call. In subsequent weeks, a friend of mine who knew of Dr. Brown's work told me not to expect any form of cooperation from him.

As I was completing my review of the cart full of documents, Mr. McKinney came in to the office and handed me a thick envelope filled with additional records and told me that they were copies for me to take with me. He said, "Tell me what you think after reading these." I put the envelope in my bag and headed out. As a commuter, I spend a lot of time in trains and try to use this "quiet time" for reading whenever possible. On the ride home, I pulled out the envelope to examine its contents. It was filled with photocopies of a mixture of diaries, letters, greeting cards, and records of legal activities from the mid-1980s. As I examined these materials, a very disturbing story began to emerge.

The relationship between Maldonado and Martin apparently got off to a rocky start in 1985. After meeting at Crate and Barrel, the two began dating. In Martin's diary, there were indications that she did not take the relationship very seriously. Cultural differences had a negative effect on the relationship. Her family was Irish American; his parents had moved to the United States from Cuba in 1960. Maldonado eventually stopped working at the store; Martin discovered that he had a serious problem with cocaine addiction. Within a few months, he made an unexpected marriage proposal and gave her a ring. She was not prepared to make any form of commitment to him at that time. She told him that she wanted him to receive help for the cocaine addiction. He failed a few attempts at rehabilitation. He eventually talked her into letting him move in with her, to help him "get straight."

There are indications that Martin attempted to break off the relationship on several occasions, which apparently resulted in emotional and, at times, violent exchanges with Maldonado. She eventually reported his behavior to the police and asked him to leave her apartment. In a diary entry in October 1985, she wrote, "My instincts tell me that this is just the beginning of a long and laborious relationship with the judicial system." She later wrote that she was "terrified of what might come next."

Materials from 1985 and 1986 document a tumultuous period during which Oscar Maldonado continually harassed and threatened Kim Martin, as well as many of her friends and coworkers. Police reports describe complaints of Maldonado yelling and screaming in the vicinity of Martin's apartment. He mailed her a number of threatening letters and called her frequently at her place of employment. On one occasion, he was seen throwing a filled garbage can through the window of the store where she was working as a manager. He was caught writing bad checks, using her address as a place of residence. On one occasion, he sent a telegram to her employer, stating that she had resigned. On another occasion, he sent the employer nude photos he had taken of her in the past. Orders of protection were issued in 1986.

During Kim Martin's "laborious" relationship with the judicial system, she developed a good working relationship with the ADA who had been assigned to her case. Maldonado violated the orders of protection repeatedly. At one point, he is quoted as saying that he would get a gun and shoot the ADA if Martin called the police. Similar threats were made against her employer and fellow employees. Notes from the ADA describe Maldonado as "obviously dangerous and acts in conscious disregard to lawful court orders."

Kim Martin had provided the DA's Office with a large bundle of letters that Maldonado had written to her. Some indicate how much he loves her; others indicate his contempt for her, as in "Kim I hate you. Your [sic] nothing but a low life whore." He later wrote that he loved her and that he would be buying her another ring. There are numerous indications that he was feeling disappointed and slighted by her. In one instance, he wrote, "You always treated me cold, so cold." Other letters state, "You lie to me you used me up then threw the unwanted part away." He continues with, "Everything you touch goes bad" and "You were too selfish to share anything, much less yourself." In a Christmas card with a happy-looking exterior, he writes, "I'll give anything for your death" and "You are a scumbag bitch."

In subsequent communications, Maldonado asks for forgiveness. At one point, he stated that he had a job and was beginning to "act like a man." The records indicate that he pleaded guilty to several misdemeanors related to his harassment of Martin and his threats against others. These included criminal contempt of court and tampering with a witness. He threatened to take his own life, as well as the lives of several others, including Martin. In one note he stated that he would kill her and, if charged with manslaughter, he "could get off after 2 years with an insanity plea." In a presentence memorandum, the ADA stated, "The defendant poses a threat to Ms. King and to the numerous others he has threatened as well as to the community at large." He served a sentence of 6 months of confinement at Rikers Island.

NEUROPSYCHOLOGICAL EVALUATION

Interview Information

I was first introduced to Oscar Maldonado on November 20, 2002, as he was escorted in handcuffs into an examination room on the ninth floor of One Hogan Place by two NYPD detectives. He had curly black hair that needed trimming and a scruffy "salt-and-pepper" beard. He was outfitted in a gray sweatshirt and sweatpants and a pair of black Converse All-Stars. It was apparent that he was once a very handsome man, although it looked like time in prison had taken a toll on him. He had very dark eyes that could be piercing at times. He was approximately 5'9" and was somewhat overweight. He told me later that he had gained 35 pounds since his incarceration. The handcuffs were removed, and he was seated in a chair across a table from me.

Also seated in the room was the defendant's attorney, "Mr. Albert Gunderman." I had met this man for the first time earlier in the day and was struck immediately by his unruly mop of gray hair and disorganized manner, resembling the stereotype of the New York defense attorney portrayed in the movies and on TV. Vincent McKinney and his trial assistant filled the two other chairs in the room. All were seated behind the defendant. The lawyers had agreed that they would observe the interview only. The detectives would sit outside of the room in an adjacent vestibule. It had been determined that the interview would be videotaped through a two-way mirror and transcribed by a court reporter. Copies of the transcripts would be available to all relevant parties. I actually welcome situations where I can obtain transcripts of my interview, because it frees me from taking such copious notes and allows me to go "with the flow" of the defendant's responses. Consistent with standardized procedures, none of the individuals mentioned would be present for either of the next two sessions, when I would be administering a battery of neuropsychological tests and recording responses on appropriate test forms.

I began with the formalities of explaining my role in the legal proceedings, the nature of the examination, and the limits of confidentiality. The defendant indicated that he understood the charges against him and the issues that I had presented. He comprehended the need to answer my questions in a truthful manner and to give his best effort during subsequent testing. I began the formal questioning by ascertaining his current state of mind. He responded to my questions with brief answers, with his head slumped. There was little eye contact. His facial expression and comportment appeared mildly depressed. (My impression was that he was an intelligent and articulate man.) His speech was organized, and his behavior was totally appropriate for the situation.

Maldonado stated that he felt bad about a number of things and gave a vague description of transgressions from his past. He admitted to having an explosive temper that had gotten him into trouble on a number of occasions. He described a couple of fights that he had had in jail, in response to others laying a hand on him. He reported "hearing things" in the past. He stated that he began to experience auditory hallucinations approximately 2 years earlier. Most of the content of his report referred to "crazy things" he had done in the past to his family and friends. The defendant admitted to saying things to get into the hospital in August

2001. These "things" included reports of hearing voices and stating that he was going to kill himself. He felt at a point where he was "getting crazy," thinking that people were out to get him. He admitted to telling the psychiatrist that he had hurt somebody, even though it was not true. He had been treated with Risperdal and Effexor since his incarceration. He had not heard any voices since March 2002.

During the course of the 2-hour interview, I learned more about the defendant's past history. He provided details about his family and his education. However, I was not able to validate any of this information, as his family refused to speak with anybody related to this case, including the defense attorney. In subsequent calls to local colleges and business firms, I was unable to confirm many of the educational and occupational entries that were listed on Maldonado's resume and discussed during the interview. I was also unable to find any information to support his description of a previous psychiatric hospitalization at the Bronx Psychiatric Center for an alleged psychotic break when he was in his 20s.

I turned the topic of questioning to his relationship to Kim Martin. He finally raised his head and, for the first time, looked me in the eye. He described how they had met and "fallen in love." He stated that the thing he liked best about her was that she was "smart." He indicated that there was "nothing wrong" with her. When I brought up the records on harassment and his previous incarceration, he responded with insistence that he had never hit her. He chalked up those experiences to a number of unfortunate misunderstandings and emphasized that he and Kim had had a "deep and loving relationship," until the end.

In response to inquiry about the events of October 2001, the defendant stressed that he was taking a number of medications after the discharge from St. Vincent's. He reported that the voices were continuing, but they never told him to hurt anybody. He denied having any anger toward, or arguments with, Kim on or around the time of the murder. He stated that he had not been getting much sleep and was not feeling well as a result of hearing things. He felt that the medications had messed him up badly. He stated that he remembered grabbing her on that day and that she responded by stating that he was hurting her. He said that he let her go and could not remember anything else from that point onward. He simply denied all discrepancies from his current story when confronted with the information obtained from records and other interviews. We concluded the interview. On his way out of the room, Mr. Gunderman shook my hand and complimented me on my interview style and my use of "open-ended" questions. The defendant was taken back to

Rikers Island. I returned to my office to digest the information obtained during that afternoon.

Up until the time of the interview, I had been considering a number of ways to conceptualize what had happened in this case. A few aspects had become more apparent to me after the interview, as a result of seeing the defendant in person and hearing his responses to my direct questions. As I saw it, this was a man with the redeeming features of reasonable intelligence and good looks, who had a bad drug problem. He was clearly using Kim Martin as a meal ticket, whether or not they truly loved each other. While she worked hard and saw her career progress, he was able to hang around and do whatever pleased him. The major unanswered question was, what did *she* get out of the relationship?—which is probably something I would never find out, given the information with which I was working. Information from a number of sources would later indicate that she had finally had enough of him in the summer of 2001 and was trying to force him out of her life. Some of the facts pointed to a conclusion that she was murdered once another man came into her life.

Looking back, it was clear that Maldonado was not the mentally deficient individual depicted in Dr. Sandelson's psychological report for the defense. I was struck, however, by Dr. Sandelson's use of the term "pseudo-neurotic schizophrenia" to describe the defendant's behavior. As a result of my prior education in psychoanalytic theory as a graduate student in New York, I remembered that this was one of the early terms used to describe what is now commonly known as borderline personality disorder. Behavior of this nature was clearly evident in the materials that I had reviewed for this case. Maldonado had proposed to Martin rather unexpectedly and prematurely, by most standards. There was evidence in the letters of a "love–hate" relationship, representing the effects of splitting. I was also very struck by the degree of idealization that Maldonado held for Martin, even after he had killed her. But the most significant evidence was seen in the degree of rage he exhibited during the course of his harassment of Martin in the 1980s. For some reason, this rage apparently remained "bottled up" for a long period, as long as he was getting what he wanted. It obviously surfaced again when she renewed her interest in ending the relationship.

I had been bothered by the psychiatric admission 2 months prior to the murder. I had to determine whether Maldonado was, in fact, experiencing symptoms of psychosis at that time. Given the specifics of the law, a documentation of psychosis within weeks of the offense would not necessarily address the legal question of insanity at the time of the murder, but it would be important to know whether there was any semblance of validity to the defense's argument. In my opinion, the nature of the episode described in the hospital record was atypical for schizophrenia. For example, the episode appeared to have come from "out of the blue." From my initial reading, I had wondered whether Maldonado's hospitalization represented something similar to what had been described in the famous study by Rosenhan (1973), wherein graduate students were able to get themselves admitted to the psychiatric unit of a local hospital simply as a result of reporting to hear voices. I was rather surprised during the interview when Maldonado admitted to me that he had, in fact, fabricated the report of voices to get himself into the hospital. I remembered reading that, in the 1980s, he had threatened to kill Martin and use the insanity defense to get off. He had said it all before. I could not believe that now he might actually be trying to pull it off.

Behavioral Observations

I take a hypothesis-driven approach to neuropsychological assessment. My belief is that the neuropsychologist develops a series of initial hypotheses based on records and other available information. The goal of the interview and testing is thus to confirm or, importantly, disconfirm these hypotheses. One should also leave open the possibility for other theories to emerge during the examination. My impression in this case was that Maldonado was a manipulative, drug-abusing guy who had murdered his long-term girlfriend once she wanted to get rid of him. Faced with the results of the defense's examination, the goals of my testing were to attempt to replicate the findings of mental subnormality, demonstrate the presence or absence of neuropsychological impairment, and determine whether the defendant exhibited any form of psychotic illness. All along I would be paying close attention to the possibility that this may be someone who is malingering the presence of mental illness. As a result, my battery included a number of tests for assessing motivation and effort.

In my next two encounters with the defendant, I administered a series of 14 neuropsychological tests. I also conducted a structured interview for assessing the validity of his psychiatric complaints. He completed three self-report questionnaires. I reminded him about the limits of confidentiality prior to each test session. He was interested in knowing how long each test session would last and what types of materials he would be using. He was outwardly cooperative. There were no obvious difficulties with comprehending or following test instructions or with manipulating any of the test materials. There were initial remarks that he was having difficulties with visualizing the stimuli. These ceased after I pointed out to him that he had not reported any such difficulty when working with similar materials in the previous psychological examination. He approached some of the tests in a hasty or impulsive manner. In some cases, he remained expressionless when giving what appeared to be outrageously wrong responses to easy questions. I repeated the need for him to give his best possible level of performance on every test.

During the second day of examination, Maldonado was presented with the MMPI-2 at 3:30 P.M., after completing other tests over the previous 2 hours. We were scheduled to continue until 5:00 P.M. on that day. He expressed a concern about missing the bus back to Rikers Island, which would mean, according to him, that he would not receive dinner that night. I informed him that the 567-item questionnaire would likely take 60–90 minutes to complete. I gave him the option of stopping at that point, emphasizing that we would then need to return to complete the examination at another time. Hearing that, he decided to proceed with the questionnaire, as scheduled. I monitored his progress over the next 45 minutes. At one point, I observed that he was filling in the responses rather quickly. I repeated to him that it was in his favor to complete the inventory as accurately and as truthfully as possible. He gave me a disdainful look and proceeded to mark the questions in a rapid and seemingly more haphazard manner. He decided that he was finished and that it was time to make it to the bus. I was struck by how the immediate interest in dinner, getting out of testing, and possibly working against his defense were more important to him than facing the much longer-term consequence of a life sentence in prison on a murder conviction. I realized that this focus on short-term gain is also likely to be the cause of his propensity for drug abuse, violence, and murder.

Test Results

The neuropsychological test data are listed in Table 14.3. To supplement testing of intelligence, I administered the Validity Indicator Profile (VIP). Maldonado's scores were invalid, with a performance curve indicating that he had approached the test in an inconsistent and careless manner. As I suspected, the defendant's performance was not an accurate indication of his true ability. I recalled that similar findings were apparent in his performance on Dr. Sandelson's administration of the Raven

Matrices. Now I had evidence in both examinations that the defendant's low scores on IQ tests were the result of poor effort, rather than any purported limitation in his level of intelligence.

The defendant's scores on other neuropsychological tests were variable. Scores providing additional evidence of insufficient effort were not obtained using commonly employed "malingering tests," such as the Rey 15-Item Memory Test and the Test of Memory Malingering (TOMM). The defendant obtained a reliable digit span score of 5, which is in the range associated with reduced effort, similar to what was observed in the previous examination.

Scores from measures of mood and personality are presented in Table 14.4. The defendant completed the Structured Interview of Reported Symptoms (SIRS), which is a measure developed for evaluating the validity of an individual's reported symptoms of psychopathology. This measure exemplifies the difference between attempts to malinger a mental illness, such as schizophrenia, and attempts to portray oneself as having some form of neurocognitive impairment, such as memory loss. Maldonado's profile of verbal responses was considered to be "honest" on seven of the eight scales, which generally means that he denied having many unusual symptoms that are rarely seen in patients with bona fide psychiatric illness. The only exception was a score in the "indeterminate" range on a measure of selectivity of symptoms. When administering this test, I was struck by the observation that Maldonado was close to smiling or laughing in response to some questions regarding outrageous symptoms.

On standard self-report indices, Maldonado endorsed an extremely high level of depressive affect with minimal feelings of anxiety. The MMPI-2 profile was invalid as a result of extreme elevations on the standard F scale and similar elevations on the additional F(B) and F(p) scales. When examining this profile, I recalled Maldonado's haphazard approach to responding to the items at the end of this test and its likely effects on the final profile of scores. He therefore failed to reproduce the profiles of response exhibited in Dr. Sandelson's administration of standardized personality inventories obtained 6 months earlier.

I administered the Rorschach Inkblot Method, consistent with Exner's Comprehensive System. The result was a total of 11 responses, which is well below the number required for obtaining a valid profile of scores. Remember that the same behavior was observed in response to the Rorschach during the previous examination. After presenting the cards personally, it was again my sense that Maldonado wanted nothing to do with these inkblots.

TABLE 14.3. Cognitive Test Results for Defendant O. M. Obtained from Prosecution Expert

	Raw score	Norms
Wechsler Abbreviated Scale of Intelligence		
Vocabulary	53	$T = 44$
Matrix Reasoning	11	$T = 34$
Estimated Full Scale IQ		78
Validity Indicator Profile		
Verbal Subtest		Invalid/Careless
Nonverbal Subtest		Invalid/Careless
North American Adult Reading Test		
Estimated Full Scale IQ	51 errors	88
Wechsler Adult Intelligence Scale–III Digit Span	5 F, 3 B	Scaled score = 4
Symbol Digit Modalities Test	32	$Z = -2.4$
Stroop Color–Word Test		
Word Score	77	$T = 38$
Color Score	58	$T = 38$
Color–Word Score	37	$T = 37$
Color Trails Test		
Color Trails 1		
Time	41	$T = 48$
Errors	0	
Color Trails 2		
Time	49	$T = 49$
Errors	2	
Controlled Oral Word Association Test	20	$Z = -2.3$
Wisconsin Card Sorting Test		
Categories	5	11–16%
Total Errors	38	$T = 37$
Perseverative Responses	20	$T = 39$
Failure to Maintain Set	1	> 16%
Hopkins Verbal Learning Test–Revised		
Total Learning	16	$Z = -3.3$
Trial 3 Recall	7	$Z = -3.3$
Long Delay Free Recall	3	$Z = -4.3$
Recognition Discrimination	9	$Z = -2.0$
Brief Visuospatial Memory Test–Revised		
Total Learning	15	$T = 30$
Trial 3 Recall	6	$T = 27$
Long Delay Free Recall	4	$T = 22$
Recognition Discrimination	6	
Rey 15-item Memory Test	12 correct	
Rey Word Recognition Test	9 correct	
Reliable Digit Span	5	

(continued)

TABLE 14.3. *(continued)*

	Raw score
Test of Memory Malingering	
Trial 1	46
Trial 2	50

TABLE 14.4. Personality Test Results for Defendant O. M. Obtained from Prosecution Expert

Structured Interview for Reported Symptoms

RS	1	Honest
SC	3	Indeterminate
IA	0	Honest
BL	3	Honest
SU	7	Honest
SEL	7	Honest
SEV	3	Honest
RO	3	Honest
DA	4	
DS	15	
OS	0	
SO	2	
INC	5	

Beck Depression Inventory–2   Raw score = 36

Beck Anxiety Inventory   Raw score = 4

Minnesota Multiphasic Personality Inventory–2

VRIN	15	$T = 88$
TRIN	12	$T = 72T$
F	26	$T = 116$
F(B)	25	$T = 120$
Fp	15	$T = 120$
L	9	$T = 74$
K	17	$T = 54$
S	28	$T = 53$
FBS		
Scale 1 (Hs)	9	$T = 68$
Scale 2 (D)	32	$T = 78$
Scale 3 (Hy)	26	$T = 61$
Scale 4 (Pd)	28	$T = 79$
Scale 5 (Mf)	17	$T = 32$
Scale 6 (Pa)	14	$T = 79$
Scale 7 (Pt)	17	$T = 98$
Scale 8 (Sc)	17	$T = 98$
Scale 9 (Ma)	3	$T = 65$
Scale 0 (Si)	28	$T = 54$

Rorschach Inkblot Test
  Number of responses = 11
  Psychotic Thinking Index = 1

Mr. McKinney informed me that he had a court date in 2 weeks, and he would need to have my report in hand before that deadline. I informed him that I needed to complete one last part of my examination. I had reviewed records, conducted an interview, and obtained test data from the defendant. However, I had not yet conducted any collateral interviews. I explained to Mr. McKinney the importance of speaking with those who had known both the defendant and the victim before and at the time of the murder. This kind of contact would enable me to obtain important information about the defendant's behavior that may or may not corroborate what is depicted in the psychological reports. In this case, Dr. Sandelson's contact was limited to a telephone conversation with one of Oscar Maldonado's sisters, who had said that she knew her brother was eventually going to get into "big time" trouble. The rest of the family refused to get involved in this case. Mr. McKinney called me with a list of phone numbers of individuals who had agreed to speak with me. All of them were family, friends, or neighbors of Kim Martin. Mr. McKinney reminded me that he still needed my report in 2 weeks.

I made a telephone call to "Mr. Evan Martin," the victim's brother, who is a member of the fire department of a medium-sized city in another state. He informed me that he is the only surviving member of his family; his parents had both passed away over 20 years ago as a result of cancer. He told me that he had never met Maldonado, even though his sister had been seeing him for a number of years. The defendant had refused to accompany her for yearly holiday trips to see him and his family. She would never give many details about their relationship. She stated at one point that he was a Vietnam veteran who was taking medication. At another point, she said that he was a mental health counselor. Mr. Martin told me that the Maldonado always sounded "loaded" when he picked up the phone. He said that the guy sounded like a control freak, making his sister feel guilty about any source of contact with her family. He apologized that he did not have any more detailed information for me. He also thanked me for working on behalf of his sister.

I made several telephone calls to the numbers remaining on my list and had to leave messages. I was surprised that nearly everybody returned my calls. Ms. Martin's coworkers described her as an excellent worker who was "very professional." She kept her personal life very separate from them. None of them had actually met Maldonado; some thought that she was married to him. From the different accounts, it appeared that she had given different stories to different people. One particular individual had been working with Ms. Martin during the period of harassment in the 1980s. She said that it was a very bizarre period of time and that Kim had been fearful for her life throughout its course. Those who lived in the same building as the couple had noted a decline in Maldonado's appearance and behavior over the past 10 years, which they generally attributed to the influence of drugs. His behavior was described as erratic: He could be helpful at times, carrying bags into the elevator for them; at other times, he could be menacing. He had once threatened to kill an old man for giving him a "funny look." These residents gave the impression that everyone in the entire building was scared of this guy, including Kim Martin.

I had now obtained all of the information that I was likely to get. It was time for me to get to work on the report. The majority of my clinical reports are three pages long, whereas medical–legal reports may reach 10 pages. Criminal reports, especially those involving the insanity defense, are typically much longer. In this case, it took me a very long time to review pages of my notes and copies of records that I had obtained. I needed to examine carefully the results from both psychological evaluations. I had to come to some form of organization of all of this material. Over the course of a long weekend (Thursday through Sunday), I produced a 17-page report.

It has been my observation that the diagnoses proffered by many defense experts consist of vague terminology, such as "neuropsychological impairment" or "emotional distress." I try to counter these with a full DSM-IV diagnosis, in order to provide the court with something more tangible. I was not in a position where I could simply offer a description of "insufficient effort" to characterize the defendant's performance in the examination. In the end, I concluded that he was malingering the presence of cognitive and mental impairment. This opinion was based primarily on the many irregularities present in the records and on the data obtained from both psychological examinations.

I felt that there was also sufficient evidence to indicate some form of depressive reaction, in the form of an adjustment disorder on Axis I. There was also evidence to support a diagnosis of polysubstance abuse, with abstinence in a controlled environment. Information from numerous sources indicated the pattern of idealization, splitting, and rageful outbursts that are seen in individuals with borderline personality disorder. In this case, I gave an Axis II diagnosis of personality disorder not otherwise specified. I concluded, finally, that Maldonado's behavior was not consistent with someone who was not able to appreciate the nature and consequences of his actions at the time of the murder. I believed that he was acutely aware of what he was doing on the date of October 29, 2001.

TRIAL TESTIMONY

Mr. McKinney called to thank me for the comprehensive report. He informed me that I would need to leave some time open in my schedule in March for the upcoming trial. According to the prosecution's trial strategy, I would be called as a witness in rebuttal to Dr. Sandelson's testimony. In some cases, when serving as a rebuttal witness, the court allows me into the courtroom to be present for the testimony of the defense witness. As a result, I am able to observe the testimony directly and offer advice to the prosecutor, if needed, regarding points to be covered in the cross-examination. Mr. McKinney informed me that he would be asking for permission to allow me to observe Dr. Sandelson's testimony.

At the beginning of the trial, the judge granted the prosecution's request to allow me to be present in the courtroom for the defense expert's testimony. I arrived at the criminal courthouse at 60 Centre Street on March 12, accompanied by one of my postdoctoral fellows. I encountered Mr. McKinney. He introduced me to Ms. Martin's brother, who had come from out of state to attend the trial. I met Dr. Sandelson and exchanged pleasantries in the outer hallway. He was accompanied by his college-age daughter. We all entered the large courtroom together, then proceeded to sit on opposite sides of the room. There were approximately 10–15 people seated in the audience, including a reporter from the *Daily News*. The defendant was brought into the courtroom in handcuffs and was seated at the defense table. The judge and jury entered the room. We were ready to begin with the day's testimony.

Dr. Sandelson was called to the witness box. He gave his oath and was accepted quickly by the court as a psychological expert for the defense. Copies of any notes taken in the courtroom must be given to the opposing counsel. I listened attentively, without taking notes, as Dr. Sandelson responded to 2 hours of questions issued to him by the defense counsel, Mr. Gunderman. The testimony started with an account of the defendant's "terrible" childhood. Maldonado was depicted as an intelligent and accomplished man who had battled mental illness in the form of a "pseudo-neurotic" schizophrenia for much of his life. He relayed to the jury information that Maldonado had given him in the interview, including the hospitalization at Bronx Psychiatric Center and his college education. I sat there knowing that none of this information was supported in the records. The testimony proceeded with a detailed description of the psychiatric hospitalization in August and the sequence of events that eventually led to the murder of Kim Martin 2 months later.

According to the defense expert's analysis, Oscar Maldonado had suffered from severe anxiety for most of his life. He was able to manage it for the most part, although there were occasions when the response to stresses in his life resulted in a psychotic break and psychiatric hospitalization. He eventually turned to drugs to cope with this anxiety. For undetermined reasons, the anxiety became more severe in the Summer of 2001, causing another psychotic break. This culminated in the hospitalization in August. Maldonado continued to hear voices from that time onward. These voices eventually commanded him to hurt Kim Martin. On October 29, he had simply succumbed to these voices and killed Martin out of an "unfathomable" level of anxiety. The psychological test data were described to be supportive of the fact that Maldonado continues to be confused and anxious, much as he was at the time of the murder. There was no mention of the history of harassment that occurred in the 1980s.

Mr. McKinney conducted a 2-hour cross-examination, with requests for Dr. Sandelson to provide information from the records supporting the history of mental illness. He queried the expert on the validity of the defendant's psychological test data. Dr. Sandelson admitted that he had turned down an opportunity to review the forensic records, including the correspondence between Maldonado and Martin, because he felt that it would not be relevant to the case. He countered that he felt strongly about the quality of the psychological data and felt no need to go beyond that. The prosecutor guided him to an admission that his conclusion was based largely on his personal interpretation of many qualitative aspects of the defendant's test responses, rather than any empirically validated data.

I entered the witness stand at 10:00 the following morning. Mr. McKinney reviewed my credentials for the court. The defense counsel argued that I was not a real "forensic psychologist" and stipulated that I be entered in the trial simply as a "neuropsychological expert" for this case. The prosecutor felt no need to argue against this stipulation. In the following hours, he conducted a direct examination covering my review of the medical records and additional material. I highlighted the previous harassment and the history of drug abuse; however, I was not able to discuss the defendant's past criminal record. I gave the jury a description of the fear depicted in Martin's letters. I expressed my skepticism about the details of hospitalization in August 2001.

I find that there are a number of similarities between teaching a class and testifying before a jury. In both settings I do my best to explain my ideas using simple terminology. There are those who are either attentive or inattentive. Some make consistent eye contact and nod in acceptance of what I am saying. Others look cranky and skeptical. Mr. McKinney asked me to explain to the jury how a neuropsychologist looks for evidence of malingering. He asked me to specify the similarities and differences between the test results obtained from my examination and those obtained by Dr. Sandelson. He concluded by asking me to review the diagnostic conclusions offered in my test report. The prosecution completed the direct examination by the 1:00 lunch break. Instructed by the judge not to discuss the case or my testimony with anybody during the break, I proceeded to have a lonely lunch in nearby Chinatown.

I returned to the witness stand at 2:00 in the afternoon. When given the cue, Mr. Gunderson greeted me and began with the cross-examination by attacking my ability to be sympathetic to the defendant and asked if I was "that way" with all of my patients. The latter, of course, was met with an objection by Mr. McKinney and was sustained by the judge. The attorney questioned the depth of my experience with psychotic patients. I informed him that I had not only worked with such patients clinically, but I had also been involved in many years of research on schizophrenia. The questioning turned to the topic of why I had rejected the claim that the defendant was psychotic at the time of the murder. The questioning continued until adjournment at 5:00. It would be necessary for me to return to following day for additional testimony.

The defense counsel began the following day's questions with details on the hospitalization at St. Vincent's. He became angry when I told him of many of the atypical features of that hospitalization and the number of contradictions that were present in the record. He raised his voice a number of times, resulting in warnings from the judge. Many members of the jury were smiling at this display. At one point, Mr. Gunderson asked me directly if I thought that the hospital admission had been orchestrated by the defendant intentionally. I simply told him that I could not exclude that possibility. This was followed by more details regarding the psychological test data. The cross-examination was concluded by 11:30 A.M. The judge thanked me for my time and told me that I was dismissed from the courtroom.

OUTCOME OF THE CASE

I find that attorneys rarely take the time to contact me after I leave the witness stand. I often find out about the resulting verdict through word of mouth or, in some cases, by reports on the radio. In this case, Mr. McKinney called me a few days after the trial to inform me that the jury had convicted Maldonado of murder in the second degree. He thanked me for all of my efforts and told me to send my time sheets and expenses to the DA's office for processing. He told me that a sentencing hearing would be held on April 29. I returned to my office and cleared the crowded windowsill behind my desk of the piles of records and files from this case and sent them for filing, then turned my attention back to the clinical reports that had accumulated during the time I had spent at the trial.

I have attended sentencing hearings for a few of my criminal cases. In this case, I was facing a number of deadlines at the end of April. I was cognizant of the fact that Maldonado was to be sentenced at that time. I scanned the newspapers to see if anything was reported, but found nothing. I did not let my curiosity go far enough to making a call to the DA's office to find out what happened. A few weeks later, I received a letter signed by the Manhattan District Attorney. It informed me that Maldonado had been sentenced to a term of 22 years to life in state prison. I was thanked for my cooperation in the case. I thought about the fate of Kim Martin and the finality of it all as I placed the letter in the file, put it away, and closed the file drawer.

LESSONS LEARNED

I was struck by the fact that two people could live together for many years in one of the world's largest cities, yet nobody around them really knew much about their life together. Much of the hardest work in this case resulted from having to reconstruct the lives of both the defendant and the victim through available records. The task would have been much easier if I had been able to obtain more information from individuals who had known both of them, saw them interacting, and had some sense of what kind of relationship they had. The individuals I contacted provided only limited information. Others who had potentially more useful information refused to speak to me.

Looking back, I wish that I had been able to find at least one person who had some understanding of why Martin and Maldonado had stayed together for so many years. Contacting Maldonado's treating psychiatrist would have provided greater insight into his drug history. He also might have given me names of individuals with whom he interacted "on the street." A discussion with the treating physicians at St. Vincent's might have resulted in learning more about the hospital admission occurring in the months prior to the murder. I often wonder who it was that drove Martin home in the van on the night before the murder. What did he or she know? All of these questions make it clear to me that forensic work involves an integration of much more information than is provided in a series of test responses.

REFERENCES

Rosenhan, D. L. (1973). On being sane in insane places. *Science, 179*, 250–258.

15

Murder in Chicago
Insanity and Tragedy

ROBERT E. HANLON
MICHAEL W. MAYFIELD

BACKGROUND INFORMATION

On August 28, 1999, a family of six, including four adults and two children, were walking down 35th Street on the south side of Chicago on their way to a White Sox game at Comiskey Park. It was approximately 4:30 on a sunny afternoon, and they were going to stop at O'Malley's for hot dogs before going to the game. Upon reaching the corner of 35th Street and Lowe, about four blocks from the ball park, a 19-year-old man stepped out of an alley and attacked the family with a large wooden table leg. Eleven people witnessed the assault, including two children and nine police officers. The police station of the 9th district of the Chicago Police Department is located on the corner of 35th Street and Lowe.

Following the attack and the arrest of the offender, the investigation report of the Chicago Police Department documented the following:

> The offender in custody attacked the victims. He struck Victim #1 with a long, large table leg. Victim #1 fell to the ground with a massive head wound and was lying next to a white Dodge auto. The offender then struck Victim #2 with the large table leg. Victim #2 also had a massive blunt trauma to his

head. He then turned to the other victim (Victim #3), and stated "do you want some." He then struck Victim #3 with the table leg. Victim #3 also fell to the ground, next to Victim #1. At this time the other victim (Victim #4) was attempting to run to the north side of 35th Street. The offender chased her into the street and struck her in the head. During this time the witnesses, police officers came to the victims' aid, subdued the offender, and summoned medical aid for the victims.

After the offender was subdued and handcuffed, he was taken into the police station on the corner. He was advised of his rights at approximately 5:30 P.M., but he refused to talk. At 6:30 P.M., he was advised of his rights again, but he refused to talk. At approximately 11:30 P.M., he was advised of his rights again, and he reportedly stated that "it was personal." At 11:30 A.M. on August 29, he was advised of his rights and acknowledged that he understood his rights. With regard to previous arrests, the offender stated that he had been arrested twice, for traffic violations. According to the report of the police investigation, the 19-year-old offender stated that he lived with his aunt. He had left her house the morning of August 28 and "just walked," stopping to have a Big Mac. He subsequently found a table leg under a railroad viaduct, picked it up, and carried it with him. In response to questioning regarding the reason for the attack, he reportedly stated that all he wanted was their money. He was subsequently charged with four counts of attempted murder and four counts of aggravated battery. Figure 15.1 is a crime scene photograph of the weapon (i.e., wooden table leg) used in the attack. Figure 15.2 is a photograph of the crime scene; the police station is in the foreground, and Comiskey Park, home of the Chicago White Sox, is in the background.

I originally became aware of the crime through television news reports and articles in the *Chicago Tribune*. The media focused on one pertinent aspect of the crime: the fact that the victims were white and the attacker was a black male. On August 31, 1999, a writer for the *Chicago Tribune* wrote that "an ugly racial incident happened in Chicago's Bridgeport neighborhood over the weekend" (Kass, 1999a). However, he also noted that both the police and the Cook County State's Attorney had stated that they did not believe it was a hate crime. Subsequently, Richard Daley, the mayor of Chicago, announced that he did not believe that the attack was a hate crime. On September 1, 1999, Mr. Kass of the *Chicago Tribune* wrote "if the races were reversed [i.e., whites attacking blacks] the

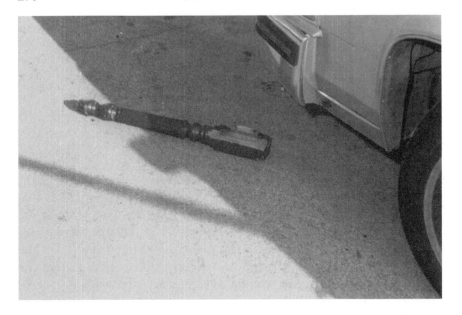

FIGURE 15.1. The weapon (i.e., wooden table leg) used in the attack.

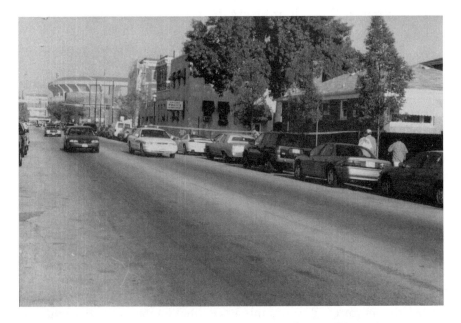

FIGURE 15.2. Crime scene: Police station is in the foreground and Comiskey Park is in the background.

activists, the politicians, the media, all of us would have reacted differently" (Kass, 1999b).

Two months following the attack, Victim 2 died of injuries sustained in the beating. He died in coma, having never regained consciousness following the assault. As a result, the charges against the offender were upgraded to first-degree murder. Ultimately, he was charged with three counts of first-degree murder (i.e., due to different legal classifications of the same crime), three counts of attempted first-degree murder, and eleven counts of aggravated battery.

At the time, I had been conducting forensic neuropsychological evaluations for 10 years. During the first few years of my involvement in forensic cases, I was frequently asked to testify as a treating neuropsychologist in traumatic brain injury cases that resulted in personal injury or workers' compensation litigation. Gradually, I was asked to serve as an expert in forensic cases involving traumatic brain injury. After about 5 years of extensive involvement in traumatic brain injury cases, I began accepting more diverse civil cases, such as medical malpractice, fitness for duty, and guardianship.

As I expanded my forensic practice, I was increasingly approached by criminal defense attorneys and prosecutors requesting neuropsychological evaluations of criminal defendants facing charges of insurance fraud and Social Security fraud, related to allegedly fraudulent claims of disability. Later, I became involved in violent criminal cases, involving capital murder, attempted murder, and sexual assault. Initially, I conducted evaluations of death row inmates at the request of appellate defenders, primarily for purposes of mitigation. Shortly thereafter, I was increasingly requested to evaluate capital murder defendants to address issues of competency to waive Miranda rights, competency to stand trial, and insanity. At the present time, I have been performing forensic neuropsychological evaluations for 15 years.

LEGAL DEFENSE

The defense attorney appointed to the case was Michael Mayfield, Assistant Public Defender, Murder Task Force, Office of the Cook County Public Defender. Mr. Mayfield is a veteran defense attorney in the Public Defender's Office, who has represented many murder defendants. Following the death of Victim 2, Mr. Mayfield was appointed to represent the offender. When he first met him, the defendant was housed in Division 8 (psychiatric division) of the Cook County Jail. The defendant's handshake was limp, and he moved very slowly. His facial expression was blank and he appeared drugged. The defendant was unable to describe the crime. He stated that he wasn't clear about what had happened and that he wasn't sure why he was in jail. He repeatedly asked about going home and did not seem to understand that he would not be going home. The attorney tried to explain that the state was seeking the death penalty and that it was important for the defendant to understand that Mayfield was his attorney and that he should not talk to anyone else about the crime. The attorney's initial impression was that the defendant did not comprehend what he had been told and that he did not appreciate his current legal situation.

Given the fact that the defendant had attacked a family in broad daylight with many witnesses present, the attorney knew from the start that he would be using an insanity defense.

There was no indication that the defendant acted in self-defense or that he was provoked by anyone. In Mayfield's view, the attack was, on the surface, the act of a person who was insane.

After compiling all of the documentation available, including police reports, school records, records from the Department of Child and Family Services, and reports of the psychiatrists in the clinical forensic services division of the Cook County Jail, Mr. Mayfield began to search for mental health professionals to evaluate the defendant. Considering the high profile nature of the incident and the publicity that had ensued, he wanted mental health professionals with no official ties to the criminal justice system. During our initial discussion about the legal issues of the case, the attorney explained that he was pursuing an insanity defense. However, in addition to my opinion regarding the defendant's mental status at the time of the offense, my findings would also be used for mitigation purposes.

HISTORY

I had loosely followed the case in the local media. As such, I was familiar with the crime, the subsequent death of Victim 2, and the media's view of the defendant. With the exception of a couple of the death row inmates whom I had evaluated, this case had received much more media attention than any of the previous capital cases in which I had been involved.

Prior to my evaluation of the defendant, I received most of the relevant records from Mr. Mayfield, including the list and description of offenses, police reports of the incident and interrogation, records from the Department of Child and Family Services (DCFS) that included a previous psychological assessment, mental health records from Division 8 of the Cook County Jail, and other jail records. Additionally, he provided me with a letter to the Cook County Department of Corrections that would allow me access to the defendant, specifying that I would need to bring a laptop computer and electronic recording equipment into the jail, in addition to standard test materials.

A review of the relevant records revealed that the defendant had become a ward of the state at 9 years of age, as a result of neglect and chronic drug abuse by his biological mother. At the age of 10, he was referred for a psychological evaluation by the DCFS. Results included a Wechsler Intelligence Scale for Children–Revised (WISC-R) Full Scale IQ of 83, a Verbal IQ of 75, and a Performance IQ of 93. Academic grade levels, as assessed on the Wide Range Achievement Test (WRAT), were as follows: reading (3.3), spelling (2.7), arithmetic (3.1). Although he was not diagnosed with psychosis, the examination reportedly revealed borderline reality testing, poor frustration tolerance, and poor impulse control. At the age of 11, he was placed in the home of his aunt, who eventually became his foster mother. He grew up on the south side of Chicago in a neighborhood ravaged with gang violence and drug abuse. By age 13, he had joined a gang and begun selling crack cocaine.

The defendant completed the 11th grade, but he failed the 12th grade and did not graduate (GPA = 1.34). He reportedly dropped out after a friend was killed by gang members at school, and he was afraid to return to school. His legitimate work history was negligible. He had been selling marijuana and cocaine since the age of 13. With the exception of driving without a valid license, the defendant had no previous criminal charges as an adult; he had had three nonviolent criminal charges as a juvenile, but all three charges were dismissed.

Medical history was generally unremarkable. He reported that he had sustained one probable mild concussion at age 10, with brief loss of consciousness. Substance abuse history reportedly involved daily marijuana (i.e., up to 12 "black jacks" per day) and alcohol (up to a case of beer per day) beginning at age 14. However, he reported that his substance abuse had diminished significantly during the month prior to the attack.

Psychiatric history was remarkable for depression with suicidal ideation and psychosis with auditory hallucinations. He reportedly grew progressively depressed during his adolescence and on more than one occasion, he had sat alone in his room with a loaded gun, contemplating shooting himself in the head. Following the gang-related murder of his cousin in June of 1999, he reportedly began to experience auditory hallucinations. These hallucinations, which continued for several weeks, involved the voice of his cousin reassuring him that he would be OK.

According to the defendant, the next time he experienced auditory hallucinations was on the day of the attack. He reported that he heard both male and female voices that seemed to be coming from outside his head. The voices were reportedly instructive and stated: "You should kill yourself," "If you don't kill yourself, someone else will," "Someone is going to kill you," and "Leave the house." He stated that he was afraid of the voices and wanted them to stop. Additionally, he described thought broadcasting and a paranoid delusion in which he believed that the source of the voices was going to kill him.

Following his arrest and incarceration, medical records from the health services division of the Cook County Jail documented that he had an extensive drug-use history, including phencyclidine (PCP), marijuana, and heroin. However, the defendant adamantly denied a history of PCP or heroin use, and he stated that he did not understand why his jail records included such misinformation. Upon his admission to the psychiatric division of the jail on August 30, 1999, it was noted that his behavior was inappropriate, and he reported hearing voices. He was diagnosed (with rule out) schizophrenia, paranoid type, and polysubstance abuse. Two days later, on September 1, 1999, a psychologist from the criminal forensic services division of the jail diagnosed him with psychotic disorder not otherwise specified. A psychiatric examination from the criminal forensic services division 1 day later described him as paranoid with disorganized thoughts and loosening of associations. A social work evaluation on September 7, 1999, reported that the defendant stated that he had picked up the table leg because he was angry and wanted to release his anger by beating people. He also reportedly stated that he knew he was in front of a police station and that he hoped the police would shoot and kill him. During the interview, he intermittently banged his head on the table. Another social work evaluation 1 day later resulted in diagnoses of paranoid schizophrenia and polysubstance abuse. He was subsequently treated with Haldol and Cogentin.

About 2 months following the defendant's incarceration, voices reportedly commanded him to sharpen a toothbrush and stab himself. As a result, he sharpened a toothbrush on the floor and stabbed himself in the right eye and the left arm. By October 5, 1999, he required full restraints for his protection. He was subsequently treated with Zyprexa and Zoloft. Afterward, he became increasingly depressed and attempted to hang himself with a sheet, but he was discovered and placed on suicide precaution with restraints.

On May 9, 2000, he was discharged from the psychiatric division with a diagnosis of schizoaffective disorder, depressed, and returned to the general population of the jail. However, by October 2000 (5 months later), it became apparent that he was not taking his medications, and he became increasingly paranoid. He was readmitted to the psychiatric division and diagnosed with paranoid schizophrenia. The following day, he suddenly attacked correctional officers and was found to have a piece of cloth in his mouth. A mental health progress note following the attack documented that auditory hallucinations had prompted the attack.

NEUROPSYCHOLOGICAL EVALUATION

I eventually completed a neuropsychological evaluation of the defendant in the Cook County Jail in Chicago approximately 20 months after the crime. As is often the case with mental health evaluations conducted by outside examiners in correctional facilities, the environmental conditions for the evaluation were far from ideal. But, given the constraints and the inherent inflexibility of the correctional system, I was forced to accept the environmental conditions with which I was provided. The examination room was dirty and smelled of body odor, and there was considerable noise from correctional staff and other defendants outside the room. The light was adequate, but only if the examination table was placed directly beneath it.

The defendant presented as a young African American male with unresponsive and flat affect, who seemed frightened and paranoid. Although sluggish, he was alert and oriented to person, place, time, and reason for the evaluation. He ambulated independently, and his sitting posture was symmetric. Spontaneous speech was fluent and intelligible but characterized by a slow rate of production and increased response latency. His verbal responses were characterized by paucity of speech and speech content. Based on his responses, his thought content was intermittently disorganized, and he reported periodic auditory hallucinations involving suicidal ideation. Overall, his behavioral self-regulation was characterized by decreased initiation and increased response latency.

Incidentally, following my evaluation and while I waited for the guards to unlock the series of doors necessary to allow me to leave the jail, a female correctional officer unknown to me stated "there's something wrong with that one—he just ain't right."

During my interview of the defendant, he reported that he was experiencing auditory hallucinations on the day of the attack. Immediately prior to the attack, the voices reportedly told him that someone was going to kill him. He stated that "I believed everyone was against me." The voices reportedly told him to pick up a table leg that he saw lying under a viaduct. As he continued to walk, carrying the table leg, he saw some people walking down the sidewalk toward him. He stated that he believed they were going to kill him. He reported that he swung the table leg at a man in the group, striking him in the head. The man fell to the pavement. Then he struck a woman in the group, and she fell to the pavement. He stated that he did not recall if he struck the other people in the group or not. His next memory was the arrival of the police. In response to a direct question about substances, he reported that he drank one beer prior to the attack, but he denied the ingestion of any other drugs that day.

I administered the following battery of tests during one session over approximately 7 hours:

Wechsler Adult Intelligence Scale–III
Wechsler Memory Scale–III
Test of Memory Malingering
California Verbal Learning Test
Brief Test of Attention
Trail Making Test
Controlled Oral Word Association Test
Wide Range Achievement Test–3
North American Adult Reading Test
Judgment of Line Orientation Test
Wisconsin Card Sorting Test
Stroop Color–Word Test
Finger Tapping Test
Minnesota Multiphasic Personality Inventory–2 (MMPI-2).

During the course of my evaluation, the defendant appeared to be periodically distracted by both internal and external stimuli. Incidentally, I was also periodically distracted, but only by external stimuli. He periodically needed to stop and rest his head on the table.

Consistent with my impression that he was actively psychotic at the time of my evaluation, the test results revealed multiple neurocognitive deficits involving attentional disturbance, anterograde memory dysfunction that was significantly compounded by his attentional disturbance, and executive dysfunction. Based on his performance on the Test of Memory Malingering, I interpreted his test performance as valid and concluded that he had put forth sufficient test-taking effort. However, his MMPI-2 profile was invalid, due to response inconsistency secondary to thought disorganization and active psychotic symptoms. At the time of my evaluation, he was being treated with Zyprexa and Depakote. See Table 15.1 for a detailed description of the test results.

Following my evaluation and analysis of the data, I contacted the defense attorney to discuss the findings and my opinions. I informed him that I believed the defendant was actively psychotic at the time of my evaluation, and that his neuropsychological status involved multiple neurocognitive deficits. He responded that he was not surprised by my findings, but he did not want me to produce a report at that time. Rather, and in addition to the completion of the forensic neuropsychological evaluation for mitigation purposes, he wanted the defendant to undergo a psychiatric examination to assess his fitness to stand trial. Dr. James Knoll, of the Division of Psychiatry and Law at Northwestern University Medical Center and a colleague of mine, was asked to become involved in the case and examine the defendant. Dr. Knoll examined the defendant on July 17, 2001, 22 months following the crime and 10 weeks after my evaluation. Dr. Knoll completed a lengthy, detailed, and insightful fitness evaluation of the defendant.

Dr. Knoll concluded that the defendant was fit to stand trial, despite his psychiatric disorder. Additionally, his extensive interview of the defendant uncovered information of which I was unaware. He discovered that, on the day before the attack, the defendant was planning to sell some crack and had two "dime" bags of crack cocaine in his mouth, which had eventually burst. He reportedly experienced mild anxiety and rapid heartbeat. But, given the fact that the crack was swallowed rather than inhaled via smoking, as intended, the psychological effect was subdued and diminished after 20 minutes. However, several hours later he began to experience auditory hallucinations, which as previously described, continued until the attack on the family.

A few months later, Mr. Mayfield contacted both Dr. Knoll and myself and asked us to produce reports of our respective findings and opinions regarding the defendant's sanity at the time of the offenses. Dr.

TABLE 15.1. Neuropsychological Test Results

Test	Standard score
Test of Memory Malingering	
Trial 1	46/50
Trial 2	50/50
Trial 3	50/50
Wechsler Adult Intelligence Scale–III	
Full Scale IQ	80 (9th %tile)
Verbal IQ	85 (16th %tile)
Performance IQ	78 (7th %tile)
Verbal Comprehension Index	88 (21st %tile)
Perceptual Organization Index	86 (18th %tile)
Working Memory Index	95 (37th %tile)
Processing Speed Index	71 (3rd %tile)
Vocabulary	6
Similarities	7
Arithmetic	8
Digit Span	10
Information	10
Comprehension	4
Letter–Number Sequencing	10
Picture Completion	5
Digit Symbol Coding	3
Block Design	7
Matrix Reasoning	11
Symbol Search	6
North American Adult Reading Test	Estimated premorbid Full Scale IQ = 88
Brief Test of Attention	$Z = -3.4$
Trail Making Test	
Part A	$T = 36$
Part B	$T = 46$
Wechsler Memory Scale–III	
Logical Memory I	SS = 3
Logical Memory II	SS = 4
Visual Reproduction I	SS = 14
Visual Reproduction II	SS = 10
Face Recognition I	SS = 8
Face Recognition II	SS = 9
California Verbal Learning Test	
Trials 1–5 Total	$T = 9$
Trial 1	$Z = -2.0$
Trial 5	$Z = -5.0$
Short Delay Free Recall	$Z = -3.0$
Long Delay Free Recall	$Z = -3.0$
Recognition	$Z = -5.0$ (12 hits, 2 false positives)

(continued)

TABLE 15.1. *(continued)*

Test	Standard score
Controlled Oral Word Association	5th %tile
Wide Range Achievement Test–3	
Reading	42nd %tile
Spelling	34th %tile
Judgment of Line Orientation Test	56th %tile
Wisconsin Card Sorting Test	
Categories Completed	4
Total Errors	61 ($T = 33$)
Perseverative Responses	32 ($T = 35$)
Nonperseverative Errors	30 ($T = 35$)
Set Failures	0
Stroop Color–Word Test	
Word Score	$T = 31$
Color Score	$T = 26$
Interference Score	$T = 37$
Finger Tapping Test	
Dominant	$T = 29$
Nondominant	$T = 32$

Knoll and I produced our reports, independently. In addition to the defendant's neuropsychological status, which was previously described, I provided two opinions. It was my opinion, with a reasonable degree of neuropsychological certainty, that the defendant was suffering from a mental disease, characterized by auditory hallucinations, paranoid delusions, and multiple neurocognitive deficits, at the time of his offenses. Secondly, it was my opinion, with a reasonable degree of neuropsychological certainty, that the defendant's mental disease caused him to lack the mental capacity to appreciate the criminality of his conduct at the time of his offenses. The DSM-IV diagnoses I offered were as follows: 295.30 schizophrenia, paranoid type; 305.20 cannabis abuse; antisocial traits. Similarly, Dr. Knoll opined that the defendant was suffering from a mental disease at the time of the offense and that the mental disease caused him to lack substantial capacity to appreciate the criminality of his conduct. As such, our opinions held that the defendant was insane at the time of the crime and, as stated, our opinions were consistent with the legal definition of insanity in the State of Illinois. Additionally, Dr. Knoll opined that the defendant's exposure to cocaine the day before the offense had unmasked an underling schizophrenic disorder.

Following the disclosure of my opinions and the opinions of Dr. Knoll, the state's attorney requested an evaluation by a court-appointed forensic psychiatrist, who concurred with our opinions. At that point, the state hired another forensic psychiatrist who opined that the defendant was not insane at the time of the offenses.

TRIAL TESTIMONY

In advance of the trial, Mr. Mayfield updated me with regard to the legal issues in the case. He also provided me with some background regarding the presiding judge and the state's attorneys who were prosecuting the case. The judge who was originally appointed to the case was an experienced but very "state-minded" judge; Mr. Mayfield anticipated that the judge would not help the defense in any phase of the case. However, he also knew that the judge would not interfere with the defense that he wanted to pursue. The original prosecution team consisted of two of the best attorneys from the Office of the Cook County State's Attorney, both of whom were experienced with high-profile cases. However, by the time the trial began a different judge and new prosecutors had been appointed to the case. The judge was relatively new to the criminal justice arm of the courts, and he had come under tremendous media scrutiny and criticism for recent rulings and comments he had made on the bench.

Naturally, given the media attention that the case had already drawn, the local press closely followed the trial proceedings. During the trial, John Kass of the *Chicago Tribune* wrote that the defendant "in brown jail clothes, kept his eyes trained on a small patch of floor. He seemed medicated" (Kass, 2002). He added that the Chicago political community had remained conspicuously quiet regarding such a racially oriented crime. However, he also noted that Rev. Jesse Jackson had expressed a desire to oust the presiding judge, given his recent controversial ruling in another "political/racial case" (Kass, 2002).

I met with Mr. Mayfield in his office in the Cook County Jail complex prior to my court appearance, and he provided me with his opinion regarding the defendant's current mental status. He also confirmed that I was able to state verbatim the legal definition of insanity in the State of Illinois. We subsequently proceeded to the courtroom. The courtrooms in the Criminal Court Building of Cook County in Chicago have a practical design; they are divided into two sections by a wall of reinforced glass. On one side of the glass is the main courtroom, including the judge's bench, the witness stand, the jury seats, and the tables for the defense counsel and the prosecutors. Behind the glass are several rows of seats for observers and visitors, and an aisle separates the seats into two sections. At the trial, the friends and family of the defendant were seated on one side of the aisle, and the friends and family of the victims were seated on the other side.

My direct examination by Mr. Mayfield was straightforward and factual. He reviewed my credentials and proceeded to question me about the findings from my evaluation, diagnoses, the psychopathology and neuropathology of schizophrenia, and the behavioral and neurocognitive features of schizophrenia. He concluded by asking me to state the legal definition of insanity and to state my opinions with regard to the defendant's sanity at the time of the offenses.

The cross-examination by the state's attorney was aggressive and challenging. Initially, she asked me to acknowledge through repeated questions that I was not a forensic psychiatrist. The following series of questions was intended to demonstrate that I was not a physician and that I was not capable of performing surgery or prescribing medications. She questioned me regarding my ability to prescribe medications and proceeded to question me about my ability to prescribe a series of neuroleptics, including Haldol, Risperdal, Zyprexa, and Thorazine.

Following her initial line of questioning, she proceeded to question me regarding the administration, scoring, and interpretation of all the tests that I had administered to the defendant. Next, I was asked to inform the court of my fees, including the fee for testimony. Then she pulled out a copy of DSM-IV and asked if I was familiar with it. Naturally, I responded that I was, in fact, familiar with DSM-IV. At that point, she approached the witness stand and asked me to read a highlighted passage from the section on schizophrenia, paranoid type. The sentence I was asked to read was the following: "These individuals usually show little or no impairment on neuropsychological or other cognitive testing" (American Psychiatric Association, 1994, p. 287). Fortunately, I am familiar with the schizophrenia literature, particularly the neuropsychological aspects of schizophrenia. And although paranoid schizophrenics with positive symptoms are not generally characterized by global cognitive dysfunction, I tried to point out that several empirical studies have demonstrated neurocognitive dysfunction in paranoid schizophrenics, even during remission (e.g., Abbruzzese, Ferri, & Scarone, 1996; Butler, Jenkins, Sprock, & Braff, 1992; Goldberg et al., 1988; Zalewski, Johnson-Selfridge, Ohriner, Zarrella, & Seltzer, 1998).

Nevertheless, and empirical data notwithstanding, I was confronted with a widely used and respected reference that states that paranoid schizophrenics don't reveal cognitive dysfunction on neuropsychological tests. Furthermore, I was required to read a passage from DSM-IV that essentially contradicted my findings and testimony. The prosecutor continued to grill me with various hypothetical questions and inconsistencies between information that the defendant had told me versus information that he had told other experts. Although this particular line of questioning was challenging, and at times frustrating, I consistently adhered to my previously stated opinions and avoided speculation.

Fortunately, during the redirect examination by defense counsel, I was given the opportunity to elaborate on the fact that some paranoid schizophrenics manifest neurocognitive dysfunction, despite the position of DSM-IV. Furthermore, I was also given the opportunity to explain that the defendant was actively psychotic at the time of my evaluation and therefore would be expected to manifest attentional disturbance, executive dysfunction, and thought disorder. During the recross-examination, the prosecutor continued to hammer away at the fact that my findings and opinions were not consistent with DSM-IV. In a final redirect examination by the defense, I was given the opportunity to reiterate my opinion regarding his active psychosis at the time of my evaluation, as well as my position that his neuropsychological status at the time of my evaluation was consistent with a paranoid schizophrenic who was actively psychotic. I was subsequently dismissed and left the stand.

Following the completion of my testimony, the court adjourned. I walked out of the courtroom with Mr. Mayfield and observed the anger and resentment in the eyes and faces of the family members of the victims. Immediately outside the courtroom, the defense attorney briefly met with the family members of the defendant, while at the same time and just a few steps away, the prosecutor met with the family members of the victims. Mr. Mayfield graciously thanked me for my professionalism during testimony, and I promptly left the courthouse.

During closing arguments, the lead prosecutor insisted that the defendant was trying to commit suicide by police (i.e., trying to force the police to kill him). Conversely, the defense attorney argued that the defendant was unable to control the demons in his mind and was clearly insane at the time of the attack.

CONCLUSION

In October 2003, 4 years after the crime and 1 year after the trial had started, the judge found the defendant guilty but mentally ill. Jeff Coen of the *Chicago Tribune* wrote that the judge believed there was proof that the defendant suffered from mental illness, "but not enough that it left him legally unable to comprehend and appreciate the criminality of his actions" (Coen, 2003a). The prosecution praised the verdict, and the defense counsel responded that the judge had failed to consider the testimony of the experts for the defense (i.e., Knoll and Hanlon) to a sufficient degree. One month later, at the sentencing hearing, the defendant apologized to the family he had attacked in 1999. He was subsequently given two consecutive sentences of 25 years for murder and 12 years for attempted murder. With time off for good behavior, the 23-year-old could be released from prison at age 54. In an interview by Jeff Coen of the *Chicago Tribune*, Mr. Mayfield stated that because of mental illness the defendant not only severely injured the family he had attacked but also severely injured his own family. He concluded that "it's a tragedy all the way around" (Coen, 2003b). From the perspective of the defense, it was clear that the judge had not understood the nature of the defendant's mental illness—or perhaps he had succumbed to the intense pressure generated by the media.

LESSONS LEARNED

As in nearly every forensic case in which I have participated, I learned an important lesson from my experience. I should have completed an objective assessment of psychiatric symptom exaggeration, such as the Structured Interview of Reported Symptoms (SIRS). It was obvious to me that the defendant was psychotic at the time of my evaluation, and based on the nature of the crime and his well-documented psychiatric status following the crime, I believed that he was psychotic at the time of the crime. However, objective assessment of psychiatric malingering is imperative in cases in which an insanity defense is pursued. And, as a result, I complete such measures on nearly all of the capital murder cases in which I'm involved.

Finally, my opinion of the defendant was unchanged by the verdict or the sentence. In my view, he was a psychotic man who had committed a horrible crime. Regardless of his mental state at the time of the crime, his actions destroyed an innocent family. *Fact*: The defendant killed a man. *Fact*: The defendant savagely beat a young woman with a club, leaving her chronically disabled. *Fact*: The defendant's actions left the surviving members of a family to live with the tragic nightmare of a homicidal attack.

ACKNOWLEDGMENTS

We would like to acknowledge the invaluable contribution of James Knoll, MD, in the preparation of this chapter.

REFERENCES

Abbruzzese, M., Ferri, S., & Scarone, S. (1996). Performance on the Wisconsin Card Sorting Test in schizophrenia: Perseveration in clinical subtypes. *Psychiatry Research, 64,* 27–33.

American Psychiatric Association. (1994). *Diagnostic and statistical manual of mental disorders* (4th ed.). Washington, DC: Author.

Butler, R. W., Jenkins, M. A., Sprock, J., & Braff, D. L. (1992). Wisconsin Card Sorting Test deficits in chronic paranoid schizophrenia. Evidence for a relatively discrete subgroup? *Schizophrenia Research, 7,* 169–176.

Chicago Police Department. (1999). *Investigation report.* Chicago: Author.

Coen, J. (2003a, October 16). Man in fatal attack near Comiskey ruled guilty. *Chicago Tribune,* p. 1.

Coen, J. (2003b, November 13). 37-year term in fatal beating; 1999 attack near Comiskey Park. *Chicago Tribune,* p. 1.

Goldberg, T. E., Kelsoe, J. R., Weinberger, D. R., Pliskin, N. H., Kirwin, P. D., & Berman, K. F. (1988). Performance of schizophrenic patients on putative neuropsychological tests of frontal lobe function. *International Journal of Neuroscience, 42,* 51–58.

Kass, J. (1999a, August 31). Some crimes more hateful than others. *Chicago Tribune,* p. 3.

Kass, J. (1999b, September 1). Political reaction not best response to hateful crime. *Chicago Tribune,* p. 3.

Kass, J. (2002, October 3). On this beating in Bridgeport, silence deafening. *Chicago Tribune,* p. 2.

Zalewski, C., Johnson-Selfridge, M. T., Ohriner, S., Zarrella, K., & Seltzer, J. C. (1998). A review of neuropsychological differences between paranoid and nonparanoid schizophrenia patients. *Schizophrenia Bulletin, 24,* 127–145.

16

Competence to Confess
A Case of False Confession and a False Friend

JAMES P. SULLIVAN

I began conducting neuropsychological evaluations of plaintiffs for use in personal injury litigation soon after I was licensed in the early 1990s. While I was living in the Northeast, I discovered I was much more comfortable operating in the legal arena then many of my colleagues. I actually enjoyed much about the adversarial process and realized that it continually challenged me to increase my level of proficiency and knowledge base. When I relocated to Arizona in 1993, I became more involved with criminal forensic neuropsychology activities. This was a natural progression, given my comfort level with the high pressure of the courtroom, along with the high rate of death-penalty eligible cases in Arizona. Many otherwise qualified individuals did not want to perform death-penalty assessments, citing moral objections and/or a high level of personal discomfort in the death row environment.

Believing that credentials go a long way toward establishing credibility in the courtroom, I worked toward my American Board of Professional Psychology (ABPP) diplomate in clinical neuropsychology, achieving that goal in 1997. At that point my forensic involvement was upward of 90% criminal forensic neuropsychology, with probably a 60/40 split between defense and prosecution. In the late 1990s I realized this was going to be my life's work, and because I had always made such a big deal of credentials, that it was time for me to "walk the talk." I began to work toward my ABPP diplomate in forensic psychology, achieving that goal in late 2003. This process was much more of a challenge for me, because my education and training had been along traditional neuropsychology lines. One point I learned during this process was that very few professionals have had formal forensic psychology training, largely due to a lack of available programs and internships. Most professionals who are board certified in forensic psychology used a combination of self-study, continuing education, and supervision to increase their knowledge base to a point where they were ready to start the board certification process. Once I realized that, I figured I too could employ this approach.

BACKGROUND INFORMATION

I was initially contacted by the defense attorney in this case. A 36-year-old male defendant by the name of "William Johnson" had allegedly shot and killed an acquaintance while drinking, and he was facing a charge of first-degree murder. Mr. Johnson reportedly had a history that included prenatal insult, special education, numerous head injuries, and chronic alcohol abuse. The defense attorney had concerns about her client's cognitive function, specifically how it may have impacted Mr. Johnson's understanding and appreciation of his *Miranda* rights. She felt that his confession, if admitted, would serve to severely limit defense options during the trial. Mr. Johnson told the attorney 2 days after he had given a statement to police that he didn't remember what the circumstances of the evening were, and that he had given his statement because he "wanted to go home." As is usually the case, in my experience, I was told that the evaluation needed to be conducted "as soon as possible," although the defendant had been incarcerated for the last 3 months. Rather than get caught up in the urgency of the moment, I first needed to address several issues for the attorney and myself. Using Melton, Petrila, Poythress, and Slobogin (1997) as a guideline, the issues were as follows:

1. *What type of evaluation is this?* It was an evaluation focusing, at least initially, on Mr. Johnson's ability to competently confess. In other words, was he able to knowingly, intelligently, and voluntarily waive his *Miranda* rights and offer a confession without the benefit of legal counsel? This assessment was to be conducted with the foreknowledge that

the results would possibly be used to inform my involvement as a psychological expert in legal proceedings, charged with providing information to the trier-of-fact (either judge or jury). With that prior knowledge, the assessment is clearly a forensic psychological evaluation and should be guided by the aspirational model of practice offered in the *Specialty Guidelines for Forensic Psychologists* (Committee on Ethical Guidelines for Forensic Psychologists, 1991).

This is no small point. The specialty guidelines were specifically created because the American Psychological Association's "Ethical Principles of Psychologists" do not adequately address, nor are they designed to address, the unique issues and problems that confront forensic psychologists (defined as any psychologists, including clinical neuropsychologists, who regularly engage in the practice of forensic psychology; Committee on Ethical Guidelines for Forensic Psychologists, 1991; Fisher, 2003). Knowledge and proficiency in neuropsychology, no matter how impressive, are not sufficient credentials with which to enter the courtroom. I have often noticed a rather myopic perspective on the part of some neuropsychologists functioning in the role of experts. "I've been hired because of my proficiency in neuropsychology. Why do I need to know anything about the law? I'm not a lawyer." Not exactly . . . in my opinion, an expert who is not familiar with the rules and regulations governing his or her involvement as an expert loses credibility and is a less effective advocate for the data. Additionally, through some faux pas he or she may intrude into the process where he or she should not and potentially do irreparable damage to the defendant's case (e.g., not observing legal guidelines on the handling of incriminating information obtained during competency evaluations).

2. *Who will my client be if I accept this referral?* For purposes of evidentiary law, the client is always the individual who requests the evaluation, not the one being examined. In this case, the client would be the attorney, not Mr. Johnson.

3. *Am I qualified, through specialized knowledge and skill, to serve as an expert in this case?* I anticipated that this case would likely require proficiency in the areas of clinical psychology, clinical neuropsychology, and forensic psychology. Remembering that, if the case should ever go to trial, I am likely to be asked this same question during *voir dire* (i.e., expert qualification), it is important for me to rely upon external indicators of proficiency (e.g., licensure, specialized training, ABPP board certification, relevant publications, experience with similar cases) to answer this question. As an aside, it has been my experience that the profession-

als who ask themselves this question are precisely the ones that really don't need to. With high-level training and preparation comes an internalization of ethical practice.

4. *Have I clarified financial arrangements?* Fees that are dependent upon a certain verdict or finding are specifically prohibited by the specialty guidelines, because it would be professionally undesirable to engage in any behaviors that could serve to compromise, or *appear* to compromise, objectivity as expert witnesses.

5. *Have I requested all available records and collateral information?* I need to keep in mind that the defense attorney is not bound by the same practice ethics as I am. The defense attorney's main priority is to be an effective advocate for his or her client. As such, the attorney may not provide you with all the available information. If I suspect that necessary information is being withheld, I may need to have a conversation with the defense attorney detailing how a lack of information could serve to undermine my effectiveness as an expert.

6. *Have I clarified any prior relationships?* I have run into several situations in which the individual I was asked to evaluate was a codefendant with another person I had already evaluated. As such, their interests were at odds. In such a situation, I would decline involvement in the case to avoid the appearance of impropriety and would refer the attorney to a qualified colleague, using the ABPP directory if necessary.

7. *Have I clarified communication of results?* For most court-ordered assessments, a report summarizing my opinions is required. However, when an assessment is requested by defense counsel, the rules are different. The only purpose of the assessment requested by a defense attorney is to assist in the defense of his or her client. I am not the one qualified to determine whether the results, once the assessment has been completed, will serve that end. Once the report has been written, it may become a part of the record, which, in turn, may have to be disclosed to the state. Therefore, if the results are likely to hurt their case, most defense attorneys will direct you not to write a report and to conclude your involvement in the case. In fact, most defense attorneys will prefer to discuss results with you before authorizing a written report. As mentioned above, in this case the defense attorney is the client, and it is the client who will make the call.

All of these issues were able to be resolved adequately, in advance, so I agreed to evaluate Mr. Johnson. The first order of business was to review the statement Mr. Johnson had given to the police.

Transcript and Audiotape
of William Johnson Statement

Obviously, a review of the actual statement is of extreme importance in any assessment designed to determine a defendant's competency to confess. I make it a point to never rely solely on a written transcript if audio or videotape is available. Transcriptionists do make errors, and when the stakes are this high, there is a world of difference between "I did" and "I didn't." In this case, the statement was videotaped. I reviewed the video and the transcript simultaneously. My principal impressions from reviewing Mr. Johnson's statement were:

1. At the beginning of the interview "Detective Phillips" advised Mr. Johnson that "you have the right to remain silent . . . you have the right to an attorney prior to and during any questioning. If you can't afford an attorney, one'll be provided to ya [sic] at no cost. " Mr. Johnson responded "right" when asked if he understood. Noteworthy for its absence was the required warning that "anything you say can and will be used against you in a court of law." The omission of that particular warning definitely would help Mr. Johnson's attempt to get his statement suppressed, but not necessarily definitively. Historically, very few statements (< 5%; Gudjonsson, 2003) are successfully suppressed. At the suppression hearing the judge determines what the "totality of the circumstances" were (including the defendant's level of education, cognitive function, prior experience with the legal system, etc.). In the past several years some statements have been admitted, despite the absence of *Miranda* warnings, when the judge determined that the totality of the circumstances indicated the defendant had offered his statement voluntarily and with full knowledge.

2. Mr. Johnson reported that he had consumed a significant amount of alcohol. He began drinking at approximately 10 A.M. (verified by several different sources) and continued to consume alcohol until his friend was shot at about 6:45 P.M. (time of 911 call from the residence). He estimated that he had consumed "about a 12-pack and 10 or so shots." This information, while impossible to verify, appeared consistent with information obtained from other sources.

3. Mr. Johnson maintained that he couldn't remember what had happened. He did remember that he and his friend had been "shooting in the desert" earlier in the afternoon, and that he had brought his handgun back to the residence where the shooting later took place, placing it on top of the TV.

4. The interviewing officers berated Mr. Johnson, telling him they knew he was lying and that other individuals at the residence had seen them arguing. Mr. Johnson continued to deny any memory of the shooting, asking only if he could go home, or make a phone call, to which the officers responded "we have to finish this up." This type of exchange continued for just over an hour.

5. At the 1-hour and 8-minute mark, Mr. Johnson spontaneously asked if he could speak to "Sergeant Guidry," a man he had met at several Alcoholics Anonymous meetings and whom he identified as his "temporary sponsor." Mr. Johnson continued to deny any recollection of the shooting. At the 1-hour and 21-minute mark a note was brought into the interviewing officers from "behind the glass" and there was a subsequent break in the action.

6. The interview resumed after a break of unidentified duration. Sergeant Guidry, dressed in a patrolman's uniform, is in the room. He begins by saying "I heard you wanted to talk to me, how can I help you?" Mr. Johnson reports what has been happening, saying he can't remember any shooting. Guidry responds, "You know me, I know you from the streets, we both know that blackouts are bullshit, they're just an excuse we alcoholics use to get out of trouble." They begin to discuss what could have happened, with Guidry offering various hypotheses. At 1 hour and 41 minutes Guidry takes a note from behind the glass. The note is later found to have been written by one of the two officers, saying, "Use the AA stuff if you have to." At 1 hour and 44 minutes Guidry says "It's important that you come clean about what happened; that you make a searching and fearless moral inventory, and that you tell someone about it, that you say it out loud, man. . . . " (Subsequent investigation revealed that these were paraphrases of steps 4 and 5 of AA's 12 steps.) Mr. Johnson begins to cry, putting his head between his hands on the table. Guidry moves his chair closer, touches Mr. Johnson on the shoulder, and says " I know you're hurting, get it out, you'll feel better."

7. Mr. Johnson says he thinks he "might remember a part of what happened." Guidry responds, "That's how these things go, a little at a time." Guidry reminds him that the deceased was known to be quite aggressive at times. Mr. Johnson responds that they'd had their arguments. Guidry tells Johnson, "These guys are good, they're going to figure it out."

8. At 2 hours and 12 minutes Guidry threatens to leave; 30 seconds later Mr. Johnson says "I guess I could have shot him." Guidry replies, "Good, were you angry with him?" Mr. Johnson says, "I think I was."

Guidry responds, "So you're saying you shot him?" Mr. Johnson says, "Yes, my life is over." Guidry reassures him that it's not over, then gets up to leave. The last thing Mr. Johnson asks is if they'll be able to stay in touch. Guidry says, "My number's in the book," and exits the room.

9. At 2 hours and 16 minutes Mr. Johnson, again crying with his head on the table, is advised by Detective Phillips that "We have to follow all these rules. You have the right to remain silent, anything you say can and will be used against you in a court of law. You know, you have the right to an attorney prior to and during any questioning, and if you can't afford an attorney, one'll be appointed to you."

10. At the end of the interview Mr. Johnson is informed, apparently for the first time, that the deceased was dead and that he was being charged with first-degree murder.

During the course of listening to the statement and taking notes, a few issues immediately became apparent to me. Organizing my thinking along the lines of the pertinent psycholegal topics, I was concerned whether or not Mr. Johnson had been able to make a knowing, intelligent, and voluntary waiver of his *Miranda* rights and whether his free will was overcome at any time during the interrogation. The knowing and intelligent prongs would have to be more fully evaluated by cognitive and neuropsychological testing. However, the following seemed clear to me:

1. Mr. Johnson had been consuming significant amounts of alcohol during the time leading up to the arrest, and he was quite likely intoxicated at the time of the statement, possibly compromising his ability to make a knowing and intelligent waiver.

2. Mr. Johnson was much more concerned with immediate gratification of his needs (e.g., "Can I go home? . . . I need a drink") than with making a careful appraisal of his situation, also compromising his ability to make a knowing and intelligent waiver.

3. Although there was no indication that Mr. Johnson's will had been overcome during the initial waiver of the *Miranda* rights (incomplete as they may have been), there was a significant concern on my part that the introduction of Sergeant Guidry into the mix really complicated matters. I knew of a U.S. Supreme Court Case (*Spano v. New York*, 360 U.S. 315, 1959) in which the court found that the use of a "false friend" (an individual previously known to the defendant and considered a friend) in the service of securing a confession had served to overcome the will of the

defendant, and the justices had ruled to suppress the statement. This current case was even further complicated by the fact that the police had capitalized upon Mr. Johnson's membership in a known special-interest group (Alcoholics Anonymous) in an attempt to influence him, another practice previously frowned upon by the U.S. Supreme Court (*Brewer v. Williams*, 430 U.S. 387 1977).

Making note of these issues was critical for me in conceptualizing my evaluation of Mr. Johnson. Was he cognitively impaired to the extent that it would place him at increased risk to be influenced by these police strategies? It was time to meet with Mr. Johnson.

RECORD REVIEW

I wanted to prepare to corroborate some of the information I expected to acquire from Mr. Johnson. I chose the most effective way to establish the credibility of defendant information: record review and information from collaterals.

In addition to the statement Mr. Johnson had given to police, the rest of the records were limited to police reports and my interviews with Mr. Johnson's wife, mother, and 13-year-old daughter. I requested educational and medical records, but they were reportedly unavailable. I handled this apparent unavailability of necessary records by documenting my request and noting in any subsequent communication of results (through report or testimony) that the records were requested and that without them, my impressions and results were qualified. Creating written records of any verbal communication with the retaining/authorizing party is a practice I would recommend for all forensic evaluations.

My impressions from the clinical interview with Mr. Johnson and interviews with his wife, daughter, and mother are listed below. Source attributions are in parentheses. Over the years I have found source attribution to be an efficient and effective way to communicate information in forensic reports. I believe that it makes it easier for me to organize my thinking in a linear fashion and that it increases my credibility in the minds of the individuals reading the report. Source attribution makes it clear that these assertions are not just my subjective impressions but are based on verifiable information.

1. Mr. Johnson's mother consumed alcohol regularly during the time she was pregnant with William. (Defendant/Mother/Wife)

2. Mr. Johnson's mother was physically abused while she was pregnant with William. (Mother/Wife)

3. Mr. Johnson started drinking alcohol as a youngster. (Defendant/Mother)

4. As a child, Mr. Johnson was diagnosed with dyslexia and borderline mental retardation (Mother/Wife), and he was in special education classes throughout school. (Defendant/Mother/Wife)

5. Mr. Johnson was severely injured in a train accident in 1977, sustaining head and multiple systemic injuries. (Defendant/Mother/Wife)

6. Mr. Johnson was in one (Mother)/multiple (Defendant/Wife/Daughter) motorcycle accidents involving loss of consciousness. He was in a severe motor vehicle accident that involved loss of consciousness in 1997. (Wife)

7. Lisa Thomas married William Johnson in 11/88, gave birth to Courtney in 1990, divorced in 11/97, but cohabited with Mr. Johnson and their daughter from 6/98 to the time of the 1/03 arrest. (Defendant/Wife)

8. Lisa Johnson has been responsible for all household finances since she and Mr. Johnson married. He has not been able to have a bankcard because he was unable to understand "how they worked." (Wife)

9. When their daughter was being home-schooled in the fifth grade, Mr. Johnson was responsible for supervising her but was unable to assist her with any of her work because he "didn't know how." (Defendant/Wife/Daughter)

10. Although there have been some periods of abstinence, Mr. Johnson has abused alcohol throughout most of his life since age 9, often drinking to the point of passing out. (Defendant/Mother/Wife/Daughter)

11. Mr. Johnson reported that, as a child, he had received instruction in gun safety.

12. Mr. Johnson reported that he had shot himself by accident in 1992.

13. Mr. Johnson reported that he did not remember but was sure he had not intended to shoot the deceased.

My initial impressions regarding Mr. Johnson's alcoholism and low cognitive function seemed to be supported by information from these collateral sources. It was now time to conduct the formal assessment.

NEUROPSYCHOLOGY EXAMINATION

Clinical Interview

I met with Mr. Johnson, introduced myself, and conducted a structured clinical interview. Structured interviews are superior to unstructured interviews in forensic settings because they decrease examiner bias. Asking the same questions in the same order, regardless of whether you are working for defense, prosecution, or the court, is one way to control your own bias. It is also one way to answer the question, "Well, Doctor, you just asked the questions that would help you establish a diagnosis of _____, didn't you?"

The first order of business during the initial meeting was to review a forensic-informed consent contract. I use a three-page document that explicitly and repeatedly states the fact that I am not the defendant's doctor and he is not my patient; that there are cases of mandated reporting, but besides those instances all information will be controlled by his attorney and is protected by attorney–client privilege. I make sure that no one is forcing the defendant to participate against his will. Assessments often take place over several occasions. Before each session I review the consent contract with the defendant and then have him or her initial and date it. Mr. Johnson appeared to have great difficulty reading, so the form was read to him.

Mr. Johnson presented as extremely cooperative, even submissive, during the initial interview session. He was a marginally adequate historian. He reported he was extremely distressed, that he "shouldn't be here," and that he cried himself to sleep every night. Mr. Johnson was one of the more sympathetic characters I have met. Consequently, I found it necessary to remind myself (and him) that I was there in an evaluative capacity, not to offer him advice about how to deal with his difficulties.

TEST RESULTS

I formulated an assessment that was designed to evaluate Mr. Johnson's general cognitive abilities and briefly assess his neuropsychological functions. Once this foundation had been established, a more specific assessment of functions pertaining to the waiver of *Miranda* rights was performed. In doing forensic neuropsychological assessments, it is important to tailor the evaluation to the issue in question. It made no sense for me to do a comprehensive, 8- to 10-hour neuropsychological assessment when, even after all that, I wouldn't have the information needed to answer the relevant psycholegal questions. When selecting the measures I will use, I remind myself that there is such a thing as having too much information. I wanted to make sure I knew what I would do with the answer and how I would use it to address the psycholegal issues before me, before I even asked the question. By way of review, the questions before me were these:

> Was Mr. Johnson able to make a knowing, intelligent, and voluntary waiver of his rights at the time of his arrest?
> Is Mr. Johnson likely to be particularly suggestible?
> Is there anything about Mr. Johnson's cognitive or personality function that makes it easier for his will to be overcome than for a normal person?

I selected the following assessment procedures. For present purposes, results are briefly presented and discussed.

- Structured Clinical Interview (administered in first session)
- Trail Making Test (TMT)
- Wechsler Adult Intelligence Scale–III (WAIS-III)
- Wechsler Memory Scale–III (WMS-III)
- Wide Range Achievement Test–III (WRAT-III)
- Booklet Category Test (BCT)
- Peabody Picture Vocabulary Test (PPVT)
- Gudjonsson Suggestibility Scales (GSS)
- M-FAST Test of Malingering(M-FAST)
- Test of Memory Malingering (TOMM)
- Instruments for assessing understanding and appreciation of *Miranda* rights

Behavioral Observations

Mr. William Johnson is a 36-year-old right-handed Caucasian male with 8 years of formal education. In addition to the information detailed above, Mr. Johnson reported that he has worked intermittently in the construction industry for almost 20 years, most recently as a "job foreman" for a "friend." Reportedly, Mr. Johnson had been placed on Doxepin, an anti-depressant used to treat depression and anxiety, by the psychiatrist at the jail 2 weeks after his arrival.

Mr. Johnson presented as motivated and cooperative throughout the testing sessions. His pattern of responding reflected maximum effort. Formal measures designed to detect feigning of cognitive impairment and/or psychiatric dysfunction were administered during the sessions (BCT, TOMM, M-FAST). I design my assessments so that measures of response bias are administered in each session, rather than only in one session. I have found this can help address questions such as "Well, Doctor, you can confidently say he was trying his hardest in session one when you administered those measures, but what about 2 weeks later, in session 2?" There were no indications of feigning at any time. Thus, obtained findings were considered to be an accurate estimate of Mr. Johnson's level of function at the time of the assessment.

Cognitive and Neuropsychological Measures

Mr. Johnson was administered the WAIS-III. Results were consistent with low-average to borderline function (Verbal IQ = 72; Performance IQ = 80; Full Scale IQ = 74.) Some measurement error is inevitably included in all test scores. Therefore, confidence intervals can be used to report Mr. Johnson's IQ scores in terms of a range that is 95% likely to include Mr. Johnson's true scores. The 95% confidence intervals for Mr. Johnson's IQ scores are: Verbal IQ = 68–78, Performance IQ = 74–88, Full Scale IQ = 70–79. Individual subtest and index scores identified significant impairment in processing speed (Processing Speed Index = 72) and working memory (Working Memory Index = 69).

Mr. Johnson was administered the WMS-III. The index scores were variable, ranging from a low of 72 (Auditory Delayed) to a high of 88 (Visual Immediate). On the WRAT-III, reading was at the third-grade level, arithmetic operations at the second-grade level, and spelling at the first-grade level. Mr. Johnson was administered the PPVT-III, a measure of receptive (hearing) vocabulary that did not require him to respond verbally, but allowed him to select a drawing capturing the meaning of the presented word. I included this measure to see if Mr. Johnson's receptive vocabulary was as impaired as his expressive vocabulary, as observed during the WAIS-III and in conversation. Mr. Johnson's score fell at the third percentile for his age group, marginally better but still quite impaired, clearly enough to compromise his ability to understand what he was being asked to do when the police read him his rights.

Since time was a consideration, I had to select my neuropsychological measures carefully. Two specific neuropsychological measures were administered. The TMT comprises two timed tests requiring sustained attention, sequencing of visual material, and mental flexibility. The second of these two tests (TMT-B) has been found to be highly sensitive to brain damage. Mr. Johnson's performance on the first of the two tests (TMT-A) was in the low-average range. However, his score on the second measure (TMT-B) was in the severely impaired range. Mr. Johnson was also administered the BCT, a very demanding, language-free measure of abstract conceptualization and problem solving. The BCT is also sensitive to brain dysfunction, comparable to the full Halstead–Reitan Neuropsychological Battery (of which it is a part) for determining the presence or absence of brain damage. Mr. Johnson's performance on this measure was in the moderately impaired range for someone of his age and education, falling at the 2nd percentile.

In summary, Mr. Johnson's performance on several different measures of cognitive function was consistent with borderline cognitive function. Memory was in the low-average range but declined precipitously when Mr. Johnson was required to manipulate information under time constraints. Measures of academic achievement indicate that Mr. Johnson's abilities in reading, spelling, and arithmetic range from the first- to third-grade levels. Receptive vocabulary is similar to expressive vocabulary, in the lowest 3rd percentile and at about the 6-year-old level. Finally, performance on two neuropsychological measures that are very sensitive to brain dysfunction was consistent with organic impairment. The obtained results, combined with Mr. Johnson's authentic effort on measures designed to detect feigning, were consistent with brain damage sustained through prenatal complications and/or subsequent brain trauma and/or chronic alcohol abuse. The results are also consistent with reports of longstanding difficulties in school. As mentioned earlier, my impressions were tempered by the lack of additional corroborating records (e.g., medical, educational records).

Personality Assessment

Mr. Johnson completed the Gudjonsson Suggestibility Scales, which are specifically designed to identify individuals likely to demonstrate decreased resistance to subtle pressure or suggestion. Individuals identified as more suggestible on the GSS often provide less accurate, more erroneous material in statements to law enforcement personnel. The Gudjonsson Suggestibility Scale-1 (GSS-1) provides a story about an event and then includes questions about the event. The defendant is asked a series of subtle leading questions about the story, interspersed with nonleading questions. The extent to which the defendant modifies his or her answers in response to the leading questions is taken as an index of suggestibility. On the GSS-1, Mr. Johnson obtained a total suggestibility score of 14, which places him at the 90th percentile of the sample of "normal subjects," meaning that he is more suggestible than approximately 90% of the normative sample. The Gudjonsson Compliance Scale (GCS) is a 20-item true–false measure that was constructed to measure compliance in an interrogative situation. The GCS is intended to assess individuals who manifest an eagerness to please and attempt to avoid conflict with people in authority. Given Mr. Johnson's low reading level, the GCS items were read to him, as suggested in the test manual. Mr. Johnson's score on the GCS was 18/20, placing him above the 95th percentile of the normative sample of "normal subjects." My inclusion of these scales is an example of adapting my assessment to the situation, rather than forcing the situation to fit my assessment. The next measures provide further evidence of that type of adaptation.

Instruments for Assessing Understanding and Appreciation of Miranda Rights

These four assessment instruments, developed by Thomas Grisso, PhD, have been used since 1981 and have been commercially available since 1998.

Comprehension of Miranda Rights

The CMR was designed to assess the defendant's understanding of the four primary *Miranda* warnings by asking him to paraphrase each warning after it is read to him. On the CMR, Mr. Johnson obtained 6 of 8 points, falling at the 12th percentile when compared with a normative sample of adult offenders. An example of Mr. Johnson's responses in this section: When asked, "Anything you say can and will be used against you in a court of law—what does that mean?", Mr. Johnson responded, "You're in trouble."

Comprehension of Miranda Rights—Recognition

The CMR-R as developed to assess comprehension of *Miranda* rights without requiring the defendant to produce verbal responses on his or her own. The defendant is asked to determine whether each of three options is the same or different from the specific warning. Mr. Johnson scored 8/12, equal to the 7th percentile compared to the normative sample. An example of Mr. Johnson's responses in this section: When presented with "Anything you say can and will be used against you in a court of law. Now . . . If you won't talk to the police, then that will be used against you in court. Same or different?", Mr. Johnson responded, "Same."

Comprehension of Miranda Vocabulary

The CMV was included to evaluate a defendant's ability to define six critical words included in *Miranda* warnings. Not surprisingly, Mr. Johnson had pronounced difficulty on this measure, obtaining only 3 of a possible 12 points, at about the 1st percentile. An example of Mr. Johnson's responses in this section: When presented with "*Right.* You have the right to vote. What does *right* mean?", Mr. Johnson responded, "I know what it means, it's your God-given right. . . . I can't tell you, it's yours, you should do it."

Function of Rights in Interrogation

The FRI was designed to evaluate the defendant's beliefs about the rights described by the *Miranda* warnings and how they apply to a particular situation. The defendant is presented with sketches of different scenarios (e.g., a man sitting at a table in a police station with two police officers who are taking notes) and asked specific questions about the drawings (e.g., "What is it that the policemen will want Joe to do?") FRI scores can be further delineated into three areas. On items concerning the nature of interrogation or whether the defendant is aware of the adversarial nature of interrogation, Mr. Johnson obtained 10/10 points. On items assessing the right to counsel, or whether Mr. Johnson was aware of the function of counsel and the advocacy nature of the attorney–client relationship, he obtained 5/10 points, placing him below the 1st percentile in the normative sample. An example of Mr. Johnson's responses in this section:

When presented with a sketch of a man meeting with someone identified as his lawyer, and asked why the lawyer might want to know whether the man committed the crime he's suspected of, Mr. Johnson responded, "So he can tell the truth. Lawyers should always tell the truth about everything. That's their job." Finally, on items evaluating the right to silence, or whether Mr. Johnson was aware of protections related to the right to silence and the role of confessions, Mr. Johnson obtained only 1 of 10 possible points, suggesting a severe level of impairment, again below the 1st percentile. An example of Mr. Johnson's responses in this section: When presented with a sketch of a man sitting at a table, being interrogated by two individuals identified as police officers, and asked "if the man decides not to talk, what is the most important thing the police are supposed to do?", Mr. Johnson responded, "Take him to jail. They always get the truth. One looks mad. He has to talk or he'll go to jail." Of note, Mr. Johnson's obtained scores on both right to counsel and right to silence items were below even the average scores obtained by juveniles in the normative sample.

Following completion of the formal Understanding and Appreciation of *Miranda* Rights instruments, an interview was conducted, focusing on the specific events leading up to the statement and Mr. Johnson's understanding of what was happening during the interrogation. Mr. Johnson reported that he was held in a vehicle at the scene for several hours and then transported to the sheriff's station. He said that he had been asking to go home and that he asked "again and again." The detectives told him that he had to talk first. Mr. Johnson is not sure when his rights were read to him: "I think I talked for a while and then he read me my rights." Mr. Johnson reported that he didn't request a lawyer because "it was 3:00 in the morning, who would come?" When asked why he spoke to the detectives, Mr. Johnson responded, "I wanted to be helpful, but I really couldn't remember. I wanted to tell the truth. If I talked to them, I might be able to go home. They told me I could use the phone after I talked to them. A uniform told me I could use the phone if I talked. I thought it would help." Additionally, Mr. Johnson reported that he felt a personal connection with Sergeant Guidry. "I was so glad to see him. I gave him my hand." Of the detectives Mr. Johnson said, "They were real friendly. One guy was saying him and Bob [Johnson's boss] was buddies. I thought they cared about what happened to me. . . . They kept telling me I could call Lisa, but I never did." Finally, when asked if the police ever specifically told him he would be able to go home if he provided a statement, he responded, "I'm not sure, I just thought if I told the truth it would all be OK."

Conclusions

Results of cognitive and neuropsychological testing were consistent with impaired functions in several domains. Mr. Johnson's IQ is in the border-line range, and he has particular difficulty with the rapid processing of verbal material and holding that material in memory while actively manipulating it. Results of neuropsychological screening suggest the likelihood of significant neuropsychological impairment. These results, along with indications of sustained effort on multiple tests of malingering, are consistent with the available history of likely prenatal insult, developmental delay, multiple brain injuries, and a history of substance abuse. These impairments cannot be satisfactorily accounted for by depression or by the effects of psychoactive medication. Actually, Mr. Johnson's level of function during this assessment was likely higher than during the interrogation, given that he had been abstinent from alcohol for several weeks prior to this assessment.

Results of personality assessment specifically intended to evaluate his likely behavior in an interrogative setting describe Mr. Johnson as a very suggestible and compliant individual, especially with authority figures. Similar individuals are more likely than others without these characteristics to accede to subtle (as well as not so subtle) interrogative pressure. His performance on a specialized measure for Assessing Under-standing and Appreciation of *Miranda* Rights was consistent with pro-nounced difficulties in the areas of comprehending the vocabulary used in the actual *Miranda* warning and understanding the advocacy inherent in the attorney–client relationship. Mr. Johnson also had profound diffi-culty conceptualizing the implications of the right to silence, believing that if he did not provide a statement, he would be immediately pun-ished. Mr. Johnson apparently does not understand that the right to silence is an absolute entitlement that cannot be modified by individuals in positions of authority.

The obtained results offered converging evidence, drawn from mul-tiple sources, that Mr. Johnson's ability to offer a knowing and intelligent waiver was likely compromised. Similarly, his will is likely to be more eas-ily overcome than that of the normal person.

Additionally, review of the statement, as detailed earlier, raised some very significant issues about Mr. Johnson's ability to withstand interrogative pressure when the "false friend" appeared on the scene. Mr. Johnson's existing cognitive impairment, along with the fact that he was likely intoxicated and highly anxious, all combined to make it extremely difficult for him to decipher what it was he should do. It appears quite likely that Mr. Johnson agreed to the fact that he had shot his acquaintance because Sergeant Guidry encouraged him to do so, rather than him having an actual memory of that act. As such, Mr. Johnson's confession was not based on a true recollection. It was very likely based on something other than actual recall and, in essence, was a false confession.

I felt the evaluation was thorough and well conceptualized. I used the experience of writing the report as an opportunity to organize my thoughts and prepare for the suppression hearing.

TESTIMONY

When the validity of a confession is in question, a hearing will often be scheduled to determine whether the statement will be allowed into evidence. In many jurisdictions this is called a suppression hearing. The stakes are high. In many cases, and definitely in this one, confession to the crime is the most convincing piece of evidence to the trier-of-fact. The additional evidence against Mr. Johnson was weak, certainly not enough to warrant a first-degree murder charge. All the players were "ready to roll" on this day.

The state and the judge had already been given a copy of my report. During voir dire, my qualifications as an expert were agreed to by the state without challenge, a clear advantage of having a history of working for both the state and the defense. On direct questioning, my testimony followed the outline of my report. Things went very smoothly. The questions had been reviewed in advance with the defense attorney and testimony went off without a hitch. On cross-examination the biggest challenge was the area of feigning. How could I say that Johnson hadn't created these problems to avoid responsibility? As I mentioned above, in anticipation of this line of questioning I had administered multiple measures of feigning (both psychiatric and cognitive impairment) at different times. I had not relied solely on Mr. Johnson's report but sought to corroborate his statements through available documents and collateral interviews. Additionally, evidence of dysfunction was arrived at through convergent assessment results, not just one or two tests.

Finally, the fact that I had included measures specific to the psycho-legal questions at issue served to increase the face validity of the results, and to avert a very common line of questioning on cross-examination: "Doctor, so he has a low score on the _____. What does that have to do with Mr. Johnson's ability to waive his rights intelligently?" With all the available information, I was able to make a solid connection to the test data and answer this question to a reasonable degree of psychological certainty.

The judge ruled that Mr. Johnson's statement to the police was inadmissible. Without the statement to rely on, the state made an offer of manslaughter, a significantly lesser charge to which Mr. Johnson elected to plead guilty about 2 months after the hearing. Although I continually try to not become invested in the outcome of cases, but rather to focus my energy on providing accurate information to the court, I do occasionally find myself particularly interested in how a case turns out. This was one of those times. When it was all over, I really felt that my efforts had been useful in helping justice to be served.

LESSONS LEARNED

In many respects, this assessment experience served to further emphasize the importance of several guidelines that I have adopted over the years. I wish I could say otherwise, but many of these lessons have been learned through trial and error.

1. *The design of the assessment determines its effectiveness.* Familiarize yourself with specialized instruments. There are several excellent forensic psychology measures available; there is no reason that a neuropsychologist cannot acquire the necessary training to incorporate these measures into his or her evaluations.
2. *Be your own toughest critic.* Anticipate cross-examination and difficult peer review (from opposing experts) every step of the way.
3. *Know your territory.* You probably wouldn't go to an unfamiliar city without trying to acquire a map. In the same way, you shouldn't undertake a forensic evaluation, in which you are charged with providing specialized information to the trier-of-fact, without familiarizing yourself with the psycholegal constructs at issue.
4. Finally, *be well aware of the Specialty Guidelines for Forensic Psycholo-*

gists. Be informed by them in all your dealings. You may be a clinical neuropsychologist, but if you are presenting yourself to the court or some other legal body as a psychological expert on psycholegal issues, you are, by definition, engaging in the practice of forensic psychology (Committee on Ethical Guidelines for Forensic Psychologists, 1991).

AUTHOR NOTE

Potentially identifying information has been altered to protect confidentiality.

REFERENCES

Committee on Ethical Guidelines for Forensic Psychologists. (1991). Specialty guidelines for forensic psychologists. *Law and Human Behavior, 15,* 655–665. Available at www.abfp.com/careers.asp.

Fisher, C. B. (2003). *Decoding the ethics code: A practical guide for psychologists.* Thousand Oaks, CA: Sage.

Gudjonsson, G. H. (2003). *The psychology of interrogations and confessions: A handbook.* West Sussex, UK: Wiley.

Melton, G. B., Petrila, J., Poythress, N. G., & Slobogin, C. (1997). *Psychological evaluations for the courts* (2nd ed.). New York: Guilford Press.

17

Gambling, Money Laundering, Competency, Sanity, Neuropathology, and Intrigue

ROBERT L. DENNEY

Sitting on a cement pedestal, in a locked 4′ × 6′ × 8′ cage, "Mr. Small" was not your typical appearing criminal defendant. At 69 years of age, he was a gray-haired, chipper fellow, even when viewed through cold metal mesh. I have seen a handful of men through this mesh whom I would consider to be some of the most dangerous men in the world, but not this day. The only information I had about Mr. Small indicated that a federal jury recently found him guilty of illegal gambling, money laundering, and racketeering. The United States District Judge requested opinions regarding his competency to continue with proceedings, whether he was suffering from a mental disease or defect requiring treatment in a suitable facility, and what sentencing alternatives would best fulfill his treatment needs. In essence, it was a competency-to-be-sentenced question. All forensic study cases come into our facility in this secure manner, until we are able to ascertain their recent history of violence and current mental status. We also need to become reasonably comfortable that there are no significant risks in placing these individuals on a ward with other criminal defendants. After explaining to Mr. Small the nature of this court-

305

ordered evaluation and the fact that there was no usual doctor–patient relationship or confidentiality, I was able to talk with him briefly about his life and recent experiences. It was clear he would not pose a substantial physical risk of harm to others. He also appeared savvy enough to handle himself around other potentially manipulative men, so I wrote the order to move him to ward restriction. In this status, he had access to other patients, a television room, and a small recreation yard. I had no idea this simple appearing, gray-haired man would turn out to be one of the most complicated forensic cases of my career.

MY WORK SETTING

I never planned to get into the work of criminal forensics. I fell in love with neuropsychology's emphasis on neuroanatomy and neuropathology during graduate school in clinical psychology. I knew then that I wanted to work in clinical neuropsychology. I knew I needed inpatient experience beyond my clinical rotations in an inpatient head injury rehabilitation hospital, so I applied for a clinical internship at the U.S. Medical Center for Federal Prisoners. I never imagined working with criminals, but I had no aversion to it either. It was simply a great training environment in which to learn about a wide variety of severe mental and neurological illnesses. As it turned out, I loved it and was offered a full-time position performing mental health evaluations of pretrial criminal defendants for U.S. District Courts. I was able to continue my training in neuropsychology and learn the skill of criminal forensic assessment at the same time.

The U.S. Medical Center is a rather unique work setting. I am the only neuropsychologist in a 1,000-bed maximum security forensic hospital that serves the needs of medical, surgical, and psychiatric patients. The mental health professionals here also perform forensic studies for the U.S. District Courts throughout the United States and U.S. Territories. Typically, these referrals focus on such issues as competency to stand trial, sanity (mental state at the time of the alleged offense), risk of future dangerousness, and need for mental health treatment—all of which occur in the context of federal criminal charges. As a neuropsychologist, I tend to receive those cases that involve the suspected presence of neuropathology. This case is an example of such a court referral.

Criminal forensics is typically a stressful type of work because you need to answer questions that have potential for substantial impact on a person's life (often dealing with U.S. Constitutional rights) in a generally less than optimal environment (e.g., county jail), and under a tight time frame. The great benefit of my setting is that we see these individuals for a longer period (e.g., 30–120 days), and they are in an inpatient setting with around-the-clock supervision. This setting is ideal for forensic evaluations. There are two significant differences between forensic and typical clinical neuropsychological evaluations: multiple data sources and a healthy level of cynicism regarding what the evaluee tells you. Inpatient evaluations allow you to address both of these issues more easily. It is not unusual for a criminal defendant to act strikingly different when he or she is in the television room or recreation area as compared to your office during interviews and testing. Acquiring information from corroborative sources is generally quite important and can oftentimes be priceless. Corroborative information is also relevant to the healthy cynicism. As the late President Reagan said, "Trust, but verify." Inpatient evaluations help you incorporate surreptitious observation by others, prolonged observation, and the opportunity to perform more testing than what might otherwise be feasible. This case exemplifies how corroborative information can impact an opinion.

BACKGROUND INFORMATION

Because this evaluation was court ordered, my role was as a nonpartisan evaluator. All forensic evaluators are charged with the duty to remain objective in their evaluations, but there is less tendency to feel obligated to one side or the other when you are court appointed. I contacted both the prosecutor and defense counsel and requested whatever information they had about Mr. Small. Ideally, this information should include investigative records, prior medical and mental health records (hospital records and records of past evaluations), educational records and military records (if there are any), and anything else that would pertain to the defendant's current or past mental state. I received 30 different documents, which included considerable investigative information and medical records.

I learned that Mr. Small had been evaluated by an out-of-state neuropsychiatrist 2 months previously. As part of that evaluation, he had a magnetic resonance imaging (MRI) of the brain and an electroencephalogram (EEG). A well-known neuropsychologist who was called in from out of state also tested him. His defense team was looking for anything they could use in making a case for diminished capacity at the upcoming sentencing hearing. I acquired the neuropsychiatrist's report, received the raw neuropsychological test results, but the neuropsychologist never wrote a report (I confirmed this with a quick telephone call to the neuropsychologist). Mr. Small had a history of adult-onset diabetes mellitus and was on insulin during the period of the trial. MRI results revealed he had mild diffuse atrophy and one "probable lacunar infarct" in the white matter of the left posterior frontal lobe. In looking at the neuropsychologist test results, I did not think the results indicated much in the way of neurocognitive compromise, which was probably why the neuropsychologist did not write a report. Nevertheless, I received reports that Mr. Small was confused and misunderstanding events around him at the time of the sentencing hearing. This apparent confusion precipitated the referral for inpatient assessment regarding his competency for sentencing.

PERSONAL HISTORY

Mr. Small was the youngest of five children born to his parents. He had no developmental or apparent learning disabilities. He enlisted in the U.S. Army after completing high school and served as a diesel mechanic in the South Pacific from 1943 to 1945, received an Honorable Discharge, and returned to the western United States to start an antiques business. He eventually began buying and selling real estate. He has owned a variety of antiques businesses over the years and at one time owned about $6 million worth of property.

Mr. Small had no drug or significant alcohol history. He did not smoke. He has been healthy throughout his life until he was diagnosed with diabetes mellitus at 61 years of age. It was controlled with oral medication and diet initially, but during his most recent trial, he was treated with insulin. He developed phlebitis with two blood clots in his leg at 62 years of age and was placed on blood thinners. He had no mental health treatment history.

Three years prior this referral, he reported noticing a period of general weakness, which resolved in just a "couple of weeks." By all reports, things were well with him until a couple weeks before his recent trial. He was frustrated that his defense team was not focusing on the facts that he thought they should focus on. He wanted to testify on his own behalf (always a serious risk for a defendant to take). Mr. Small said that he was having trouble keeping facts straight in his mind. His defense team put him through a mock testimony, during which he supposedly demonstrated confusion about facts such that his lawyers would not allow him to testify. He said, "My recall was not good enough to satisfy them." He became even more irritated and frustrated at not being allowed to assist in his own defense, as he desired. He had to watch his defense unfold in a manner he did not like, and he was ultimately convicted of gambling and money laundering. As noted, his referral to this facility occurred because he appeared confused on the day of his sentencing hearing.

Mr. Small quickly learned the rules of ward living and progressed to open population status, where he had access to institution-wide facilities (such as the dining hall, recreation center, and main recreation yard). During this time, I received another court order from another federal court in the same jurisdiction. This time the judge wanted an opinion regarding Mr. Small's sanity *during the most recent trial* because he had acquired new charges. These charges were for jury tampering and obstruction of justice: He was alleged to have contacted a juror in an attempt to change the outcome of his gambling trial. This case instantly became complicated.

I interviewed Mrs. Small on the telephone. She indicated that she had observed her husband quite closely throughout the trial preparation and trial itself. She was part of all attorney meetings and sat next to her husband during court proceedings. She noted that his mental acumen had dropped 1 month before the trial. At that time she reportedly told the defense attorneys that her husband was not telling them accurate information. Consequently, the attorneys began asking her for dates and figures rather than her husband. She noticed that he started having a hard time sorting dates, amounts, and places. She thought it was simply frustration on his part, but it began to worsen as the trial neared. By the time the trial started, she believed it was useless to talk with her husband about important events. He was also getting increasingly frustrated with his defense team, because they would make decisions he did not like and shrug him off when he tried to provide his own input. She said that his confusion had worsened during the trial, as evidenced by the fact he went to court one day wearing one brown sock and one black sock.

At home, Mrs. Small noticed her husband having difficulties as well. He was usually an active person who rose from bed quickly in the morning. She recalled one morning when he was particularly groggy and could not stand up. His blood sugar read 300 on the glucometer. He also complained of headaches. She called his primary care physician, who told her to "play with it" in regard to adjusting his insulin dose. Her husband was not eating regularly, and his sleep pattern was strange. He would take "cat naps" but not sleep through the night. Normally a sociable person, he now wanted to be left alone. He felt like he was being "rail-roaded" in the court case and was quite frustrated. On one occasion, she found her husband sitting by himself crying.

Although he was not demonstrating accurate recall of facts and events, she did not believe that he was "out of control." She just believed his judgment was poor. She further viewed his behavior in regard to the juror as irrational and unexplainable for a man who clearly understood that contacting a juror was impermissible.

I interviewed "Mr. Calvin," the defendant's trial attorney who had represented him during the tax trial a year previously and the gambling and money laundering case most recently (the trial during which he allegedly contacted the juror). Mr. Calvin originally viewed Mr. Small as an elderly man who did not have "perfect" memory, but he did have "normal" memory. During the summer just before this most recent trial, however, he became concerned about Mr. Small's ability to recall events and keep them straight, and to deal rationally with what was going on around him. For example, Mr. Small did not deal rationally with the plea-bargaining process and did not even realize that he was behaving irrationally. His responses to offers extended by prosecution were fanciful and served no purpose beyond angering the prosecution and worsening his situation. The case moved to pretrial hearing, for which Mr. Small was present but not particularly involved. Consequently, Mr. Calvin focused his attention on the government rather than Mr. Small directly. Mr. Calvin viewed this change in focus as the likely reason why he did not realize Mr Small's worsening condition at the time. He said it was very difficult to deal with Mr. Small during September, as they moved in to the trial, because he could not remember facts and keep the different cases straight in his mind. For example, he did not realize the role of the arraignment and acted as if he were going to present his defense against the charges at that moment in court.

Mr. Calvin indicated that Mr. Small had good days and bad days. He said that the juror issue was utterly irrational and had served no positive purpose for his defense. Mr. Calvin had viewed this particular juror as an asset to the defense because he had a similar professional position in the community as the defendant and would likely have been sympathetic with their case. Mr. Calvin said that Mr. Small's behavior was the "most self-destructive, self-defeating, irrational behavior I've ever seen."

Mr. Calvin continued to represent Mr. Small during the sentencing phase of his gambling case and requested to be present during my "competency" interview, in which I would ask him about his understanding of his legal situation, proceedings he is facing, roles of courtroom participants, and his plans for dealing with the case. I have never been asked to allow an attorney to sit in on an interview before, and at the time I perceived no problem with it. Out of courtesy and fairness, I contacted the prosecuting attorney about the situation. He wanted to be present as well, but his schedule did not allow it. He asked if I would videotape the interview for him. Because it was a court-referred case, I had this arrangement approved by the court. Although I had never completed an interview with an attorney present, I had a sense of the potential disruption it could cause. As a result, I asked Mr. Calvin to remain quiet during the interview, and he agreed.

Mr. Calvin arrived on the day of the interview and came into the institution to the visiting room where attorneys can visit with their clients privately. I had the video equipment set up and everything seemed ready. Mr. Small arrived and the interview commenced. I realized this was not a typical interview once I started. Although Mr. Calvin stayed true to his word not to say anything, the entire flow and pace of the interview was "off" in such a way that it was much more difficult to get the information I needed. I had trouble getting Mr. Small to open up about his ideas and understanding of the case. I completed the interview and asked the questions I had planned on asking, but it was not until after several short, less formal, interactions with Mr. Small on the evaluation unit that I became fully comfortable with his understanding of the nature and consequences of his current legal situation. I also found out rather quickly after the interview that the video camera battery had not been charged sufficiently. The video recording had stopped shortly after I started the interview. I felt like the whole interview had been a waste of time. It was not until that interview that I realized the significance of "involved" third-party observers during clinical interviewing. Having psychology interns and post-doc fellows present is one thing, but having an attorney and a camera present was something else entirely. Even though Mr. Calvin did nothing intentionally to disrupt the interview, I decided then that I would not allow third-party observers again unless forced to do so. I have since become aware of the literature on the subject, which demonstrates exactly what I experienced—that third-party observers can change the nature of the interview in a significant manner (Binder & Johnson-

Greene, 1995; McCaffrey, Fisher, Gold, & Lynch, 1996; McSweeny, et al.,1998; National Academy of Neuropsychology, 2000). This learning experience prepared me to deal with a much more explosive third-party observer encounter that was going to occur later on this case.

NEUROLOGICAL CONSULTATION

As part of this evaluation, Mr. Small underwent a neurological consultation, which included a neurological examination and MRI study of the brain. During this examination, he was fully oriented, had appropriate free-flowing speech, his serial 7's were accurate, and he remembered three objects for 5 minutes. His strength, reflexes, and sensations were normal. The bicep jerk may have been just slightly greater on the left than the right, but it was within normal limits. Toe signs were flexor, and his gait, station, and stance were normal. The MRI revealed mild diffuse atrophy, a probable lacunar infarct in the left posterior frontal lobe white matter consistent with previous studies, but no cortical infarcts or other disease. The neurologist concluded, "This man has mild changes in his mental status, probably due to small vessel disease, diabetes, and age—at this point, it is more inconvenient than disabling."

NEUROPSYCHOLOGICAL TEST RESULTS

Several measures were used to evaluate test-taking motivation (see Table 17.1). Results revealed no indication that Mr. Small was attempting to appear disingenuously impaired. I use age- and education-corrected scoring for neuropsychological tests, an issue which was particularly important for a man of Mr. Small's age. He demonstrated no impairments in attention or concentration. There was some indication of mild motor slowness. He had no trouble with receptive or expressive language. Results suggested no significant deficiencies in his learning or retention. His performance was normal for executive function tasks when using the age corrections. His overall intellectual efficiency fell in the superior range. On the Minnesota Multiphasic Personality Inventory–2 (MMPI-2; Butcher et al., 2001), he maintained no atypical test-taking attitude. Further, validity scales suggested a reasonable amount of internal emotional distress. He produced significant elevations on scales indicative of marked physical health and body concerns, although he produced a Lees-

TABLE 17.1. Neuropsychological Test Data for Mr. Small

Cognitive Validity Tests

Validity Indicator Profile:	Nonverbal: Valid–Compliant Verbal: Valid–Compliant	*Rey 15-item*: 12 items/4 rows *Rey Dot Counting Test:* Grouped/Ungrouped: 0.22	
Rey Word Recognition Test: 24/30 (weak but within normal limits)		*Miscounts:* 1	
Wechsler Memory Test–Revised: Forced-Choice Recognition Z = +3.94		*Abbreviated Hiscock Digit Memory Test:* 12/12/12	

Halstead–Reitan Neuropsychological Battery

	Raw	Heaton T
Halstead Impairment Index:	1.0	22
Booklet Category Test:	71	50
Trail A:	25 seconds	62
Trail B:	87 seconds	55
Tactual Performance Test		
Dominant:	10.0 minutes	45
Nondominant:	5.2 minutes	59
Both:	4.0 minutes	55
Total:	19.18 minutes	51
Memory:	5	42
Localization:	3	58
Finger Oscillation Test		
Dominant:	38.67	37
Nondominant:	35.67	33
Grip Strength Test		
Dominant:	31 kg	37
Nondominant:	22.5 kg	28
Grooved Pegboard Test		
Dominant:	81 seconds	52
Nondominant:	89 seconds	48
Seashore Rhythm Test:	24 correct	48
Speech Sounds Perception Test:	9 errors	44

Aphasia Screening Test: Clear

Construction: Perfect

Sensory–Perceptual Exam

Tactile:	Dominant: 0 errors Nondominant: 0 errors
Auditory:	Dominant: 2 errors Nondominant: 0 errors
Visual:	Dominant: 0 errors Nondominant: 0 error
Tactile finger recognition:	Dominant: 0 errors Nondominant: 0 errors
Fingertip number writing:	Dominant: 2 errors Nondominant: 3 errors
Tactile form recognition:	Dominant time: 10 seconds T 52 Nondominant time: 9 seconds T 52

(continued)

TABLE 17.1. *(continued)*

Wechsler Adult Intelligence Scale–Revised		
Full Scale IQ:	123	T 64
Verbal IQ:	114	T 55
Performance IQ:	133	T 73
Information:	9	T 41
Picture Completion:	9	T 55
Digit Span:	10	T 52
Picture Arrangement:	15	T 79
Vocabulary:	9	T 42
Block Design:	10	T 60
Arithmetic:	14	T 63
Object Assembly:	10	T 61
Comprehension:	16	T 71
Digit Symbol:	8	T 60
Similarities:	7	T 43

Wechsler Memory Scale–Revised

LM I: 28th %tile
LM II: 52nd %tile

Minnesota Multiphasic Personality Inventory–2

	Raw	T		
L:	4	52	Hs:	75
F:	10	67	D:	68
K:	11	41	Hy:	69
FB:	2	51	Pd:	40
VRIN:	6	54	Mf:	46
FBS:	15		Pa:	72
			Pt:	53
			Sc:	62
			Ma:	45
			Si:	56

Wisconsin Card Sorting Test

	Raw	Heaton T
Categories:	6	
Perseverative Responses:	10	61

Rey–Osterrieth

Copy: $Z = 1.15$
Recall: $Z = 1.65$

Haley Fake Bad Scale (Lees-Haley, English, & Glenn, 1991) of only 15. These results did not suggest that he was trying to overreport somatic symptoms. He also produced an elevation on a scale indicative of paranoid ideation. In the context of a criminal forensic evaluation, however, this scale elevation is more indicative of significant distrust of those around him, particularly government authorities. Most of the items he endorsed on this scale were consistent with the fact that he was being prosecuted criminally. There were no indications on Mr. Small's MMPI-2 profile that were out of the ordinary for an individual with a recent history of physical ailments as well as criminal prosecution. There was no evidence to suggest he had a severe mental illness.

CLINICAL FORMULATION

Mr. Small had ho history of psychotic mental illness or hospitalizations for mental health reasons. He did have a history of multiple white matter infarcts; that is, small strokes in the deep areas of the brain. Results of MRI scanning done during this evaluation supported the past results and indicated further white matter changes. There was no way to identify the exact time of onset for those small strokes. Given the sequence of events and the dates of the previous scans, however, it was clear that the strokes had occurred some time prior to, or during, the fall trial. Both he and his wife described his episodes of weakness and possible blackouts during October, November, and December, a period of intense physical and mental stress. The most likely culprit of this weakness and possible blackouts was difficulty managing his blood sugar levels, because low blood sugar levels can create weakness, confusion, and even blackouts. Weakness, however, is also a likely outcome of small subcortical infarcts. Mrs. Small's report of his blood sugar level being 300 on the morning of the weakness actually suggests stroke as the more likely cause, because a blood sugar level of 300 would not cause such a problem. The truth is, no one could say, in retrospect, exactly what had caused those weaknesses.

Added to Mr. Small's medial scenario was a psychological syndrome of exhaustion, frustration, discouragement, sleep disturbance, and appetite disturbance, culminating in a legitimate depressive episode. Such a depressive reaction can cause learning and memory impairment, secondary to loss of attention and concentration ability. In the elderly, particularly, it is more common and is typically called "pseudodementia." Overall, it appeared that the concentration and memory deficits described by him, his wife, and his attorney over the course of much of the year were due to a combination of events. It was impossible to definitively attribute those deficits to either stroke, uncontrolled blood sugar level, or depression, in isolation; they were likely due to the combination of those factors. Nonetheless, he appeared to have been suffering from a mental disability at the time of the recent trial.

Mr. Small's condition changed over the course of the last 2 months as a result of decreased levels of stress, better controlled blood sugar levels, and increased time since the actual strokes. He clearly did not show the confusion and misunderstanding he had demonstrated at the recent sentencing hearing. All available clinical information and test data accumulated during this evaluation indicated that he was no longer experiencing cognitive compromise. I diagnosed him with cognitive disorder, not otherwise specified, resolved. This diagnosis was meant to communicate that although he had had a mental defect previously, it has since resolved. He had no current diagnosable mental illness or defect at this time.

OPINION REGARDING COMPETENCE TO PROCEED

Mr. Small did not currently have a mental illness or defect and, as a result, did not meet the criteria for incompetency under the federal standard. In addition, he demonstrated significant intellectual abilities, which further supported a conclusion of competency to be sentenced. He was able to accurately describe significant events in his recent legal history in an articulate and intelligent manner. During discussion of his current legal issues, it was clearly evident that he understood the roles of courtroom participants, such as judge, jury, defense and prosecuting attorneys, and witnesses. He understood that he was recently found guilty by a jury and faces sentencing for that conviction. He demonstrated the intellectual and cognitive capacity to assist his attorney throughout this hospitalization, which I was able to observe in some of his interactions with counsel. He had the current capacity to sit down and discuss important issues with his attorney, such as the presentence report, and provide information helpful to his attorney in arguing specific points in the presentence report. Lastly, Mr. Calvin agreed that there had been a significant improvement in the defendant's mental status during the last 2 months. Overall, there appeared to be no reason to suggest that Mr. Small lacked the prerequisite abilities to assist properly in his defense at this stage of the proceedings.

I also addressed the other questions of the court order by opining that he did not need inpatient hospitalization at this time, and that his treatment needs could be met on an outpatient basis. This information was included in a report to the judge who sent the original order addressing his competency to be sentenced. I then needed to deal with the second court order asking for an opinion about his competency to stand trial and his sanity regarding the jury tampering and obstruction of justice charges.

THE ISSUE OF MR. SMALL'S SANITY

Addressing his competency to stand trial was easy, because it was basically the same question about his current functioning as that of the original order. On the other hand, identifying Mr. Small's exact mental status during the trial in the fall of the year was a particularly difficult endeavor because of the complex diagnostic situation occurring at the time. Available evidence suggested that he was experiencing a mental illness at the time as a result of the culmination of factors, including significant stress, recent subcortical stroke, poorly controlled blood sugar, and depression. The presence of a mental illness or defect, however, did not automatically eliminate his ability to appreciate the nature, quality, or wrongfulness of his actions. One must review accounts of actual and alleged behavior and the motivation that went with it in order to answer that legal question.

Investigative material alleged that Mr. Small requested a business associate to acquire the juror's license plate number, and in fact, the associate did so. Mr. Small then allegedly telephoned the juror at his residence and later met with him at the man's business property. Mr. Small's business associate then telephoned the judge to report his contact with the juror and later drafted a letter outlining the contact. The associate reported that he had told Mr. Small that he had contacted the judge and written the letter, and Mr. Small allegedly instructed him to destroy the letter while being careful not to put it in the waste can outside the courtroom. The FBI case agent also contended that she overheard Mr. Small comment at the time of the trial that he was not supposed to talk to jurors.

I interviewed Mr. Small about these issues, and he discussed his alleged behavior in detail. I did not include the details of his statements in my report and noted in my report that they were not included so as to not inadvertently violate the Fifth Amendment rights of an individual who has not yet been found competent by the court to make decisions regarding his defense. I went on, however, to write that he was able to discuss details of his behavior without difficulty. He further noted clearly that he understood that contacting a juror on one's own case would be considered a criminal offense.

Overall, there was evidence that Mr. Small was suffering from a mental illness of defect at the time of the alleged offense, which significantly affected his concentration, memory, and judgment. Although his judgment was impacted to some degree, he was not so incapacitated by illness as to cause him not to understand what he was doing or what was going on around him. On the contrary, his behavior, as outlined in the investigative reports, suggested that he made comments and acted in a manner consistent with someone who knew his or her actions were wrong and/or potentially illegal. I included this opinion, as well as an opinion that he was competent to stand trial on jury tampering and obstruction charges, to the second court in response to that court order.

A NEW COURT ORDER AND THE REST OF THE STORY

Two months after completing that evaluation, I received an order from the original court asking me to evaluate Mr. Small's mental status and competency to stand trial for the time of the past gambling and money laundering charges. In other words, the court wanted me to "go back in time" and figure out if he was, in fact, competent to stand trial when he was going through the last trial—a retrospective competency assessment. Just when I thought I was done with an already complicated case, it got even more complicated! As it turned out, the defense motioned for this opinion because of my previous opinion to the other court saying he was mentally ill at the time of the jury contact but not insane. Of course! That opinion focused on his mental state at the time of the jury tampering, which was during the last trial. My opinion just opened the door to the possibility that Mr. Small's recent conviction could be overturned based on him not being competent during the trial. The legal standard for competency is different from the standard for sanity. It is quite possible that a person could be legally sane yet considered incompetent to stand trial.

I was asked by the judge, via an assistant U.S. attorney, whether or not I needed Mr. Small returned to me to provide that opinion. Given the fact I had recently evaluated him so thoroughly and the opinion dealt with retrospective competency for the same time period I had previously evaluated him, I determined it was not necessary for him to be returned to my facility. But I would need all the court transcripts for that trial and any other information that would reflect his mental state for that time. For reasons I did not understand, this new case required a special prosecution team from Washington, DC, to become involved, and a whole new defense team was assembled. As a result, I received lots of new information—information I wish had been provided for my earlier evaluations.

It became clear why Mr. Small had a new defense team. His previous attorney (the one who flew here to sit in on the interview) motioned for the evaluation of Mr. Small's past competency and outlined his view that he had been an ineffective counsel because he had not noticed Mr. Small's "tremendous debilitation" at the time. He indicated that he was so focused on trial strategy that he did not notice that his client was "confused and unable to understand what was going on around him to such an extent he could not assist properly in his own defense"—an interesting admission, particularly coming from a nationally known defense attorney, and one who did not seem ineffective when dealing with me and my past evaluation of his client. But that was not my call. My job was to evaluate the client's mental state, and for that, I needed lots of documents.

I received the court transcripts, which were not directly helpful because Mr. Small was rarely allowed to speak in the courtroom. They also included an affidavit from one of his co-defense attorneys, "Mr. Townsend," indicating that, in retrospect, he thought Mr. Small was indeed too impaired to fully comprehend events going on around him or assist properly in his defense. Other than that, the transcripts received from the defense contained little helpful material, certainly no "smoking gun" or "Rosetta Stone." That changed with the arrival of a little package from the prosecution.

It was a box that included videotapes. I love videotapes. Videotapes allow me to travel back in time and evaluate the defendant's mental state *in vivo*, as events were actually unfolding. And these tapes were bombshells! As it turned out, Mr. Small was going through divorce court the exact same week he was going through the criminal trial on gambling and money laundering. He was out on bond during his trial, at least until he was suspected of jury tampering, when he was placed in jail. Believe it or not, this particular divorce court videotapes all its proceedings. When I viewed the tapes, I saw Mr. Small testifying in a court of law under the examination of Mr. Townsend, who was examining him on property boundaries! I saw Mr. Small answering rapid-fire questions and clarifying misunderstandings while drawing out property lines with his finger on a large map on a table. He never missed a beat under intense questioning. His responses were quick. There were no signs of slowed mentation or confusion. And the best part was the fact that he was being questioned by the very same attorney who had written the affidavit stating that, in retrospect, his client had been too impaired to properly assist in his own defense! Although the videotapes were fantastic, there was something even better tucked in the bottom of that box.

In the bottom of the box was a set of court transcripts—transcripts of Mr. Calvin speaking to the judge in a postconviction detention hearing. This is a hearing in which the defense asks the judge to let the defendant remain out on bond until the sentencing hearing. Keep in mind that this hearing occurred immediately after the trial—just a couple of days after the time in question for my retrospective competency assessment. Mr. Calvin was making an argument for why he needed Mr. Small to be released from jail. When asked by the judge how it would be helpful for Mr. Small's case for him to be released from jail, Mr. Calvin said that they needed Mr. Small's help in preparing for the sentencing hearing. He said that Mr. Small was so helpful during the trial that he was like a "paralegal" for the defense! He said he needed him out collecting information and researching like a paralegal. "Wait a minute," I said to myself. This is the defense attorney who wrote an affidavit declaring that he was ineffective because he did not notice how terribly impaired Mr. Small was during the trial. Wow! Amazing the things that turn up sometimes. And this transcript was just days after the trial, not 2 months after the fact. The tapes and this transcript opened the window for me to see more clearly how well Mr. Small was actually functioning at the time of that trial.

Now I had a tough job to do. I had to write a report explaining that new information had changed my opinion regarding Mr. Small's past functioning. I was lucky in that it did not change my opinion about the legal standard of sanity, but it would have been all right if it did, because it is important to remain flexible and willing to admit when new information changes our opinions. I wrote a report, referencing my previous reports, that said there was indication, solely from the defense, that Mr. Small was suffering some type of mental illness at the time of the trial. Given the new information made available for this analysis, I was less willing to conclude that any neurological, neuropsychological, or psychiatric condition existed at the severity level needed to hinder or markedly alter Mr. Small's thinking ability and capacity to assist counsel. I wrote, "The undersigned evaluator had what has proved to be an inadequate data base when formulating the prior opinions."

I wrote an opinion that Mr. Small was experiencing some mild mental health condition at the time of the trial as a result of combined recent neurological events, stress, and uncontrolled diabetes, but available evidence indicated that it did not rise to the level needed to eliminate his ability to appreciate the nature and consequences of proceedings against him or eliminate his ability to assist properly in his defense.

MY DAYS IN COURT

About 3 weeks later, I received a subpoena to testify in court about Mr. Small's competency to stand trial on the jury tampering and obstruction charges. When I arrived, I found out that the defense was putting their defense neuropsychiatrist on as well as Mr. Calvin. The neuropsychiatrist was to testify about how the subcortical lacunar infarct eliminated Mr. Small's competency to proceed, and Mr. Calvin was going to testify about his client's debilitation since the trial. I did not get an opportunity to see that testimony because the defense invoked the "rule." This rule refers to Federal Rule of Criminal Procedure 615, which allows the exclusion of the witness so that he or she cannot hear the testimony of other witnesses, as a means to lessen the likelihood of fabrication, inaccuracy, and collusion. This rule seems illogical to me when applied to experts, because our opinions are already spelled out in our reports. Also, it is often helpful for experts to be provided with the opportunity to testify as to whether or not anything in the other expert's testimony changes their opinion. I also enjoy seeing other people testify because I believe it helps me improve my testimony skills. Nevertheless, I was relegated to the witness room adjacent to the courtroom for 6 hours! These are small rooms with hard seats and a couple of magazines. They are typically uncomfortable. By the time I was called to testify it was late afternoon, and I was already tired. My direct examination went fine, but I was relentlessly cross-examined until evening. I noticed that because I was tired, I was not thinking as clearly. I started to get "wishy-washy" in my opinions. I finally looked to the judge at about 6:30 P.M. and told him I was too tired to continue. He was about to stop the hearing when the defense attorney interrupted and said he had "just a couple more questions." After 45 more minutes of misery, I turned to the judge and said I really cannot continue, because I am too tired to think straight after my flight into town and sitting in the courthouse all day. By this time it was nearly 7:30 P.M. The judge, thankfully, called a recess until 8 the next morning.

I went back to my hotel room, grabbed something quick to eat, and went to bed. I woke up early in order to review the case. It was amazing how much clearer my mind was after sleeping, "stepping back," and reviewing the basis of my opinion. I returned to court and was able to state my opinions clearly and definitively without the dreaded wavering. I realized that when I was tired, it was so much easier to be manipulated by artfully crafted and aggressive questioning. My testimony went quickly and smoothly. The judge found Mr. Small competent to proceed with the trial. I then realized why we went so late the previous evening. The judge had scheduled the trial to start this very day, and the jury selection was to begin immediately!

After the judge made the competency ruling, the defense actually stood and stated that although they respected the judge's decision, they still believed that their client was incompetent and motioned for further competency evaluation. The judge said no, of course, but there was much discussion. The judge finally agreed upon a plan—a plan that included me. Since I was present in the courtroom for this exchange (and the defense expert had flown out of town), I was the lucky winner! The judge asked me to stay in town and reevaluate Mr. Small's competency to proceed each morning before the start of that day's portion of the trial. Far be it for me to say "no" to a U.S. District Judge, so I changed my flight and hotel reservations to stay the entire week.

The wrangling was not over, however. The defense team argued that they should be present during my interviews with the defendant to make sure he did not inadvertently violate his rights by disclosing incriminating information. The judge asked me what I thought about this idea. I stood in the back of the room and said I would not perform the interviews if any attorneys were present. I didn't waiver; I just said it as a matter of fact. The judge and defense attorneys negotiated to the point of a compromise. A live audio/video feed would be run from a camera in the room to a monitor in an adjacent room, where the attorneys would remain without disturbing my interview. I did not like this much more (remembering my experience with such equipment previously), but I felt like I needed to agree.

There was a delay the next morning as the technical people arranged the video equipment. Eventually it was arranged, and I was sitting with the defendant in a room with a camera. We chatted a little bit, and I began asking questions about how he was doing since I had seen him last. He noted that he felt fine and that there had been no additional difficulties since that time. Now I needed to verify that he had a rational understanding of his current legal situation and a reasonable plan for a defense. I had made it through the questions concerning his understanding of the charges and roles of courtroom participants and had just asked him about his plans for the trial when my world spun around. The door flew open and in ran his attorney, yelling, "Stop! stop! Don't saying anything!" Well, I am sorry to have to admit it, but my patience had completely run out. I stood up, ushered the attorney into the adjacent room, and literally "came unglued" all over him verbally. I told him in no uncertain terms (and with rather harsh words) that he did not seem to understand my role. I had no intention of disclosing incriminating information or the defense's strategy to anyone—my only job to was to verify that this man was competent to proceed. The fact is, there is no way to verify competency unless those areas are addressed. The interview was over, and I went back upstairs to talk to the judge.

In 10 minutes I found myself, along with defense counsel and the prosecuting attorney, standing in the judge's chambers. I told him exactly what had happened and stated that I would no longer allow such intrusion during my interviews. Further, if he wanted me to evaluate the defendant, there would be no cameras or attorneys present. Otherwise, I would get on a plane and fly home. The judge was a gracious man. He allowed me to interview the defendant in private from that time on. Each morning, I would sit with the defendant and discuss his case with him. And each morning he was just as competent as he was the previous day. I would then enter the judge's chambers and he would say, "Well? What do you think?" with a big smile. I would tell him, "He's competent, your Honor," and he would give me a thumbs up and an "Okay, then! Let's get this trial going!" I stayed the rest of the week and evaluated Mr. Small each morning, until the attorneys rested after closing arguments. Oh, I also apologized to the defense attorney for "going off" on him; he was gracious, too.

Mr. Small was convicted of obstruction of justice related to jury tampering in addition to the previous convictions for illegal gambling, money laundering, and racketeering. He was found competent to stand trial retrospectively for that first trial, without testimony from me. I later found out he was sentenced to 97 months for the first charges with an additional 35 months for obstruction. He recently went into home confinement due to his age and general health concerns.

LESSONS LEARNED

I learned several lessons from this complicated case. The most important lesson for neuropsychologists involved in forensic practice is the necessity of corroborative sources. It is clear that expert opinions are only as good as their information sources. The difficulty in this regard is that you don't know what unique information or source is out there. It is hard to request the unexpected. It is easy to request medical records, school records, investigative records and the like, but it is tough to make sure you have everything. This case taught me to make sure I ask for everything the attorneys (both defense and prosecuting) have on the case. I also try to run down some basic issues, such as the possibility of any other court proceedings going on simultaneously or any atypical activities by the defendant that would potentially shed light on the person's mental state during the past time in question. Even then, you must be mindful that there might be something more out there. This case demonstrated that sometimes attorneys do not provide you will all the information. Whether by accident or intent, sometimes they withhold important facts.

Relatedly, it is important to be flexible in your opinion. Expert opinions are based on information sources (which include interviews and test data). If new information becomes available, it is fine to alter your opinion. Likewise, if inadequate information is available, the expert should limit the opinion. Never go beyond the data. The *Specialty Guidelines for Forensic Psychologists* (Committee on Ethical Guidelines for Forensic Psychologists, 1991) address these issues more thoroughly and should be familiar reading for every neuropsychologist involved in forensic work.

I also learned firsthand that having attorneys present during interviews is a disruption. Likewise, videotaping can be disruptive, although I know of forensic examiners who use video recording during interviews. I prefer not to use it at this time. I further concur with the literature in this regard, certainly during testing (Binder & Johnson-Greene, 1995; McCaffrey et al., 1996; McSweeny et al., 1998; National Academy of Neuropsychology, 2000). Related to this issue is the fact that we need to remain free from emotional involvement—"It's a job" is the operative motto. Under stressful conditions, emotions run high. I was totally out of line exploding at the defense attorney, and I was thankful for his gracious acceptance of my apology. Nonetheless, it was still unprofessional of me. Not all events are under our control when we become involved in forensic matters. We need to remember this fact and not become emotionally involved in the case, yet keep true to our opinion and the scientific/clinical truth as we see it.

Lastly, it is important to be rested and prepared for testimony. Each expert must know what it takes for him or her to function optimally. I believe it is also important to be able to recognize when you are not performing well due to fatigue. Hopefully, this will not occur early in the day! I have traveled across state to court on the day of my testimony and find that I am not always at my best. I prefer to arrive at court rested and ready to go to work, which typically requires travel the previous day; in addition, unexpected travel delays can always occur, whether driving or flying longer distances. Experts need to know the case well and be pre-pared for aggressive cross-examination, even though it may not happen. Testifying well requires intense concentration and mental acumen. In the absence of significant new information, it is best to stick to your opinion as outlined in the report in a straightforward, unwavering, manner. I believe that in this way, we can be most helpful to the trier-of-fact.

AUTHOR NOTES

This case is based on a true account, but names and details have been changed to protect the identity of individuals involved. Opinions expressed in this chapter are those of the author and do not necessarily represent the position of the Federal Bureau of Prisons or the U.S. Department of Justice.

REFERENCES

Binder, L. M., & Johnson-Greene, D. (1995). Observer effects on neuropsycho-logical performance: A case report. *The Clinical Neuropsychologist, 9*, 74–78.

Butcher, J. N., Graham, J. R., Ben-Porath, Y. S., Tellegen, A., Dahlstrom, W. G., & Kaemmer, B. (2001). *MMPI-2 (Minnesota Multiphasic Personality Inventory–2): Manual for administration and scoring* (2nd ed.). Minneapolis: University of Minnesota Press.

Committee on Ethical Guidelines for Forensic Psychologists. (1991). Specialty guidelines for forensic psychologists. *Law and Human Behavior, 15*, 655–665. Available at www.abfp.com/careers.asp.

Lees-Haley, P. R., English, L. T., & Glenn, W. J. (1991). A fake bad scale on the MMPI-2 for personal injury claimants. *Psychological Reports, 68*, 203–210.

McCaffrey, R. J., Fisher, J. M., Gold, B. A., & Lynch, J. K. (1996). Presence of third parties during neuropsychological evaluations: Who is evaluating whom? *The Clinical Neuropsychologist, 10*, 435–449.

McSweeny, A. J., Becker, B. C., Naugle, R. I., Snow, W. G., Binder, L. M., & Thompson, L. L. (1998). Ethical issues related to third party observers in clinical neuropsychological evaluations. *The Clinical Neuropsychologist, 12*, 552–559.

National Academy of Neuropsychology, Policy and Planning Committee. (2000). Presence of third party observers during neuropsychological testing. *Archives of Clinical Neuropsychology, 15*, 379–380.

IV

ASK THE EXPERTS

18

A Dialogue with Jerry J. Sweet

1. *How do you control for the effects of bias on your part when you offer opinions as a treating expert and when you offer opinions as a retained expert?*

All experts, regardless of discipline (e.g., engineering, medicine, psychology) are subject to the same forces that may diminish objectivity in rendering opinions in a particular case. These forces are both internal (e.g., related to one's own personality) and external (e.g., related to interactions with attorneys and other experts involved in the case).

Awareness of the forces that act on expert witnesses is essential, whether one is serving as a treating expert or as a retained expert. The treating expert has an additional force to be aware of: the force coming from having held, or perhaps continuing to hold, the role of trying to help the plaintiff recover from some emotional or physical injury or illness. This is not to say that all treating experts can be expected to drop their objectivity in order to "help" their patients, but experience suggests that this is a possibility. Most neuropsychologists who have been retained as defense experts have faced the testimony of a treating expert whose opinion defied logic and literature, and likely reflects this bias.

Over the years, it has been my assumption that the only defense against bias is self-awareness, first, that factors exist that can affect objectivity and, second, that a witness's best defense against unwitting bias is to consciously examine the bases of opinions as they develop and as they are maintained or evolve across the life of a case. Expert witnesses must base opinions on the facts of the individual case, as they relate to the facts developed in scientific literature relevant to the case and to the expert's field of practice. There is a need to constantly compare developing opinions against facts. A witness needs to be aware of the all-too-human tendency for error in making judgments, such as forming an opinion too soon (i.e., before sufficient data are available). As new facts become available, a witness needs to be open to the possibility that original opinions may need revision. It perplexes me when reading in a deposition that an expert who has just been introduced to new credible evidence, which offers a relevant and diametrically opposed idea to his or her own opinion, steadfastly denies that such information is cause to at least consider modifying a previously formed opinion. Can such a response be, in any way, rational? Conversely, opinions that change without the introduction of new facts should be examined closely for evidence of diminished objectivity. It is important to ask oneself whether the evidence that forms the basis of an opinion would lead to a different opinion if the retaining party were on the opposite side of the case. Related, it is important to consider whether prior testimony in similar cases, when retained on the opposite side of a case, led to similar or different opinions.

All experts are fallible human beings, no matter whether they are oblivious to their own biases or are attuned to themselves and the forces at work in a forensic consultation and, in response, attempt to maximize their objectivity. That said, it is essential to consciously work on checking one's possible biases by painstakingly checking the objective bases of one's own opinions. Being objective on one case does not ensure an absence of bias on the next case. In fact, overconfidence in one's ability and knowledge is likely to ensure diminished objectivity. A reasonable comparison would be that an expert witness should be like an airplane pilot, checking and cross-checking the integrity of the aircraft and its operational readiness at every takeoff and landing. No clear-thinking pilot would simply trust that the details of the prior takeoff and landing provided assurance of safety for future flights.

2. *What do you think is the best route for graduate psychology students to pursue if they are interested in preparing for a career in forensic neuropsychology?*

Unlike applicants to postdoctoral residency, whose interests are more developed, it is a relatively rare occurrence to come across a graduate student who has already concluded that his or her career will be exclusively in forensic neuropsychology. Much more common is the growing realization among graduate students with whom I have contact that forensic neuropsychology is an interesting practice area about which they would like to learn more. This may, in part, be an adaptive response to my strong suggestion to trainees that if they engage in any area of clinical practice as a neuropsychologist, they will not be able to avoid at least some involvement in forensic activities. After all, almost all neuropsychologists will eventually have patients who have been injured in some manner and pursue an injury claim either during or after treatment. Although not all clinical neuropsychologists will be retained specifically as expert witnesses, nearly all will provide testimony as "treating" experts.

It seems that there are not many U.S. graduate schools offering coursework in forensic neuropsychology. However, if available, taking formal graduate coursework would be a great start. For most, the opportunity of choosing clinical practica and internship and residency sites that offer relevant training is more likely to be present and for interested students, also a great idea. As soon as interest in forensic neuropsychology is identified, participating in relevant clinical research and publishing on topics related to forensic neuropsychology helps build the type of knowledge base, evident to others on one's curriculum vitae, that helps a clinical expert become a forensic expert. Additionally, there are often relevant continuing education opportunities at state, regional, or national meetings. Finally, if one's educational path does not contain sufficient learning opportunities, then the remaining option would be to arrange individual supervision with a local expert after entering practice. Learning from individuals who have already become recognized as forensic experts is important in a practice area that may be best conveyed by good mentoring.

3. Do you think that it is important for neuropsychologists who aspire to engage in forensic practice to do both plaintiff and defense work?

Yes, I do think this is important, if local referral patterns make it possible. Noting the exception that not every expert has the opportunity to do both, I believe that when experts in civil cases are retained by both defense and plaintiff and experts in criminal cases are retained by both defense and prosecution, then there is an increased likelihood, though by no means a certainty, that the expert will be focused on the merits of the

individual case and not the general position of the retaining side. To say
it differently, if retained by only one side of the case year after year, I
think it is human nature to overlook the individual merits of a case and
instead adopt a previously held, reflexive viewpoint or position. To me,
this is a context in which bias, even if unwitting, can develop. In writing
on this issue, I have specifically stated that retention by only one side of
cases does *not*, in and of itself, indicate that an expert witness is biased
and could, in fact, be the case history of an expert witness who is quite
objective. However, human nature being what it is, I believe the risk of
losing objectivity across time, in such a scenario, is a potential problem.

It has been suggested that in addition to lack of opportunity in a particular area of practice (e.g., in a rural locale in which all plaintiff or all
defense work goes to the only other neuropsychology expert), perhaps
some areas of expertise will only be attractive to one side of a case. However, ask yourself this question: What area of expertise is only *ever* of
interest to one side of a case? I believe there is *no* such area of expertise—
which to me means that at some point, even individuals with very narrow
expertise that appears of disproportionate interest to one side of cases,
ultimately is attractive to both sides in at least some cases. That is, even if
disproportionate interest leads to retention in many cases for the same
side of the case, there will be exceptions. The most extreme example I
can think of would be an individual who is recognized as having special
expertise related to malingering, which might, at first blush, be considered of interest to the defense side of a case (at least in civil law). However, malingering can be either "ruled in" or "ruled out" and hence has
interest for *different* reasons to both sides of the case.

There are at least two scenarios in which plaintiff attorneys may have
a very strong interest in retaining an expert in malingering behavior. The
first is when an honest plaintiff attorney really wants to know—usually
early in a case, before too much time and money have been invested—
whether his or her plaintiff is presenting a valid claim. Discussions with
defense and plaintiff attorneys in Illinois suggest that they are both aware
of the fact that better plaintiff firms tend to screen their cases carefully in
order not to be surprised down the road. The second is when the plaintiff attorney has a legitimate acquired brain injury case and expects that
his or her own retained expert will need to be able to effectively address
the predictable and reasonable question from the defense regarding
whether the plaintiff is malingering. Thus, at some point, even special
expertise such as that of an expert on malingering, should be of interest
to attorneys on both sides of cases.

4. *How do you handle a request for raw data from an opposing attorney who does not have a psychologist consultant? Does it matter if the retained consultant is a psychiatrist?*

This type of request most often occurs at some point after a patient seen for a clinical evaluation is involved in a civil lawsuit. It occurs less often when I have been retained to provide an expert opinion. In either instance, we have a stock letter that informs the attorney who made the request that Illinois law and ethical considerations do not allow release copies of test *materials* to someone who is not a licensed clinical psychologist. If we have already been given an appropriate release of information, which specifies mental health and psychological records, we release the test *scores*, which are not protected. In my experience, it has been rare that a psychiatrist has agreed to be named as the recipient of copies of test materials. My response would be the same if a psychiatrist were named. However, if a judge orders that I must release the materials or I will not be allowed to continue serving as an expert in the case, I will release the materials to the psychiatrist. These circumstances arose only once. As I recall, the psychiatrist eventually acknowledged, under oath and after not being able to answer traditional psychometric questions, that his training and clinical practice did not give him the requisite knowledge to independently administer or interpret the raw data. In fact, in his own practice he referred his clinical cases to psychologists for neuropsychological testing and relied upon their judgments. At this point in the history of neuropsychology, there are too many contrary precedents, clinically and forensically, for physicians, regardless of specialty, to simply claim independent expertise with our formal testing procedures. In almost all instances, arguing against this precedence would likely be "lethal" to the physician's opinion in the case at hand.

5. *When retained as an undisclosed consultant on a case, what type of information do you consider worthy of providing an attorney? Include in your answer whether it is appropriate to provide the attorney who has retained you as a consultant with (a) personal information about the other expert that could be used against him or her just to gain an advantage, and (b) information you have (but the attorney does not) about the other expert's opinions in a case that resembles the case currently at issue.*

Ask yourself this question: Why should it matter that the other expert would never know your identity? The type of information that is "worthy" of being shared with an attorney is the *same*, whether a neuro-psychologist is retained as a *disclosed* expert (i.e., identity revealed to the judge and attorneys) or an *undisclosed* expert (i.e., identity known only to side of retention). There should be no difference. If information is perti-nent to the material substance of a case, then it should be shared with the attorney. It is the question of what information should be shared in *all* cases that warrants our attention!

For the sake of discussion, let us assume that I know of *personal* facts about the opposing expert that are in some sense negative; for example, drawing from actual case experiences I have had, that the other expert (a) has been the subject of ethical complaints not relevant to the present case, (b) has had tempestuous relationships with colleagues, or (c) has obvious diagnosable psychiatric problems. Such *personal* facts do not bear on whether this expert has arrived at the correct opinion in the case pres-ently at hand. However, the personal facts could serve to undermine his or her opinion if used in an ad hominem attack during cross-examination. To be sure, most attorneys are very willing to use such information to discredit a professional. However, it is the role of expert witnesses to educate those involved in the case regarding substantive mat-ters and to render objective, competent, and relevant opinions. I believe strongly that it is *not* appropriate for one professional to facilitate ad hominem attack of the opposing expert, whether as a disclosed expert or as an undisclosed expert.

Now, let's consider facts about an opposing witness that may be rele-vant to material substance of the present case and are therefore "worthy" of sharing with an attorney. For example, again drawing on past case experiences, consider: (a) relevant research of the other expert cited in the present case has been criticized by peers; (b) the other expert's claims of extensive experience with condition X appear grossly inaccurate, based on personal knowledge of his or her career; (c) the person's pres-ent opinion is very much at odds with his or her opinion in a recent simi-lar case when he or she was retained by the other side; or (d) the other expert was not allowed to testify in a similar case after a *Daubert* eviden-tiary challenge ruled against him. If such facts are relevant to the substan-tive opinions of the other expert in the present case, then they are appro-priately "grist for the mill."

This question actually addresses the issue of bias again. If one is not biased, why not limit all attention and discussion to facts pertinent to the opinions of the experts in the case at hand? After all, a formerly unethical psychologist who does not get along well with colleagues and requires psychiatric treatment may nevertheless have a meritorious opinion in the case at hand. Therefore, why would we bring up that which is not relevant, other than for reasons associated with bias? Let the merits of the case determine the outcome.

6. *If, while operating as an undisclosed consultant, you became aware that a retained expert whose work you reviewed was acting unethically, how would you address your concerns about the ethical violation?*

Most often, I would wait until the end of the case and then address my concerns in the same fashion recommended for all ethics complaints. Namely, we are instructed within the American Psychological Association ethical standards to attempt informal resolution with the psychologist, if appropriate, and if that fails to submit a formal complaint to the relevant state or national ethics committee or licensing board. The forensic context does not change this basic approach. Importantly, an ethics charge filed during a forensic matter can introduce a type of negative bias toward the complainee that can seriously, and perhaps unfairly, damage that person's ability to render an opinion. Waiting until the close of a forensic proceeding can allow the complainant the opportunity to determine whether the issue is indeed one involving ethics or whether it instead grew out of feelings of antagonism toward the other expert generated by involvement in the case itself. Based on numerous conversations with peers, it seems that many professionals have concerns about the ethical conduct of an opposing witness during a forensic proceeding, but upon conclusion of that proceeding, they view the matter with greater objectivity and no longer consider it as an issue of ethics.

7. *Are evidentiary standards a problem for forensic neuropsychologists? Include in your response (a) how one defends against a cross-examination that intends to criticize the use of a flexible battery on the basis that it has not met the* Daubert *standard of admissibility (even if you do not practice in a* Daubert *jurisdiction); and (b) whether you believe that neuropsychologists need to be familiar with error rates of tests that they employ in order to ensure that the tests they use meet current, or perhaps future, standards of admissibility?*

Evidentiary standards are not ever a problem for an expert, regardless of discipline, *if* that expert's opinion is scientifically grounded. It has been a self-selection, of sorts, for clinical neuropsychologists to be scientist-practitioners. Psychologists who do not have a strong comfort with scientific hypothesis testing and quantitative research typically do not specialize in clinical neuropsychology. I believe strongly that clinical neuropsychologists, as a class of expert witnesses, are in one of the strongest positions to meet current and future evidentiary standards. There is no health care specialty with a stronger tradition of scientifically based practice than clinical neuropsychology.

With regard to the first subquestion, the logic of *Daubert* actually implies that no single rigid battery could be expected to meet the criteria for every case. It is difficult to imagine that any serious experienced neuropsychologist could entertain the notion that a single inviolate constellation of tests would be the *only* battery that would be scientifically acceptable for *all* possible clinical conditions across *all* possible demographics.

To be clear, there is no special requirement within the *Daubert* ruling that should lead anyone to believe that only a rigid, fixed battery can meet criteria. If there were, then the vast majority of clinical neuropsychologists in this country would not be allowed to provide expert witness testimony, given that approximately 70% of U.S. clinical neuropsychologists self-identify as adhering to a flexible battery approach. The notion that such exclusions have occurred in prior *Daubert* rulings is a myth that is *not* supported by reading the actual decisions of relevant cases. As of 2003, when my colleagues and I were writing a book chapter and reviewed all such cases that could be identified by legal search engines, I can say with conviction that no expert neuropsychology witness had *ever* been excluded from testifying on the basis of having used a flexible battery. Exclusions of neuropsychologists from testifying occurred, to be sure, but none for that reason. Such a general exclusion of the entire category of all possible flexible batteries would, in fact, not be in keeping with the *Daubert* criteria. Also, for a judge to make such an exclusion in the absence of scientific evidence—because it certainly does not exist within the profession—would go against the long-held tendency of judges not to dictate to professions that which is best left to professions to determine. This is a very unlikely event, indeed.

With regard to the second subquestion, in keeping with scientific practice and with particular relevance to the *Daubert* criteria, neuropsychologists need to be familiar with the error rates of the tests they use. Neuropsychological procedures for which scientific evidence suggests that decisions based upon their results would have unacceptably high error rates should not be used, or, if compelling reasons exist for their use, should serve only a limited role in decision making within a battery of tests and other relevant information.

8. *What kind of information is needed for an expert witness to conclude that a claimant is malingering (i.e., not just "insufficient effort," but really malingering)?*

This is the most complex of the 12 questions we have been asked to answer. To be sure, there is an answer, but it varies so much from case to case and requires so much detail and context to ensure the understanding of the reader that I am tempted to say, read a more extensive treatise or attend a 3-hour lecture on this subject. I am very wary that any answer provided in this abbreviated format will not serve to convey a reasonable and full perspective. In general, forensic opinions regarding malingering are probabilistic, with the probability increasing as the amounts of symptom exaggeration, unrealistic versus expected deficits, evidence of insufficient effort, false reporting of accident information and other history, discrepancy with real world functioning, etc., increase.

9. *How would you go about responding to a request for a third-party observation of an independent medical examination (IME)?*

We have carefully constructed a letter that outlines our opinion, and the bases for that opinion, which states that we do not allow third-party observation for fear of introducing invalidity to test results and also to maintain test security so that future evaluations will be valid. In a minority of instances, after we send this letter we nevertheless receive a court order to allow an observer. The court order most often indicates that the observer will not speak or interfere with the examination.

In years past, we refused to go forward when observation was required and, when necessary, withdrew from the case. However, attorneys subsequently convinced me that this response can be counterproductive. Therefore, we now proceed with the case, noting that the observation was court ordered. In the subsequent report, we document any observed effect on the testing process (e.g., an attorney interrupting the interview) and also indicate that unknown negative effects may have compromised some of the plaintiff's performances. The reality is that third-party observation of a litigant has only been shown to degrade performances, not to improve them. Thus, the plaintiff's own attorney is introducing a plausible *alternative* hypothesis, if subtle to mild impaired performances are found. It seems clear that if plaintiff attorneys understood that the impact of observing neuropsychological evaluations had only the potential of undermining their position, and no potential to help their case, such requests would disappear.

10. *After all the years you have practiced in the forensic arena, what have you found to be the best way to prepare for trial testimony?*

Just before the trial begins, I spend time refreshing my memory regarding the important details of the case for easy recall while on the stand. To me, the important details include (a) what allegedly happened to the plaintiff; (b) what treatments and effects are known to have occurred following the incident at issue; (c) what was evident on prior evaluations of the plaintiff (including my evaluation of the plaintiff); (d) what relevant literature has been brought into the case at depositions of experts; (e) what I have already said in my discovery deposition (which could have been a year or more earlier); and (f) what I expect to be asked by either side while I am on the stand. Finally, if exhibits will be used, I review these in detail.

Past experience in court has made it clear to me that experts can only respond to questions asked by an attorney. I may end up leaving the courtroom not having presented all the opinions I intended to provide, *if* the right questions are not asked. Therefore, I want the attorney to know all the opinions that I wish to express, so that he or she will know to ask questions that offer the opportunity for me to express my full opinion clearly. Either a meeting in my office or a discussion by telephone at some point close to the trial date will address this area. Attorneys decide for themselves how much detail to share with me in advance regarding the specific questions that they will ask. Some prefer to type out the questions and send them to me; most simply make notes of all the opinions I want to offer at trial.

11. *Imagine the following cross-examination questions. How would you respond?*

a. *Doctor, do you regard neuropsychology as an exact science?*

As with other health care practice fields, such as radiology and neurology, neuropsychology is not an exact science. Nevertheless, as in all medical specialties, the basis of our practice is scientific. For the benefit of readers, related questions asked by attorneys often juxtapose neuropsychological test data as *subjective* and radiological data as *objective*. My response to such a characterization is to point out that there is a subjective element involved in both instances, in that experts ultimately interpret the objective test data in neuropsychology and radiology, with that interpretation involving some degree of subjectivity. An informative jux-taposition involves age-related changes that are addressed more straight-forwardly (i.e., quantitatively) on most widely accepted neuropsychologi-cal measures, through relevant standardized norm transformations, than are data from computed tomography (CT) and magnetic resonance imag-ing (MRI) scans of the brain, which continue to be subjectively inter-preted by expert radiologists who do not rely upon quantitative adjust-ments.

b. *Doctor, isn't it true that two different neuropsychologists looking at the same data can come up with completely different explanations? How do you account for that divergence?*

Judgments in all clinical practice areas ultimately rely on humans. So, yes, as is the case with any two radiologists or any two neurologists, two neuropsychologists looking at the same data can come up with differ-ent interpretations. There is nothing unique to neuropsychology in this regard.

c. *Doctor, you only spent an hour and a half interviewing the claimant, and your assistant spent the rest of the time doing the testing. How can you com-pare your results to our expert, who spent the entire day with the claimant? Or to Dr. X., who has worked with the claimant in rehabilitation for over 9 months?*

As with many neuropsychologists, I use an assistant who is highly trained in administering the tests and observing the person being exam-ined. I determine what tests will be administered, and I am in touch with the testing assistant throughout the evaluation. This procedure has been our norm for many years and is no different from what we do for routine clinical referrals from physicians. Your own expert has admitted that this is common in our field. An effective evaluation does not depend on the amount of time spent but rather on the comprehensiveness and quality of the information obtained. I know from experience that I can rely upon the day-and-a-half-long evaluation we performed.

Regarding your second question, information learned in a rehabilita-tion context may or may not be relevant to answering the questions relat-ing to validity of presentation, diagnosis, and etiology that are important to lawyers. It is also the case that in a treatment context, a clinician accepts the patient's history and motivation to get better, and confirmation of facts is typically not possible. As you know, I have had boxes of historical documents available in forming my opinions, much of which likely would have made a difference in treatment, but was simply not available to Dr. X.

d. *Doctor, do you consider [insert any text title here] to be an "authoritative text" in clinical neuropsychology?*

The answer to this often-asked query depends upon the particular book. For example, there is a small number of books for which the answer might be "No, I do not consider that book authoritative." Alternatively, there are some books for which the answer is "I am not familiar with that text." Finally, among the more likely titles that will be brought up by attorneys, most will be familiar and well known in the field. In that case, a reasonable answer to this question is "I am familiar with that book and, in fact, have a copy on my shelf. It is considered generally authoritative, which as you know does not mean that all facts and opinions stated within it are correct or accepted by my peers or by me."

e. *Doctor, isn't it true that on a previous case in 2001, you testified that the plaintiff's symptoms were a result of brain dysfunction, yet here, with the same injury-related variables (e.g., loss of consciousness, posttraumatic amnesia), you are saying that the patient's symptoms are not due to brain dysfunction? Tell the jury how you can have a different opinion when the results are essentially the same?*

As a person who values and strives for consistency of opinion, if I am asked this question, I am hoping that this characterization of my current and prior testimony is inaccurate. Otherwise, unless the knowledge that anchored my prior opinion is no longer current, which could explain any professional's evolution of opinion across time, I have indeed erred and will have to admit it.

This is a question that needs to be taken very seriously. In attempting to impeach a witness, an attorney may deliberately distort or omit facts that would, if reported accurately, actually illustrate that inconsistency of opinions has *not* occurred. This possibility, coupled with the fact that two different patients rarely are truly "comparable" at baseline, in terms of age, education, premorbid health, and premorbid cognitive capacity, should lead a witness to form a well-considered response.

I have not been asked this question very often, but when it has come up, the facts of the cases being compared were actually not all that similar. The response to this question then becomes educating the judge or jury regarding the salient differences that reasonably lead to different conclusions. For example, compare the expected outcomes of two individuals who are comparable in age, education, and prior good health, who both experience a motor vehicle accident in which no loss of consciousness occurs. Both experience 15 minutes of altered consciousness. However, one of these two individuals develops a subdural hematoma that requires surgical intervention. The surgery is followed by medical complications and a second surgery. Two weeks later this same individual develops posttraumatic seizures, which become difficult to control. It is not too difficult to imagine that despite similar initial injury parameters, subsequent outcomes could differ. One year later the individual who suffered an uncomplicated injury has a reasonably good chance of being neuropsychologically normal, whereas the individual with the delayed but related complications may demonstrate persistent neuropsychological dysfunction. This example serves to show that, at minimum, the witness should ask for a clear identification of the prior case so that sufficient relevant details can be recalled before providing a substantive answer.

RELEVANT READINGS

Grote, C., Lewin, J., Sweet, J., & van Gorp, W. (2000). Responses to perceived unethical practices in clinical neuropsychology: Ethical and legal considerations. *The Clinical Neuropsychologist, 14*, 119–134.

Slick, D., Sherman, E., & Iverson, G. (1999). Diagnostic criteria for malingered neurocognitive dysfunction: Proposed standards for clinical practice and research. *The Clinical Neuropsychologist, 13*, 545–561.

Sweet, J. (1999). Malingering: Differential diagnosis. In J. Sweet (Ed.), *Forensic neuropsychology: Fundamentals and practice*. Lisse, Netherlands: Swets & Zeitlinger. Reprinted in I. Schultz & D. Brady (Eds.). (2003). *Psychological injuries at trial* (pp. 672–705). Chicago: American Bar Association.

Sweet, J., Ecklund-Johnson, E., & Malina, A. (in press). Overview of forensic neuropsychology. In J. Morgan & J. Ricker (Eds.), *Textbook of clinical neuropsychology*. New York: Psychology Press.

Sweet, J., Grote, C., & Van Gorp, W. (2002). Ethical issues in forensic neuro-
    psychology. In S. Bush & M. Drexler (Eds.), *Ethical issues in clinical neuro-
    psychology* (pp. 103–133). Lisse, Netherlands: Swets & Zeitlinger.
Sweet, J., Moberg, P., & Suchy, Y. (2000). Ten-year follow-up survey of clinical
    neuropsychologists: Part I. Practices and beliefs. *The Clinical Neuropsycholo-
    gist, 14*, 18–37.
Sweet, J., & Moulthrop, M. (1999). Self-examination questions as a means of iden-
    tifying bias in adversarial cases. *Journal of Forensic Neuropsychology, 1*, 73–88.

19

A Dialogue with
Manfred F. Greiffenstein

1. *How do you control for the effects of bias on your part when you offer opinions as a treating expert and when you offer opinions as a retained expert?*

The question treats "bias" as a clearly defined term with a single meaning, but as used by attorneys, it blurs important distinctions between types of bias. We are experts on "bias," and, in reality, biases have valences. Biases can be acceptable or unacceptable. The better question to ask is "How do you control for the effects of unacceptable, harmful biases?" Harmful biases are ones shaped solely by advocacy. Acceptable biases refer to predilections toward a certain philosophy unaffected by monetary considerations. For example, there is nothing wrong with being biased in favor of peer-reviewed papers or against reliance on subjective evidence alone. Every expert witness has biases, and it is a good idea to openly state these when the opportunity arises. For example, my bias is that "extraordinary claims require extraordinary evidence."

2. *What do you think is the best route for graduate psychology students to pursue if they are interested in preparing for a career in forensic neuropsychology?*

The best preparation for forensic work is to first become a good neuropsychologist. One's clinical training must involve assessing patients

343

with clearly defined brain damage. Seek out the best internships and training possible in organized health care settings. Neurology centers that offer evaluation of persons with neurobehavioral disorders is the ideal route, although general neurology and rehabilitation services will suffice. In such a facility, you internalize good prototypes of brain–behavior relationships against which to compare future litigants. Put differently, you develop a good frame of reference that is uncontaminated by confounding variables such as compensation, education, and adversarial attitudes. Paradoxically, the worst route to take is early training experiences in private practices devoted to evaluation of litigants with minor or questionable neurological trauma. If you have never evaluated persons with true alcoholic Korsakoff, severe brain injury, or dementia diagnoses, how could you know that the 1st percentile scores produced in a 2-year-old whiplash case are implausible? How could you know that a person with organic amnesia shouldn't be able to give you any post-incident history? In my view, lack of a good frame of reference is the main source of errors in forensic reports.

Assuming adequate pre- and postdoctoral experience, you may next consider taking the annual workshops offered by the Academy of Forensic Psychology, the membership organization for those who passed the American Board of Professional Psychology (ABPP) examination in forensic psychology. These workshops provide excellent orientation to legal issues pertinent to psychologists. In addition, stock your professional library with key texts written by forensically oriented neuropsychologists, such as this volume. Jerry Sweet's (1998) edited volume *Forensic Neuropsychology* may still be in print. Glenn Larrabee's (2005) *Forensic Neuropsychology: A Scientific Approach* was recently published. The journal *The Clinical Neuropsychologist* (published by Taylor & Francis) contains a running series entitled "Courting the Clinician," which offers practical advice or updates on law and practice. You might also seek out a respected mentor with forensic experience. At the present date, there is no organized training experience specific to forensic neuropsychology.

3. Do you think that it is important for neuropsychologists who aspire to practice in the forensic arena to do both plaintiff and defense work?

No. One should aspire to do good neuropsychology, not seek an artificial symmetry of ambiguous meaning. It is more important to develop a defensible assessment philosophy and point of view. The forensic neuropsychologist has little to no control over referral sources. Referral sources find you, not the other way around. It is inevitable that your forensic work will be dominated by one referral source versus another. If you do enough of this work, you will eventually receive more prosecution than criminal defense work, more plaintiff than civil defense, etc. Neuropsychologists who boast they "always do 50/50" may just be providing favorable opinions to whomever calls first, or writing ambivalent opinions that aim to please both sides.

4. How do you handle a request for raw data from an opposing attorney who does not have a psychologist consultant? Does it matter if the retained consultant is a psychiatrist?

My philosophy, probably unpopular with many of my colleagues, is one of legal primacy. The courtroom is a place of evidence, and there should be no exception carved out for psychologists. I give all test protocols in response to a valid subpoena. This position is consistent with the United States due process ethos, and it is consistent with the new 2002 ethics code (American Psychological Association, 2002). I draw the line at test manuals and freestanding stimuli, also in accordance with the new ethics code. It does not matter if the retained consultant is a psychiatrist. Psychiatrists proceed at their own peril if they offer far-ranging opinions based on data they are not trained or qualified to interpret. That is not your problem. Some psychiatrists may have expertise in some instruments (such as the MMPI-2), but few can lay claim to broad and deep knowledge of neuropsychological measures. Keep in mind that it is easy for nonpsychologists to purchase test materials. Unscrupulous psychologists may also provide attorneys with test manuals to assist them in coaching clients on how to manipulate test results. Dissemination of raw test data through the courts to the public has not proven to be a problem, despite years of fearful predictions and slippery-slope arguments.

5. When retained as an undisclosed consultant on a case, what type of information do you consider worthy of providing an attorney? Include in your answer whether it is appropriate to provide the attorney who has retained you as a consultant with (a) personal information about the other expert that could be used against him or her just to gain an advantage, and (b) information you have (but the attorney does not) about the other expert's opinions in a case that resembles the case currently at issue.

The background consultant's role is a potentially dangerous one from a psychological standpoint. There are two issues here: (a) absence of moral hazard and (b) honest promotion of mainstream neuropsychology. Decades of social psychology research have shown that anonymity can disinhibit aggressive impulses. One need only think of Stanley Milgram's studies to come to a sobering conclusion: If anonymous students are willing to deliver near-lethal shocks to fellow human beings, what constraints are there against expressing verbal hostility toward neuropsychologists one may dislike?

The other issue is adherence to generally acceptable neuropsychological practices. The trick is to provide consultation based on generally accepted core ideas rather than extremist or personalized beliefs. For example, the need to adjust scores for age, gender, and education is beyond any reasonable dispute. Providing the attorney with "one-size-fits-all" cutting scores is intellectually dishonest. A genuinely debatable issue to raise, when appropriate, is the particular choice of normative tables. Is the normative group small or skewed in some way, or large and strongly representative? There is no reasonable dispute that symptom validity tests (SVT) are necessary in compensability disputes. Feeding attorneys questions such as "Isn't it true that only a signed confession is the gold standard of determining malingering?" is preposterous and dishonest. A signed confession is no more necessary in civil than in criminal law. As we know, even "confessions" can be coerced. What is genuinely debatable, however, is the particular choice of SVT. Is it too insensitive? Are there too many false positives? Alternative explanations for poor scores?

My two-pronged philosophy in the consultancy role is as follows: Provide (a) consultation as if your identity will eventually be revealed, and (b) raise genuinely debatable issues. The former is an effort to self-inhibit aggression and the latter, an aspiration toward intellectual honesty. Consistent with this philosophy, I never relay information about the expert's opinions in other cases with similar fact sets. This is because I do not store or compile other expert's opinions, depositions, or reports in my offices. I am a case-specific consultant, not an investigator. Only advocacy groups (such as lawyers) keep such records. Besides, every case is different, and we do not have all the pertinent facts from any given case at our disposal. There could be a good explanation why the other witness gave different opinions in two cases with *superficially* similar fact sets. Whether I relay other types of personal information about the other expert depends on the relevance. For example, if an expert is claiming board certification when, in reality, he or she purchased a vanity board over the Internet, the issue of credentialing becomes fair game. If an expert lacks board certification but does not make excessive personal claims, I do not raise board certification as an issue. Opinions should stand and fall on their own merits, not the pedigree of who made the opinions.

6. *If, while operating as an undisclosed consultant, you became aware that a retained expert whose work you reviewed was acting unethically, how would you address your concerns about the ethical violation?*

This is a difficult dilemma because of conflicting roles. As a consultant, the retaining attorney is your client and expects confidentiality. You would lose anonymity if you filed an ethics complaint. On the other hand, you are a psychologist ethically bound to report public harm at the hands of a psychologist. A third prong of this conflict is allowing yourself to be used to raise ethical issues in the service of a partisan (the attorney). Mercifully, I have never been confronted with this situation—but I have a plan if I am. The magnitude of the perceived ethical transgression dictates whether I will report the problem immediately or wait until the conclusion of trial. If I feel there is a clear and present public danger (e.g., feeding the patient ephedra plants to "cure closed head injury symptoms"), I would report it immediately. Michigan's state licensing board allows anonymous ethics complaints. If the ethical lapse does not involve imminent psychological or physical harm (e.g., billing irregularities), I would await the conclusion of litigation before contacting the psychologist to clarify. Brodsky and McKinzey (2003) offer sample letters to use as templates for these situations.

7. *Are evidentiary standards a problem for forensic neuropsychologists? Include in your response (a) how one defends against a cross-examination that intends to criticize the use of a flexible battery on the basis that it has not met the* Daubert *standard of admissibility (even if you do not practice in a* Daubert *jurisdiction); and (b) whether you believe that neuropsychologists need to be familiar with error rates of tests that they employ in order to ensure that the tests they use meet current, or perhaps future, standards of admissibility?*

I do not consider evidentiary standards a problem. I think the "threat of *Daubert*" is overblown. I believe the opposite: *Daubert* and its follow-on cases (*Joiner* and *Kumho*) actually strengthen neuropsychology's position. We are many steps ahead of mental health specialists who rely exclusively on subjective data collection and intuitive testimony (e.g., psychiatric social workers).

It is easy to defend against the rare *Daubert* challenge to flexible test batteries. I point out that *Daubert* does not require tests to be validated "as a whole." Some neuropsychologist just made up that assertion out of whole cloth. Neuropsychologists are no more required to validate batteries "as a whole" than are testifying physicians required to validate "a group of medical tests." Is there a "battery of neurological tests"? For example, the idea that the Wechsler Memory Scale is somehow invalid because it was given without the Halstead–Reitan Neuropsychological Battery is preposterous on its face. *Daubert* is applied to individual or grouped methods and requires at least one of the following preconditions: (a) evidence of potential falsifiability, (b) potential error rate, (c) a peer-reviewed study, (d) the existence of a manual controlling use, and (e) general acceptance. These preconditions do not all have to be present; two or more of these features can be proven for most standardized measures. Besides, many judges focus on the general acceptance element alone (the *Frye* element of *Daubert*), and this is easy to prove for individual neuropsychological measures. *Daubert* only addresses the *admissibility* of neuropsychological tests, not their weight. Bottom line: The issue of whether it is better to use a fixed or flexible battery in order to understand the facts of an individual case is a jury question, not a matter of law decided by a judge.

8. *What kind of information is needed for an expert witness to conclude that a claimant is malingering (i.e., not just "insufficient effort," but really malingering)?*

I use a conservative scientific approach tempered by moral considerations: A false diagnosis of brain injury does not have the ramifications of a false positive malingering label. I require extraordinary evidence from multiple sources because DSM-IV criteria are insufficiently rigorous. The "Slick criteria" are very helpful in decision making (Slick, Sherman, & Iverson, 1999). My criteria for definite malingering include (a) below-chance responding on any multichoice format, with (b) scores below floor effects for legitimately brain-injured groups. Probable malingering criteria include (a) chance level performance on multichoice memory tests in the context of minor compensable injury; (b) two or more atypical complaints (e.g., procedural and semantic memory loss claims); (c) two or more scores below floor effects; and (d) scores > 30 on the Lees-Haley Fake Bad Scale.

9. *How would go about responding to a request for a third-party observation of an IME?*

I use a multitiered approach that begins with outright refusal and ends with case abandonment. I first refuse any request for third-party observation (TPO) of the testing, although I allow attorneys to be present during the interview. If the judge grants a motion to have an observer present, I allow observation from a remote location. I purchased a wireless baby monitor with a 5" screen and remote audio for just this purpose. I warn all parties that my interpretive section will include language about the potential impact of TPO on test results. If there is a motion to videotape the whole proceeding, I provide the court with an ideal protective order outlining disposition of the videotape (e.g., all copies returned to me at conclusion of litigation). If the court still allows taping without limitation, I drop out of the case, provide a list of other neuropsychologists, and recommend that retaining counsel seek leave to appeal. The weight of legal authority across the country is against TPO of psychological tests, as opposed to physical examinations.

10. *After all the years you have practiced in the forensic arena, what have you found to be the best way to prepare for trial testimony?*

The general contours of my preparation are as follows. First, I assume that all opposing attorneys are excellent cross-examiners. I never take anybody for granted. Even unskilled attorneys can obtain canned cross-examination scripts written by better attorneys. Second, I identify the weakest parts of my opinion, if pertinent, and try to get that issue covered on direct examination. Third, if I have experience with a particular cross-examiner, I gather documents and papers in anticipation of certain questions. For example, if the cross-examiner's favorite tactic is to manufacture ethical smears, I put a copy of the ethics code in the case file for quick reference during questioning. Fourth, my forensic reports are written with trial testimony in mind: All pertinent information is in the report. For example, I incorporate very detailed records reviews into reports. I may also include commentary in parentheses to educate the reader (e.g., definition of standard deviation, significant difference versus abnormally large difference, etc.). This way, I don't have to struggle through reams of records or textbooks to find a piece of evidence. The report subheadings reflect the sequence of my cognitive activity for that case.

11. *Imagine the following cross-examination questions. How would you respond?*

a. *Doctor, do you regard neuropsychology as an exact science?*

Definitely not. Like medicine, clinical neuropsychology is a mixture of art and science. Inference and judgment will always go into any opinion.

b. *Doctor, isn't it true that two different neuropsychologists looking at the same data can come up with completely different explanations? How do you account for that divergence?*

I might respond with the admit–deny technique. "Although what you say has some truth to it, many of the differences in opinion can often be explained by the amount of records available to an expert. In this case, 'Dr. Ima Legend Owen-Mind' did not have the school records, which I did have." The records showed a long history of special education programming for dyslexia. In this example, I acknowledged a weakness in the field, but then linked the question back to the case before bar to educate the jury. The dependent clause ("although . . . ") holds the listener in abeyance.

c. *Doctor, you only spent and an hour and a half interviewing the claimant, and your technician spent the rest of the time doing the testing. How can you compare your results to our expert, who spent the entire day with our client? Or to Dr. X., who has worked with our client in rehabilitation for over 9 months?*

I term this line of questioning the "false conceit" gambit. The answer to this question cannot be formulaic. Selecting the right answer is a highly factual undertaking shaped by the particulars of the case. A good answer addresses the imprecision and conceit of the question by raising the latent issue: Evaluation time is a function of diagnostic complexity. It doesn't take long to diagnose diabetes, but it would take a long time to diagnose a rare blood disorder. What diagnosis is being considered in the legal case? If applicable, I might say this: "If your client presented with a rare brain disorder seen once in a career, I would have spent days in testing and observation. But extensive diagnostic workups are unnecessary with common or minor problems." Such an answer deflates the question's false conceit that this particular plaintiff is special or markedly different from persons with the same claimed (common) etiology. Of course, if dealing with a rare neurobehavioral syndrome, you had better have a good explanation for not increasing documentation time. If the other expert has no known formal training in neuropsychology, an answer may be, "If it takes me 20 hours to fix a car and a certified mechanic does it in 1 hour, does that mean I know more about the car? I did what was necessary to answer the questions put to me."

d. *Doctor, do you consider [insert any text here] to be an "authoritative text" in clinical neuropsychology?*

I agree with Brodsky's (1991) advice to always turn down the learned treatise gambit. Any agreement that a text has blanket authority means that every statement in it is beyond dispute. A prudent answer may be, "I consider this book (paper/pamphlet) an important contribution to the field, but I don't agree with everything that is written in there." Always ask for a copy of the document or book rather than accept what the cross-examining attorney says about it.

e. *Doctor, isn't it true that on a previous case in 2001, you testified that the plaintiff's symptoms were not a result of brain dysfunction, yet here, with the same injury-related variables (e.g., loss of consciousness, posttraumatic amnesia), you are saying that the patient's symptoms are not due to brain dysfunction? Tell the jury how you can have a different opinion when the result are essentially the same?*

I first make a mental note that the lawyer is testifying, meaning; he or she is pretending to know facts that are not in evidence. I genuinely refuse to accept the attorney's characterization that the two cases are identical, because nobody's case-specific memory is that good. One genuine answer is, "You say the cases are exactly alike, but without taking a few days to review the entire file in that old case, how could I possibly answer the question?"

REFERENCES

American Psychological Association. (2002). Ethical principles of psychologists and code of conduct. *American Psychologist, 57*, 1060–1073.

Brodsky, S. L. (1991). *Testifying in court: Guidelines and maxims for the expert witness.* Washington, DC: American Psychological Association.

Brodsky, S. L., & McKinzey, R. K. (2003). The ethical confrontation of the unethical forensic colleague. *Professional Psychology: Research and Practice, 33*, 307–309.

Larrabee, G. (2005). *Forensic neuropsychology: A scientific approach.* New York: Oxford University Press.

Slick, D. J., Sherman, E. M., & Iverson, G. L. (1999). Diagnostic criteria for malingered neurocognitive dysfunction: Proposed standards for clinical practice and research. *The Clinical Neuropsychologist, 13*, 545–561.

Sweet, J. J. (Ed.). (1998). *Forensic neuropsychology.* Lisse, Netherlands: Swets & Zeitlinger.

20

A Dialogue with Paul R. Lees-Haley

1. *How do you control for the effects of bias on your part when you offer opinions as a treating expert and when you offer opinions as a retained expert?*

Control for bias in forensic cases begins with careful screening before you agree to accept a case. This screening includes conducting a conflict check, to be sure you have not already been retained by one of the other parties in the case, and listening carefully to the potential client to determine whether you somehow have a personal interest in the outcome of the case. It also is important to make a reasonable effort to identify multiple relationships. I recommend using the same methodology, other than evolutionary changes associated with your continual efforts to improve your assessment methodology, in all essentially similar cases. Don't emulate the expert who used different norms for plaintiffs referred by plaintiff attorneys than for plaintiffs referred by defense attorneys. Avoid working on a contingency or a lien. A useful de-biasing procedure is to identify your key opinions and think of a list of evidence for and against each opinion. Another useful technique is to argue against your conclusions, searching for ways they could be wrong or should be qualified. Sweet and Moulthrop (1998) have produced some thoughtful writing on this topic, which I recommend. Finally, we all need to battle constantly against fooling ourselves, because bias is a pervasive human limitation, not a rare or necessarily obvious phenomenon. We may be affected by celebrities, emotionally moving cases, matters that touch on scientific or intellectual issues about which we feel strongly, and numerous other factors.

We should avoid accepting cases that require both treating and forensic roles with the same person. However, we may be subpoenaed unexpectedly to testify about a patient we are treating, and then we may have no choice. In treating cases, bias arises from several sources. We often lack the information in records reviewed in forensic cases and rely more on what patients tell us. In treating patients there is no reason to conduct the detailed background study we perform in forensic cases. Issues important in forensic matters (such as causation) may be of nominal importance in treatment. Based on treating a patient, we usually are missing important data from a forensic perspective. Also, when treating, many of us were taught to be advocates of the best interests of the patient, instead of striving for neutrality or feeling that our ultimate allegiance is to the court. We can strive to be objective, but if we have an incomplete or inaccurate history, our opinions are speculative at best.

2. What do you think is the best route for graduate psychology students to pursue if they are interested in preparing for a career in forensic neuropsychology?

Obtain practicum as well as academic experience so you have concrete exposure to what forensic work is like in the real world. Find out the available career tracks and discuss them with senior professionals to determine where your interests probably are strongest. For example, some experts do only criminal work or personal injury work, whereas others do virtually any form of forensic case. Some work only with children or only with adults. Even in broad areas, there are many specialized niches. For example, if you want to spend your time assessing injured persons, you could go into personal injury, workers' compensation, Social Security Disability evaluations, etc.

3. Do you think that it is important for neuropsychologists who aspire to practice in the forensic arena to do both plaintiff and defense work?

At the beginning of your career I recommend doing both so that you will gain a broader perspective and look at things from a variety of points of view. Later, after you are seasoned, it won't matter whether you do plaintiff or defense or some of each. But watch out. If you manage to be equally attractive to two adversarial points of view (plaintiff and defense), you should ask yourself whether you may have misplaced some of your intellectual integrity along the way. If you have a coherent philosophy and intellectual consistency, you are no more likely to be equally appealing to plaintiff and defense attorneys than a presidential candidate will be equally appealing to both Republicans and Democrats. The silly myth that working 50% plaintiff and 50% defense means you are objective sounds so fair-minded when you say it, without thinking it through, that some experts actually believe it. I think saying "50/50" evokes old memories of it being fair to share things with our playmates, or touches on the common feeling that it is fair to compromise so we can all have something of value. Then, because it feels right and sounds right on its face, we don't stop to examine the idea critically. Didn't someone once suggest that people who think the world is flat and people who think the world is round should compromise and split the difference? The truth is that lawyers are advocates and when they are handling a plaintiff case, they look for a liberal expert, and when the same lawyers are handling defense cases, they look for conservative experts.

4. *How do you handle a request for raw data from an opposing attorney who does not have a psychologist consultant? Does it matter if the retained consultant is a psychiatrist?*

I handle such reports painfully. The lawyers are going to get the data eventually if the argument goes before a judge, because most judges are reasonable people who do not want witnesses hiding the data on which they are relying. Because the new language in the 2002 American Psychological Association code of ethics is being debated by intelligent colleagues of good will and integrity, I am temporarily playing it safe by asking for subpoenas. I am fairly confident that leading ethics committees will eventually conclude that the correct interpretation of the 2002 ethics code is that we should turn over our data to attorneys when we are expert witnesses in litigation. I hope we can obtain protective orders requiring attorneys to return the data at the conclusion of the case. In the long run, we need concrete guidance designed by an interdisciplinary committee that includes lawyers, neuropsychologists, other psychologists, judges, and others from many jurisdictions and fields of law. For years I have argued that the American Psychological Association and American Bar Association should set up an interdisciplinary panel to design guidelines for the handling of raw test data and related materials in litigation.

I have only known a few psychiatrists who were interested enough in neuropsychological or psychological testing to interpret raw data independently. With all due respect, neuropsychological testing is usually not one of their competencies. Occasionally you will discover that a psychiatrist or other nonpsychologist expert (e.g., example, epidemiologists, statisticians, survey researchers, educational testing experts) has some well founded, thoughtful, scientific opinions about the instruments we call tests. When in doubt, I remind myself that forensic work is about the rules of the court. If the judge orders me to turn the raw data over to Mickey Mouse, I look up the address of Disneyland!

5. *When retained as an undisclosed consultant on a case, what type of information do you consider worthy of providing an attorney? Include in your answer whether it is appropriate to provide the attorney who has retained you as a consultant with (a) personal information about the other expert that could be used against him or her just to gain an advantage, and (b) information you have (but the attorney does not) about the other expert's opinions in a case that resembles the case currently at issue?*

When I happen to know personal information, such as the fact that you smoke marijuana and have affairs without telling your spouse, my view is that this is none of the attorneys' business and I don't tell them (assuming you are not doing these things at your office during your neuropsychological evaluations). On the other hand, if the attorney wants to know if the university providing your PhD has a campus, or if you scored the WAIS-III properly, or if it's true that the CV you submitted as an exhibit to your deposition is flagrantly falsified, I will tell them that.

Information I am aware of from previous cases may or may not be fair game for discussion. Was the case sealed? Is the information public record? Is it truly relevant? Is this an expert who uses different procedures depending on whether the case is plaintiff or defense? Sometimes I comment on previous reports, testimony, research or other articles by the expert. Sometimes the other expert brings up such matters first (e.g., mentioning his or her research as a basis for conclusions).

6. *If, while you were operating as an undisclosed consultant, you became aware that a retained expert whose work you reviewed was acting unethically, how would you address your concerns about the ethical violation?*

Carefully. When I serve as a work-product consultant to an attorney, there are two walls of confidentiality surrounding the work: The attorney client has rights because I'm a psychologist, and the attorney also has rights under work product, privileged communication rules. If the ethical violation is minor or unclear without hearing both sides (a situation I've seen too many times to count), and I bring up the concern with the attorney, I'm invariably asked to respect the confidentiality. I have negotiated agreements not to object if I agree to wait until the case is over before contacting the psychologist or filing a complaint. I pray that I never run across a situation in which I discover that the opposing expert is abusing a child, or something like that.

7. Are evidentiary standards a problem for forensic neuropsychologists? Include in your response (a) how one defends against a cross-examination that intends to criticize the use of a flexible battery on the basis that it has not met the Daubert *standard of admissibility (even if you do not practice in a* Daubert *jurisdiction); and (b) whether you believe that neuropsychologists need to be familiar with error rates of tests that they employ in order to ensure that the tests they use meet current, or perhaps future, standards of admissibility?*

Evidentiary standards are an important concern but not any more of a problem for us than for many other experts. I would briefly educate the judge or jury about the general state of the art in neuropsychology and then zero in on specifics. There is no test battery used by a majority of neuropsychologists, and specific tests and batteries are not always used for the same purpose. If you validated your battery or test yesterday for a different purpose, then it may not apply to today's case. To deal with the arguments over fixed versus flexible batteries, focus on the issue of what question the procedure is allegedly valid for answering. I recommend thinking of your tests as individual measures and determining their reliability and validity for specific purposes. I also recommend looking at the combined result of your various methods using a procedure such as Rohling's Interpretive Method.

The question of whether a test battery or test is valid must always be considered as part of the question, "Valid for what?" To measure the error rates for tests in a form that can be visualized as a 2×2 table, we need a criterion. We can only depict error rates in a 2×2 format when we can accurately count right and wrong answers. Let's look at a specific question as an illustration. Suppose you are challenged on the question of whether a plaintiff can work in the future. There is relatively little predictive validation research on tests related to this common question, and speculation is common. John Meyers has been looking at this important question, with impressive results (Meyers & Rohling, 2004). Using Meyers's method, you can make a statement such as, "The probability of a cooperative examinee's returning to work with this level of neuropsychological functioning is N%." This presumes you have a valid neuropsychological assessment, but Meyers's work deserves wide attention, as does Rohling's, which is used in Meyers's procedure. Another way to think about error is in terms of standard error of measurement, where we conclude that the probability of a score falling within an identified range is X%. This method interests us more than it does juries and judges, but it can be valuable when you are wondering whether a plaintiff can meet some specific minimum standard. Ironically, a third way experts sometimes cope with challenges based on error rates is to use the legal expression "more likely than not." In effect, they are saying, "My error rate is less than 51%, so I'm more likely than not right." The first time I heard this I wasn't sure whether to laugh. I'm not an attorney, but apparently this sort of answer may tiptoe into the zone of admissibility. To add insult to irony, there actually is a certain logic to this argument, so it may be a starting place before presenting more scientific data.

8. *What kind of information is needed for an expert witness to conclude that a claimant is malingering (i.e., not just "insufficient effort," but really malingering)?*

Let's start with the bottom line: If I think you are malingering, my job is to say so just as surely as I'm supposed to say so if I think you are suffering a major depression or have an IQ of 100. Those experts who avoid the term *malingering* because it is "serious"—as if other diagnoses were not serious—are making a specious argument and failing to consider the impact of their statement on the victims of malingerers. There are two or more sides in every lawsuit. I use the DSM definition of malingering, which is DSM-IV, as of this writing. The medical–legal context is a notorious red flag for malingering, and that criterion is relatively clearly defined. Lack of cooperation may or may not signify malingering in this context, depending on the nature of the lack of cooperation. For example, adolescents who openly put forth poor effort, admit not trying to do well, deny any serious injury, and say the lawsuit is their parents' idea and a waste of time, are not what I call malingerers, even though they are blatantly uncooperative in a medical–legal context. Poor effort has to be interpreted in context. I have met adults who put forth poor effort on testing during both the plaintiff and defense examinations but said they did so because the evaluations were pointless, and they were not claiming injury, they were suing on principle. I did not conclude that they were malingering. The people I most commonly conclude are malingering make implausibly severe complaints of injury relative to the alleged causal event and show signs of poor effort or nonsensical results on their testing.

In recent years, the problem of coaching has presented us with this challenge: The plaintiff experiences a trivial event, alleges profound consequences that are worse than those resulting from most severe injuries, shows an observable level of functioning that is dramatically superior to the severe level of impairment suggested by test scores at face value, fails malingering checks that are internal to tests designed for other purposes (e.g., memory, intelligence, concept formation), and passes the well-known effort tests with flying colors. I have noticed that some of our colleagues consider a confession to be the ultimate verification or gold standard of malingering. I disagree, based on the reality of false confessions. Granted, confessions are rare in personal injury litigation, but they too should be examined in the context of other data, not accepted automatically as a trump card.

9. *How would go about responding to a request for a third-party observation of an IME?*

Object. Complain. Whine. Write letters objecting. Write affidavits. Call friends to ask for permission to plagiarize from their affidavits and speeches. Give the attorney who retains me a copy of the federal case of *Ragge v. MCI/Universal Studios* (165 F.R.D. 605) and relevant state court decisions. Send my client relevant professional association documents from NAN, AACN, APA, etc. Gossip with colleagues about attorneys who don't argue vigorously against the presence of third-party observers. Tell my wife I hate lawyers. Refuse. Agree, based on requirements of applicable state law. Document my objections and potential negative effects at the beginning of my report and testimony.

My experience with third-party observers has ranged from a smooth event with no detectable problems to a complete disaster. My objection is not based on the belief that I can predict the specific consequences of a particular third-party observer in every case; it is based on the risk and the impossibility of foreseeing all the potential consequences. The problem is analogous to speeding in a car. Most of the time I probably would not have an accident driving 120 mph, but it is unwise so I avoid doing it.

10. *After all the years you have practiced in the forensic arena, what have you found to be the best way to prepare for trial testimony?*

First, read the records and discuss with the attorneys who retained me the nature of the trial from a legal point of view, so that I can focus my testimony on questions that are being considered by the court. Remember, your job is to assist the jury or judge. Second, find out if anything has changed shortly before the trial starts (e.g., sometimes plaintiffs drop certain parts of their claim, or judges dismiss some causes of action, either of which may change the nature of the trial at the last minute). Third, memorize the medical records, depositions, reports, and test data. Then ask myself "What are the questions they are likely to ask me, do I know the answers to all these questions, and what are my answers?" That tells me if I need to obtain any other information to provide fully informed answers or simply say I do not know. For the reader who has not testified before, here is the sort of thing I am referring to when I say "questions they are likely to ask me":

> Does the plaintiff have an injury?
> If so, what is the nature of the injury and how mild or severe is it?
> What caused this injury or deficit?
> What are the consequences of such an injury?
> Is the condition treatable?
> Are the effects temporary or permanent?
> Is the patient disabled? (Partially or totally? Temporarily or permanently?)

If other experts testify before I do, it is often helpful to know what they said. For example, sometimes lawyers and experts don't mention something that I would have expected them to introduce as a significant issue. In one case, one of the experts thought the plaintiff had PTSD, and I thought the plaintiff was depressed. At trial the expert who diagnosed PTSD was not called to testify, so it would have been pointless for me to testify that the plaintiff did not have a diagnosis of PTSD—when no one had said he had it in the first place. In reviewing your own opinions before testifying, bounce everything against two pervasive and fundamental science questions: What does that mean? How do I know?

11. *Imagine the following cross-examination questions. How would you respond?*

a. *Doctor, do you regard neuropsychology as an exact science?*

No.

b. *Doctor, isn't it true that two different neuropsychologists looking at the same data can come up with completely different explanations? How do you account for that divergence?*

Yes. How do I account for this divergence? There are many possible explanations. Different teachers. Different norms. Use of different definitions for the same terms. Different opinions about which data are the most important for making decisions. Reading different research articles. Not reading the research literature. Prostitution. Intelligence. Stupidity. I am confident that some other colleagues can come up with completely different explanations.

c. *Doctor, you only spent and an hour and a half interviewing the claimant, and your technician spent the rest of the time doing the testing. How can you compare your results to our expert, who spent the entire day with our client? Or to Dr. X., who has worked with our client in rehabilitation for over 9 months?*

Excuse me. You are mistaken. I was the one who spent the entire day with the plaintiff, but that is not the critical issue. The issue is, who had better quality data and evaluated it by a valid process to reach reasonable conclusions. As for Dr. X., who spent 9 months with the plaintiff: Based on my 1 day in person with the plaintiff and the records I examined, I know more about the plaintiff than Dr. X. does. I realize that this might lead some people to wonder what Dr. X. accomplished with the $100,000+ in rehab and retesting he provided, but you didn't ask me that.

d. *Doctor, do you consider [insert any text here] to be an "authoritative text" in clinical neuropsychology?*

No.

e. *Doctor, isn't it true that on a previous case in 2001, you testified that the plaintiff's symptoms were not a result of brain dysfunction, yet here, with the same injury-related variables (e.g., loss of consciousness, posttraumatic amnesia) you are saying that the patient's symptoms are not due to brain dysfunction? Tell the jury how you can have a different opinion when the result are essentially the same?*

No, it's not true at all. You get that sort of illogical testimony from experts who think it's a compliment instead of a veiled insult to characterize them as experts whose work is 50% plaintiff and 50% defense. Over here on "The Dark Side" we reach logical conclusions based on reliable data. How did you find out about that 2001 case, anyway? My parole officer told me they sealed those records.

REFERENCE

Meyers, J. E., & Rohling, M. L. (2004). Validation of the Meyers Short Battery on mild TBI patients. *Archives of Clinical Neuropsychology, 19*, 637–651.

Sweet, J. J., & Moulthrop, M. A. (1998). Self-examination questions as a means of identifying bias in adversarial assessments. *Journal of Forensic Neuropsychology, 1*, 73–88.

Index

"f" following a page number indicates a figure; "n"following a page number indicates a note; "t" following a page number indicates a table.